Discover the Healthful and Healing Properties of Herbs

Use wisdom from around the world to help yourself—with solutions to problems such as:

- VIRUSES: The mild Chinese herb *astragalus* is a remarkable cold preventive—and the spicy, aromatic cubeb berry not only builds immunity but relieves coughs, strengthens lung tissue, and helps heal asthma.

- HEADACHES: Ginger, feverfew, and rosemary are standout migraine relievers; peppermint oil dabbed on temples, scalp, and neck eases tension headaches.

- INSOMNIA: Valerian, hops, and scullcap leaf are just a few of the botanicals that can help you sleep—without the risk of dependency.

- FATIGUE: Eleuthero, fo-ti, and yerba mate are only a handful of the herbs that can energize you without overstimulation or side effects.

- EAR INFECTIONS: Discover why a few drops of mullein oil, garlic oil, or onion juice are usually more effective than antibiotics—not to mention healthier and cheaper.

❧

"Robyn Landis and Karta Purkh Singh Khalsa have written a masterful and comprehensive work that will teach readers the practical essentials of herbal medicine. Its scope is immense, yet its organization and friendly, personal style make the information extremely accessible and easy to apply. The book will undoubtedly increase one's confidence regarding herbal self-care."

—Ralph T. Golan, M.D., author of *Optimal Wellness*

ROBYN LANDIS is the author of the bestselling *BodyFueling®* and the creator of the *BodyFueling Workshop®*. She has delivered health education seminars, lectures, and workshops to thousands of people—children and adults, athletes and physicians, and executives from America's top corporations worldwide—since 1990. She has studied traditional herbal medicine with herbalist Karta Purkh Singh Khalsa for seven years.

KARTA PURKH SINGH KHALSA, C.N., A.H.G., is an herbalist and educator with twenty-five years of clinical experience. He has studied under Ayurvedic master Yogi Bhajan for two decades and also has expertise with Western, Chinese, European, and Native American herbs. His knowledge spans both traditional and modern views and practices in herbal medicine. A sought-after consultant and teacher, he travels extensively to offer his knowledge and experience through classes, conferences, and the media. He also developed Kinesionics®, a unique muscle-testing tool used widely by other practitioners. He is a licensed nutritionist, licensed massage therapist, yoga teacher, certified trainer for the International Association of Specialized Kinesiologists, and a professional member of the American Herbalists Guild and many other professional organizations.

ALSO BY ROBYN LANDIS

BodyFueling®

Visit Robyn Landis's Web site at www.bodyfueling.com

HERBAL DEFENSE

POSITIONING YOURSELF TO TRIUMPH OVER ILLNESS AND AGING

ROBYN LANDIS

WITH KARTA PURKH SINGH KHALSA

FOREWORD BY
MICHAEL T. MURRAY, N.D.

WARNER BOOKS

A Time Warner Company

PUBLISHER'S NOTE: The information in this book is not intended and should not be construed as medical advice. If you need medical attention, please seek the advice of your own health practitioner. You should have a health professional check your condition before making any changes in an existing treatment program.

Copyright © 1997 by Robyn Landis with Karta Purkh Singh Khalsa
Foreword copyright © 1997 by Michael T. Murray, N.D.
All rights reserved.

Warner Books, Inc., 1271 Avenue of the Americas, New York, NY 10020

Visit our Web site at http://warnerbooks.com

W A Time Warner Company

Printed in the United States of America

First Printing: August 1997

10 9 8 7 6 5 4

Library of Congress Cataloging-in-Publication Data

Landis, Robyn.
　　　Herbal defense : positioning yourself to triumph over illness and aging / Robyn Landis and Karta Purkh Singh Khalsa.
　　　　　p.　cm.
　　　Includes bibliographical references.
　　　ISBN 0-446-67242-4
　　　1. Herbs—Therapeutic use.　2. Medicine, Ayurvedic.　I. Khalsa, Karta Purkh Singh.　II. Title.
　　　RM666.H33L36　1997
　　　615' .321—dc21　　　　　　　　　　　　　　　　　97-1817
　　　　　　　　　　　　　　　　　　　　　　　　　　　　　　　CIP

Book design by H. Roberts
Cover design and photo by Kathy Saksa

Acknowledgments

For me, this book has been an ambitious project because I had much to say and there is so much information to be shared. To educate on this kind of scale requires enormous support and assistance from many people; thus I offer many thanks as follows:

To my family: my husband Robert, my kindred spirit of health since the early days, who has indestructible faith in me and offers a bottomless well of encouragement, constancy, and insight; my parents, Marty and Doris Weisen, for loving me no matter how downright eccentric I may seem; and my brother, Dr. Steven Weisen, M.D., for sharing my passion for health sciences, despite our different ways of expressing that passion. And of course, my special pal Bailey, herbal wonder-dog, a dear buddy who warms my feet and keeps me company during long nights of writing and editing.

To Karta Purkh, my coauthor, a gifted healer and good friend, whose articulate, graceful introduction to the wonderful world of herbal medicine started me on my own power journey to phenomenal health, which I am now privileged to share with others. His responsiveness to my insatiable curiosity evolved into a partnership that culminates in this book, which gives the world access to his twenty-five years of accumulated knowledge, experience, and insight.

I must acknowledge my love and gratitude for a cadre of special friends who bless my life with unique and unstintingly generous contributions. They listen to my ranting, send endless relevant news clippings, read my stuff tirelessly, challenge me, advocate for me, commiserate with me, believe in me—and authentically strive to be living examples of the kind of health and self-care I write about. Each has, in one way or another, inspired me to keep on with this. First, kindred spirit Amanda Bergson-Shilcock is a sainthood candidate for the huge gifts of precious time and talent she gave to this book. Among them was spending two entire "vacations" in 1996 and 1997 working in my office as my research/editorial assistant and right-hand woman. Others are Christine Carlson, Karen Tuff, Romney Gibson, and Scott, Ann, Jack, and Curtis Allen.

Dr. Michael Kinnear, Dr. Kaaren Nichols, Dr. Ann McCombs, Janice Lehrer, L.M.P., and Stacey Stevens, L.M.P., are health-care practitioners with whom I have empowering professional alliances as well as valued friendships. All have taught me a great deal about the body, medicine, and healing over the years, and the education continues. Extra, extra thanks goes to Dr. Michael Murray, N.D., one of my favorite natural healing authors and a respected researcher and professor of naturopathic medicine, for his time and assistance; and also to Dr. Ralph Golan, M.D., for his input.

I deeply appreciate my Warner Books editor Diane Stockwell's sincere interest in this project and her help in achieving the book's goals with sensitivity, clarity, and—believe it or not—brevity. I am thankful that Warner Books has again given me an opportunity to communicate with many people in this manner.

Karta Purkh's wife, Jagdish Kaur, offered tremendous assistance throughout the project, and many tasks could not have been completed without her. Melanie LeDoux is an angel for her out-of-the-blue offer of last-minute data entry. Dick Paulsen and Judy Jackson gamely took armloads of chapters home for "test-driving" and gave me honest criticism. And special thanks to Jeanmarie LeMense for being a friend and hand-holder long after the official role as editor had ended.

I could not have devoted as much attention to this project for as long as it took without Joan Lewis's understanding and flexibility regarding my commitments to other projects. And thanks to all the Bergson-Shilcocks, especially Emily, for graciously parting with Amanda (again).

Herbalist David Overton, PA-C, R.N., of the University of Washington, must be credited for his contributions providing clarity on the biochemistry of mood disorders.

Finally, I would like to thank all of the pioneering health and science professionals—far too many to name here—who study, practice, write, and speak on behalf of a new era of medicine and an authentic *health*-care system. I am grateful for their dedication, inspiration, determination, courage, visionary spirit, and love for people. For my own sake and others', I am relieved that they are out there.

—*Robyn Landis*
Vashon, WA
1996

Acknowledgments

Many friends and colleagues have shared my journey through the world of natural healing. All taught me in their own way. My heartfelt thanks to each of you.

To Yogi Bhajan, my teacher and natural healing mentor for these many years, for his vast knowledge, his compassionate nature, and his persistence in approach. Without him, my life would not have been what it is today. He taught me so lovingly that God is the true healer.

To Jagdish Kaur, my wife, for all her kindness, support, and balance, and for making it possible to juggle all the areas of our lives so effectively.

To Robyn, my co-author, whose skill, tenacity, and consistency forged such an articulate rendition of our vision. It is my honor to know her.

To Sewa Singh Khalsa, my longtime associate in the natural healing arena. His expertise, insight, and humor have kept alive the vision of bringing natural healing to "every person" for over two decades.

—*Karta Purkh Singh Khalsa*
Seattle, Washington
1997

Contents

Foreword

For many people of the world, herbal medicines are the only therapeutic agents available. While it's difficult to assess the extent to which plants are used as medicines throughout the world, in 1985 the World Health Organization estimated that 80 percent of the world's population relies on herbs for its primary health-care needs. This widespread use of herbal medicines is not restricted to developing countries; for example, it's estimated that 70 percent of all medical doctors in Germany regularly prescribe herbal medicines.

As modern medicine gains more knowledge and understanding about health and disease, it is turning to natural, nontoxic therapies such as herbs with increasing regularity. Botanical medicine, along with stress reduction, exercise, meditation, diet, and many other traditional naturopathic therapies, is pressing to the forefront of medicine.

New models of understanding are emerging in health care. While the old model viewed the body basically as a machine, the new one focuses on the interconnectedness of body, mind, emotions, and the environment in determining health. The new model recognizes that the human body has considerable power to heal itself. It focuses on ways to promote wellness, rather than dealing only with disease. And it emphasizes natural, noninvasive techniques, whether to enhance health or to heal illness.

There is increasing evidence that the healing process is enhanced with the aid of natural nontoxic therapies such as herbal medicine. Further, many drug treatments are effective only in suppressing symptoms, while many natural treatments, especially herbal medicines, effectively address the causes of disease. In fact, in most instances, natural therapies offer significant benefit over standard medical practices.

For these reasons, I have no doubt that the medicine of the future will rely on many of the herbal medicines and general health principles so well described in *Herbal Defense*. People will benefit from this expansion into concepts that are new to us, but which draw from healing wisdom that has long thrived in many cultures, including India (Ayurvedic), China (Taoist), and Greece (Hippocratic). In the throes of this movement toward natural healing, it's a good idea to become well informed about the medicines at your disposal and the issues surrounding them. If you're interested in what herbal medicine has to offer, I strongly urge you to read on!

—*Michael T. Murray, N.D.*
November 1996

For Mom and Dad

If everyone is thinking alike,
then no one is thinking.
—*Benjamin Franklin*

Americans always do the right things
after they've tried everything else.
—*Winston Churchill*

Part I

Background and History

Introduction

YOU DON'T HAVE TO GET SICK

Does it ever occur to you that it might be possible to live your life free of the sicknesses you've always thought were inevitable? Imagine a time in the future when you haven't been troubled by even a sniffle or a rash—for years. That future can become reality for you. I'm proof of it—and I'm not alone.

This is a hopeful thought at a time when our health's future is reported, by many accounts, to be grim. Amid a rising tide of increasingly ruthless "superbug" outbreaks, in a world where our health professionals themselves admit that disease appears to be outrunning the effectiveness of our standard medicines, fear is running high.

If you're like me, you want to know what you can do to protect yourself—right now—not only against increasingly hardy "bugs" and an unknown future of potential plagues, but also against the degeneration, aging, and daily irritations that undermine the quality of so many people's lives. And you want to know that, rather than shrink in fear or simply hope to stay well, you can take the initiative to create health, strength, and vitality.

Like many people, you're probably increasingly concerned about health care and its costs as well as effectiveness, about the best ways to heal, about the way you age and your quality of life throughout the process. In my experience, people have never been more interested in what they can do for themselves, by themselves—and with good reason.

This is an era of rising consumer disenchantment with and cynicism about many aspects of conventional medicine. Natural healing is of paramount interest right now. There is much talk about personal responsibility and self-care as keys to making a true health-care (not "sick-care" or disease-management) system work.

But who is teaching you what you need to know in order to live that way, and inspiring you to do it? My first book, *BodyFueling*®, gets that job done in the area of basic healthy eating and exercise. *Herbal Defense* fulfills that goal at the next level.

Herbal Defense gives you access to the mighty contents of the herbal medicine chest: the natural, cost-efficient, and powerfully effective tools you are demanding to determine your own destiny in the quest for superior health. You will learn that it *is* possible to be bigger, stronger, hardier, and smarter than the rising tide of drug-resistant threats to our health and quality of life. And you will learn exactly what you can do about it, and how.

HERBS IN THE HOUSEHOLD: MEDICINE OF THE PEOPLE

Herbs have been used medicinally around the globe for centuries, with success in a fantastically broad range of situations that should excite anyone who wants to heal him- or herself or others. Through the ages, other cultures (Native American, Indian, Asian, and European) have demonstrated ways to prevent and heal the ailments we fear and dread the most. Today, research is continually confirming what these cultures have known all along: Herbs and foods can help you enhance your health, strength, youthfulness, and immunity for as long as you live.

Herbs are not only consistently filling the void left by conventional treatments that are running aground; they are also enormously useful to help you dodge disease in the first place. It's possible to go way beyond our culture's present notion of "prevention" to a largely unexplored dimension of healing and health. Healing systems that rely on the medicinal properties of safe, natural herbs and foods can help you realize this exciting goal.

Nothing in the world can beat our country's medicine for advances in crisis and trauma care. But for the chronic, non-life-threatening and prepathological stages of disease, the natural approach works—without a doubt and without side effects. What's more, herbs are not so high-tech that they cannot be administered by you. Their use returns you to the driver's seat. Herbs allow you to care for yourself in your own home—easily, inexpensively, and effectively.

There are many good reasons (all of which will be discussed in greater detail throughout the book) to consider and choose herbal medicine in the case of most common, chronic illnesses and discomforts. Frequently, herbal medicines are safer, more effective, and less expensive for both you personally and the system (whose costs you bear in the long run anyway), have fewer side effects, if any, and are more accessible. Herbs deal with underlying issues, not just symptoms, and they help prevent health problems from advancing to crisis proportions.

HOW DID I GET INVOLVED IN HERBAL MEDICINE?

Let's go back in time for a moment to catch a glimpse of me one decade ago, at the age of twenty-one. I was young and should have been the picture of health. Youth equals health, right? Not! I couldn't have been farther from what I now consider to be "health." I had dozens of food allergies and persistent intestinal candida (yeast), as well as recurrent bladder infections (for which I took antibiotics constantly). I thought headaches were a fact of life—I had them almost every day. I had more colds and flu than anyone else I knew. I had gastritis that landed me in a hospital emergency room. I felt cold almost all the time. I had a total absence of menses (i.e., amenorrhea, or no menstrual periods) for over two years.

In 1987, I visited seven different physicians regarding the amenorrhea. I (or, rather, my employer-paid insurance at the time) spent close to $3,000 on diagnostic tests—and got nowhere trying to determine the cause of my health problems.

Though I made no connection at the time to my lifestyle—just as I see many people today not making that connection—my state of health should not have been surprising. My diet was extremely high in fat and sugar, processed and refined foods, and artificial stimulants. I ate very little fresh food and few fruits and vegetables. I exercised haphazardly—sometimes not at all, other times obsessively. The enormous amount of coffee, chocolate, and frozen yogurt in my diet displaced food with real nutrient value. I had a high-stress job to which I devoted almost all of my time, to the exclusion of relationships and nourishing hobbies. I never felt rested and slept poorly. My immune system was constantly under fire, and I wasn't doing a single thing to ease the load, let alone to nurture and enhance its functioning.

Today, I can happily say that I haven't experienced any of the conditions described above for close to nine years. In fact, my health is phenomenal and exemplary—and *the older I get, the healthier I get*. What happened?

Not long after I had made some essential changes in the way I lived, I became acquainted with Karta Purkh Singh Khalsa, a professional herbalist, kinesiologist, and educator, and a longtime student of some of the world's oldest and most respected natural healing masters, including Ayurvedic healer and author Yogi Bhajan. I'd heard wonderful things about his classes and knew people who had achieved tremendous health changes by applying what they had learned from him. I soon became one of those people.

SOMETHING FOR EVERYONE

Through my own experience, research, and extensive interviews with benefactors and practitioners of herbal healing, I have come to see that there is virtually nothing herbs cannot do—sometimes more slowly than conventional treatments, but often also more safely and surely—from easing pain to building strength and energy, to slowing or reversing the progress of serious illness.

Herbal Defense details stories of healing for everyone to identify with. You'll hear about some of the experiences shared by thousands of people whom Karta Purkh has observed over more than two decades—people just like you who have prevented, soothed, or cured common conditions using simple, inexpensive herbal remedies. And you will learn how you can share those experiences.

You'll meet people just like you who tried every typical conventional treatment for aggravating, chronic health conditions—until herbs eliminated the source of the issue along with the symptoms. You'll also meet people from traditional cultures who don't have the kinds of problems we do—and find out why.

From the everyday grievance to the serious illness, you will learn how just about every discomfort and disease known to us can be successfully averted or mended using herbs and foods. You can look forward to *naturally* reversing child hyperactivity, banishing morning sickness, lifting fatigue, curing insomnia, eliminating allergies, resolving candida issues, arresting arthritis, easing indigestion, vanquishing ulcers, shrinking enlarged prostates, sidestepping viral illness, de-stressing, clearing up skin problems, controlling diabetes, and much more. You can also expect to increase and enhance your energy and general immunity.

BEYOND SYMPTOMS

Does it ever occur to you that your headache, your indigestion, your runny nose, or your knee pain has a purpose—that it's trying to tell you something? Do you ever wonder if it might be connected to something else, buried deeper somewhere in that sophisticated network of organs and systems that makes up your body? Do you ever think that perhaps your medicine should be aimed not at your pain, but at the *source* of your pain?

To have the health you want, you must expand your consciousness beyond the small, localized site where something hurts you right this minute, to the much broader matter of the way you work, eat, think, and live. *Herbal Defense* will help you make healing, nourishing herbs a part of a whole, healthy life   not just a panacea or knee-jerk response to illness or injury.

Herbal Defense is not about using herbs or foods merely as a different kind of "quick fix" to replace allopathic "magic bullets." It is about creating health, and knowing how to make the body heal *itself* better—not just treat or manage disease. We will present *ways not to get ill*—or, at the very least, to get sick less often and less severely. The absence of symptoms is just a beginning point. *Herbal Defense* is about going beyond "normal lab results" to the exceptional health you really want.

YOUR BEST TEAM FOR THE STORY

At this urgent moment when you are hungry for answers that offer promise, when many of the superficial panaceas on which we have relied are failing, Karta Purkh and I have a unique contribution to make. I was interested in bringing Karta Purkh's specific wisdom and expertise to the rest of the world because, while I have read a lot of herb books and talked to many practitioners, I have never met anyone with more mastery of the diverse traditions of herbal medicine than Karta Purkh. His teaching represents the best in herbal healing; to me it speaks more clearly than anything else I've personally encountered on the subject. Thus, as a contributing author, Karta Purkh is a primary source for much of the factual information in this book.

We also both have track records for making health information and new health habits useful in people's everyday lives—helping them to integrate new concepts, take action, and produce the extraordinary benefits and results they always wanted. As author and teacher of *BodyFueling*®, I've been acclaimed for my way of making healthy eating and exercise not only practical and comprehensive, but actually appealing. Karta Purkh has been making Eastern healing approaches palatable to the Western mind for twenty-five years. Feedback on his teaching mirrors the comments I've received about mine: "Wow, this has never made so much sense to me." "I never really understood that before." With a subject like herbal medicine, the translation can make the difference.

I have an additional, unique advantage as an author and educator to communicate this information to you: I am not a medical professional. I am highly knowledgeable, since I have been reading about, writing about, and working with herbs for years. I am also a good gatherer and "explainer" of information. What's more important, though, is that as someone like you:

1. **I know what you most want and need to know, because I've been there, and I know how to answer your questions in our language.** One part of what made *BodyFueling*® work so well for so many people is the fact that I am a layperson who understands what kind of questions you have and the need to answer them in simple English. I am able to frame the wealth of information I have gathered in a way that makes sense and inspires action. That's why consumer-to-consumer education has become my niche. I helped basic "fueling" and its physiology make sense for the layperson. Now I translate herbal healing so that it becomes practical and applicable to *you* every day. Not only can we inform you, but we can also make herbal medicine friendly and familiar, help you find a comfort level with this form of self-care—a place where this

world of natural medicines no longer seems "way out" but rather appears as a viable alternative to be weighed seriously with other options.

2. **I can be an inspirational example.** Another reason I gained the public's attention with *BodyFueling®* was my success as a person just like you who has used—with glowing success—the facts and practices I write about. This brings an entirely new, more immediate credibility to the idea that one can really use this stuff. With *Herbal Defense*, I have not only asked hundreds of questions and researched the answers—I *live* the answers. I have "walked the walk" for many years. A hundred healers could tell you that natural medicine is the way of the future and tell you what you "should" do. I have done it—and I have the body and health to show for it. I offer myself as an example of how informed and empowered an "ordinary consumer" can be. It doesn't take a Ph.D. in physiology or botany to be extremely knowledgeable about your body and about herbal medicine.

THE GIFT I WANT TO GIVE

I have some things that a lot of people want. I feel fantastic—strong, healthy, and energetic—virtually all the time. I feel like I grow healthier and look younger every year. I don't live in fear of disease. I don't have the daily physical complaints most people do. I don't get colds and flu. I'm very clear about what keeps me this way, and it's not "luck."

I derive such tremendous satisfaction and value from living the way I do, and am so fascinated by the gentle plant medicines that help me achieve the kind of health I enjoy; how could I not want to share it? I abhor suffering, especially when I know it can be easily prevented. With *BodyFueling®*, I sought to end the needless suffering that accompanies epidemic and misguided efforts to "diet" and lose "weight," and to make sense of nutritional nonsense and "diet thinking" that confuses people and constantly contradicts itself. With *Herbal Defense* I hope to end the suffering associated not only with preventable illness, but also with the use of painful, dramatic, radical treatments—when gentle, nurturing, nontoxic treatments that you can use by yourself at home will do very nicely.

I don't have the illusion that "perfect" health is possible for all, but I am convinced that a great many people can get a lot closer than they are. That is the fundamental principle upon which I base how I care for myself, and the fundamental philosophy underlying this book. It's why I do what I do.

THE ROAD AHEAD

This book is divided into four sections, to give some order to your journey to a new level of understanding about your body, health, and healing options.

Part I, "Background and History," is designed to lay a foundation by introducing you to key concepts that will help you become a more powerful and intuitive consumer of information as well as of herbs. We'll look at what herbal medicine is, what it can and can't do, and what Eastern/alternative philosophies have to offer you, including an introduction to the Ayurvedic healing system that provides ways to address your body's own individual needs. You'll also receive an "Immune System 101" course that will help you appreciate the marvelous mechanisms that keep you well, and understand how to care for and feed that system optimally.

Part II, "Herbs for Health and Healing," deals with all of the proactive ways you can enhance and bolster your health in different areas. You'll be delighted to learn of the easy, inexpensive, and natural ways you can relieve pain and discomfort and, more importantly, work on the deeper issues that underlie your symptoms to prevent recurrence permanently. Whatever the health concern, herbal medicine deserves a place in your healing strategy, and these chapters will show you why and how.

Part III, "Dealing with Disease the Natural Way," outlines specific herbal and natural healing strategies for some of the common health afflictions and issues Americans deal with.

Part IV, "Living It: Herbs in Practice," features the chapters that will help you with the practical integration of what you've learned. We discuss how to buy, prepare, and use herbs, how to choose your sources and practitioners, quality concerns, and more. We also expose common myths, to help you get beyond the hype to where the authentic riches of responsible medicinal herbalism await you.

Following these four sections there are resource pages with names, addresses, and phone numbers of organizations and companies that may be helpful as well as an extensive recommended reading list.

If there is a common thread in all the work I do, whether writing or teaching about diet, exercise, and herbs, it is to inspire you to live life fully, vibrantly, and energetically, and to make you aware of all the available tools that give you that power. I think I live in a wonderful world, and I invite you into my world. I know you can become more deeply committed to your body, on a path toward increasing (rather than degenerating) health, creating extraordinary vitality that will let you live your life as fully as you wish. If that's what you're looking for, let us be your guides on this leg of your journey.

Note: The use of "we" in this book represents the collaborative voice of both authors. "I" represents Robyn speaking, usually reflecting personal experience or opinions.

Note: If you want to get 100 percent value out of herbal healing, we recommend that you read this entire book from start to finish before merely using it as a reference. This book is designed to be much more than a "remedy reference." If you use it to really understand the subject and its connection to your body and health, you will be able to use herbal medicines far more powerfully.

At minimum, we strongly recommend you read Chapters 1 through 6 (Part I, "Background and History") and Chapters 23 through 25 (Part IV, "Living It: Herbs in Practice"). Not all of the information on specific conditions, diseases, and issues detailed in the middle sections may apply to everyone, but these opening and closing sections provide context and contain fundamentals that are important for everyone.

1

Herbs: The Original Medicine

I am dismayed at how far apart the fields of medicine and botany have drifted. . . . 150 years ago, medicine and botany were very closely allied; today, it is almost impossible to find people from those two fields who can converse together, and this situation represents the extent to which science and medicine in this century have moved us away from, even created a fear of, nature. But healing is a natural process, so it seems to me the further we move away from nature, the further we move away from healing and knowing how to foster it in people.

—Dr. Andrew Weil, M.D.
"The Body's Healing Systems: The Future of Medical Education"
Alternative and Complimentary Therapies, September/October 1995

Herbal medicine has a bountiful history stretching back to the time of the earliest healers. In most of the world, today's use of herbal medicine represents simply a continuation of that history. According to the World Health Organization, herbal medicines are now used as primary health care for over 80 percent of the world's population—and not just in underdeveloped nations. In Europe, where much of the modern research on herbal medicines has been conducted (much of it government approved), natural medicines briskly outsell synthetic ones.[1]

But in the United States, current use of herbal medicine reflects a return to roots after a hiatus; our history with herbal medicine is a broken line. While at one time herbs were native to medicine and our culture, the field today is being resurrected from ashes. Now its popularity is unquestionably on the rise. In ever greater numbers people are finding diminishing returns in much of the current thinking in medicine, seeking milder yet equally effective alternatives, and pursuing a more active role in their own health and healing.

PHILOSOPHICAL CHANGE ON THE WESTERN FRONT

A change in the philosophical beliefs and premises of science led to the demise of herbal medicine early in this century. At the turn of the century, natural healing was well developed, highly respected, and relied upon here as much as it was in any other part of the world. There were hundreds of institutions and schools that taught methods of natural healing. Nature was respected as a primary and competent resource for health-giving and healing substances, and medical practice reflected that.

What happened? The seventeenth-century French mathematician René Descartes is largely credited with having shaped the scientific thinking accepted in the West today. The principles he introduced then—analytical, materialistic, reductionist views—formed the basis for the kind of science and medicine that became firmly entrenched here by the 1900s.

In Descartes' view, even products of nature were not more than the sum of their parts; bodies were no more than machines governed by fixed mechanical laws, science was absolute and certain truth, and the mind and body were most certainly unrelated. When Louis Pasteur in the mid-1800s "discovered" that pathogens outside the body are origins of disease, this mechanistic view of the body was further fueled.

Identifying microorganisms that could create sickness in previously "healthy" individuals led to what is sometimes referred to as the "doctrine of specific cause." It led medicine to seek and attack causes of illness outside the body, and away from considering the multitude of factors related to the health of the whole person—the host—that might affect resistance to those external pathogens. The doctrine of specific cause still very much drives medical research and treatment today. As Patrick Quillin, Ph.D., R.D., C.N.S., author of *Beating Cancer with Nutrition,* puts it, "Our reigning allopathic medical system has maintained a philosophy that most diseases have a readily identifiable enemy that can be blasted into submission."[2]

It is easy to see how, in modern conventional medicine, disease came to be divorced from the organism as a whole, how the quelling of symptoms became equated with the cure of disease, and how organs, limbs, or tissues came to be viewed as parts that could be treated separately from the rest of the body. These views came to be the underpinnings of what we call today the "scientific method," still believed by many in the West to be the only relevant and valid way to view and assess "reality."

The fate of conventional medicine, to be driven by these conceptual models (which, thanks to Descartes' influence, came to be known as "Cartesian"), was sealed in the early 1900s when, according to Oriental Medicine Doctors Harriet Beinfeld and Efrem Korngold, authors of *Between Heaven and Earth: A Guide to Chinese Medicine:*

> . . . A survey of medical schools was subsidized by the Carnegie and Rockefeller foundations. Its purpose was to find out which of the schools would be most interested in promoting "scientific medicine," therefore promoting the newly developing drug- and hospital-based technology industries. The Flexner Report, issued in 1910 by the American Medical Association following this survey, recommended that financial support from the foundations be awarded only to medical schools committed to scientific research based on models developed in the nineteenth century. All therapies not based on the Cartesian model were considered unscientific and would therefore be disenfranchised. Only 20 percent of the existing medical schools survived. The other 80 percent adhered to the "vitalist doctrine," which asserted that "man assists, but nature heals." Naturopathy, homeopathy and herbology were forced out of the mainstream and relegated to the status of folk medicine. They were ultimately driven under by lack of funds and political harassment.[3]

It was thus that a trend still very much in place today was begun, in the name of "progress." Doctors, once modest facilitators for people taking care of themselves and largely assisted by nature, became highly specialized and sophisticated mechanics and engineers, wielders of superpotent and complex technologies to be used in heroic front-page and last-minute measures.

Increasingly the balance of power shifted to the doctor, because only the doctor was expert enough to understand and work with something as technical as the body and as complicated as the implements used to fix it. Any intimacy in the relationship between healer and patient was lost as the doctor's vocabulary became too specialized for the layperson to grasp, and the doctor's role changed from facilitator to director. The patient became frequently superfluous to the healing process, nonessential to the repair of the broken part that happened to be attached to him or her.

Health was viewed as the result of external interventions—possible only with the help of the doctor and his or her highly specialized tools. The concept of stimulating or supporting the body's own innate capacity for healing was all but completely abandoned. Prevention was forsaken; since the cause of disease was external, issues affecting the body's susceptibility were disregarded.

Beinfeld and Korngold observe that while the doctor in Western medicine is essentially a mechanic, in Eastern healing philosophies such as Chinese medicine, the doctor is like a gardener. A gardener is not a "fixer" of things so much as an ally; he or she nurtures, promotes, enhances, and works with the garden, *but does not try to control it.* A garden is a system that's alive, and the rule of Chinese medicine is to cultivate life. By contrast, one of the rules of the Cartesian doctrine came to be to prevent death at all costs. In the East, healers seek to make the body well; in the West, we seek to keep it alive, running. There is a difference.

TOOLS OF THE TRADE

In Eastern healing systems, the body is viewed as a system of energy, not as a machine, and the contents of those cultures' medicine chests reflect that. Gardeners and mechanics, after all, use different implements. Natural therapies obviously are not based on the Cartesian model. Quite the opposite: They are based on "holistic" principles. That the whole is considered in the assessment of health and the treatment of disease, and reinforcement of the host internally is as important as (or more important than) eradication of disease-causing agents externally.

Thus the tools of Cartesian, or conventional, medicine are by necessity radically different. If you are interested only in patching the body back together once it is already in an advanced stage of disrepair, you need different tools than if you are interested in promoting a body condition that resists disrepair. In conventional medicine, the focus on fixing what is already broken, and on eliminating outward symptoms—simply removing the "bad"—makes drugs and surgery appropriate as tools that can cut, manipulate, and replace.

The holistic model, embodied in the healing and medical systems of the East, views prevention as the vanguard of health and focuses on the body's own capacity to heal and repair itself. Symptoms are not equated with the underlying basis of disease. The tools most valued in holistic medicine are therefore those that can promote the "good," assist the body in maintaining balance and enhance its own healing mechanisms. Those tools include the plants and foods that make up herbal medicine. These tools are usable by us because they are gentle, nontoxic, and easy to understand.

Herbal medicine has its complexities, and truly mastering it can take a lifetime of intensive study. Yet there is enough simplicity about it that you can get started with it very effectively without having a degree in horticulture (as Beinfeld and Korngold point out, it is something "Chinese children are practically born knowing"). Part of the point of natural medicine is that it is practicable by you, because in the holistic model, you are considered to have most of the power in terms of your health.

GETTING BACK ON TRACK—
WITH HELP FROM AROUND THE GLOBE

Fortunately, even as herbal medicine fell out of favor in the United States, other cultures continued to study and use botanicals liberally and progressively, and we can now reap the benefits of their experiences and their wisdom.

Interestingly, some of the cultures in which use of herbal medicine has been most prolific may be experiencing serious problems—politically, economically, environmentally—but they don't have the heart disease, cancer, stroke, diabetes, and liver disease that kills nearly all Americans. "It sounds paradoxical that immigrants from a developing country are healthier in many ways than those who grow up here, but other studies have also reached similar conclusions about other immigrants," said the *Berkeley Wellness Letter* in July 1995, reporting on a UC Berkeley study that examined how the traditional Mexican diet changes after immigration to this country.

In Europe, botanicals have long been considered an important complement to conventional drugs. There doctors routinely prescribe herbal preparations for insomnia, colds, heart problems, constipation, depression, and more. Top-selling medicines in Europe include echinacea, hawthorn berry, St. John's wort, and ginkgo biloba (all herbs we will discuss later). Germany in particular leads the way with research and regulation as well as usage. As Dr. Andrew Weil points out:

> Germany is way ahead of us. There are many German pharmaceutical companies that make high quality, standardized, stable products. The government has worked out a system of regulations and standardization. . . . In every pharmacy the window displays were 100 percent natural products: valerian for sleep; peppermint oil for irritable bowel syndrome; ginkgo for blood circulation. When you walked in, there was a revolving rack of herbal teas, and the pharmacist would tell you what the teas were for and how to use them. The German pharmacists thought it silly that we live in a country where you have to go into one kind of store to get an herbal product, and another kind of store to get a pharmaceutical product; and that herbal products couldn't say on the label what they were for or how to use them.[4]

The sophistication of herbal medicine has been heightened by advances in global communication and transportation. This connects us to peoples from all over the world who have used herbal medicine with varying degrees of sophistication and in ways that are indigenous to their cultures. As American healers and patients turn back to natural medicine with renewed interest and hope for more productive views and methods, they are returning to a field much more worldly and refined than it was just a few decades ago.

In Karta Purkh's natural healing experience spanning twenty-five years, he has used and taught many modalities, including Kinesionics®, a muscle-testing health-assessment technology based on applied kinesiology that he developed. However, the core of Karta Purkh's expertise is herbal medicine. While the heart of his training is in Ayurveda, the ancient healing science of India, he has associated with practitioners of virtually every major healing system from many other cultures. This provides a strong, diverse base of knowledge in what herbalist and author Michael Tierra has termed "planetary herbology." It could also be called global herbology.

Thanks to global herbology, the best herbs from each culture are available to everyone now, giving herbal medicine incredible power and diversity. Karta Purkh says, "In the last five to ten years, we have been able to do things with natural healing, and especially herbal medicine, that we could only dream of before that. It's become a very small world. We can get herbs from anywhere on the planet at a moment's notice. We can call China and have an herb air-freighted to us next day. We can obtain things we could only hope to read about in a book ten years ago. Thus we can create previously unheard-of combinations of herbs from China, India, Africa, and so on that may be much more effective medicine than a single herb."

The evolution of this kind of herbal medicine also challenges the modern herbalist to learn about botanicals from all over the globe, not just those indigenous to the area. The "globalization" of herbal medicine compensates for what has been lost by the fragmenting of traditional ethnic communities. This fragmenting is a downside of increased transportation and communication.

As Karta Purkh explains it, in the "old days" of herbal medicine, the lack of transportation and communication meant that people used and studied only the herbs indigenous to their particular areas. This focus did not mean a shortage of material to master. Every civilization with a sophisticated herb-based healing system was within a day's walk to a vast cornucopia of herbs—enough to treat any kind of ill that culture might encounter. Most native ethnic herbalists have repertoires of about 2,000 different substances—meaning they can not only prescribe them appropriately, but can also identify them in the wild, harvest them, process them properly, and prepare them for best effect.

So an herbalist would learn the technique or school of thought in herbal medicine specific to his or her culture—for example, Chinese, Native American, African, or East Indian. In these stable ancient cultures, the apprentice was taught by the master, and then became the master and had his or her own apprentice, and so it went generation after generation. They experimented, they made their contributions to the field, they passed on the knowledge and it continued to expand. But the systems didn't mix very much with one another.

In many places today, that stable and ancient system has broken down. In some areas there are no masters to study with anymore. North America is, unfortunately, one of those areas. Much of the herbal medicine originally developed here died with the native peoples. There certainly are some experts who continue to study what was recorded, and some knowledge has been saved. But there aren't many people left who know the indigenous native plants of this area.

Therefore, much of what North American herbalists know is a fusion of what native herbalists from all over the world have learned in the context of their local healing systems. Fortunately, because each of the systems has so much to offer, this blending has yielded a powerful brand of medicine.

WHAT ARE HERBS?

Herbs are edible plants or, sometimes, concentrated foods. They are usually extremely safe, often nutrient rich, and full of compounds that can nourish, balance, rejuvenate, and stimulate the body's own healing responses. They are often very powerful, yet not habit-forming or addictive. They are whole and complete, not isolated substances like drugs (except when their active ingredients are concentrated into standardized supplements, a topic we will cover later on).

Herbs fall somewhere in the middle of the spectrum between food and drugs. Some herbs actually are nutritive, the way food is, and can be used the way food is used—consumed because it is healthy and makes you feel good. Other herbs have high concentrations of compounds that are not nutritive in the classic sense, but which nevertheless have specific actions that can influence body processes and move them in the direction of healing. Such compounds, whose names you will see used from time to time throughout this book, include alkaloids, polysaccharides, tannins, terpenes, saponins, flavonoids, and glycosides.

From the middle of the spectrum, some herbs lean farther toward the food side of the continuum, and others are closer to the drug side. The herbs that are most foodlike—or which sometimes are literally foods or spices—are generally the ones that are more nutritive in the classic sense.

Parsley, for example, is food when we put it in salad. But if we juice it and use it to treat edema (water retention), it is considered medicine— extremely mild medicine, but still medicine.

On the continuum a little closer to the drug side is an herb such as the well-known echinacea. Echinacea is not nutritive like food, but contains its own unique "brands" of some of the compounds mentioned earlier (in echinacea's case, chiefly polysaccharides) that are considered to be responsible for echinacea's supportive and stimulating effects on the immune system. Still, echinacea is far milder than a synthetic pharmaceutical drug.

Still closer to the drug end of the continuum is a plant like foxglove, from which the heart medicine digitalis is made. A fresh piece of this plant the size of your thumbnail will kill you. There are very few herbs this close to the drug end of the spectrum, but it's important to know that they do exist.

HERBS AND DRUGS: PROS AND CONS

Pharmacology has its roots in herbalism. Many medications are purified, synthesized versions of phytochemicals (naturally occurring plant chemicals). So what's the difference between drugs and herbal preparations? People are often curious about what makes herbs more desirable to use for health and healing than drugs. There are several important reasons why herbs are a healthier and more sensible choice for treating many health conditions, and for enhancing existing health.

Our Bodies Know and Understand Herbs

One of the great advantages of herbs is that our bodies know what to do with them. They are so close to the food end of the spectrum that our bodies recognize them because we have been in contact with compounds like these for millennia. Foods are composed of the same kinds of elements that make up herbs, only herbs are more concentrated. All over the world, in every culture, people evolved being exposed to plant foods and the building blocks of plants. Our bodies know how to metabolize, digest, and excrete waste from plant compounds. Our bodies do not react negatively to most plant compounds, as if they were foreign, because they aren't foreign.

Drugs, on the other hand, are new to our bodies. They've only been around for a couple of generations, and some drugs now being prescribed have only been on the market for months or years. Compounds like this are totally unfamiliar to our systems, and our bodies don't know what to do with these unrecognizable foreigners because they haven't had millennia to evolve specific mechanisms for dealing with them.

Because drugs are unlike anything our bodies have seen and dealt with before, they almost always produce what we call "side effects." While undesirable, side effects are the body's normal reaction to a foreign invasion—which is what ingestion of a drug represents. The body may mount an attack on the invader, just as it does on anything out of the ordinary. A drug may also produce toxic buildup because of the body's lack of built-in ability to process, assimilate, and eliminate such substances.

Dr. Andrew Weil in *Spontaneous Healing* calls drug toxicity "the most common sin of commission of conventional medicine today" and asserts, "In whatever form and for whatever reason you take drugs, you are increasing the workload on your liver, since it is the task of the liver to metabolize most foreign substances."

For this reason, most herbs are appropriate for long-term use, while most drugs are not. The medical model in which drugs are created and used is itself focused on the short term, so it should not be surprising that modern medicine yields only treatment devices made for short-term use.

Herbs Have All Their Parts Intact

Another great advantage of herbs, when used traditionally in their whole forms, is the action of a wide range of complementary components. Each medicinal plant can be shown to have from dozens to hundreds of component ingredients, like those named earlier, which act synergistically to restore health. Some would be considered primary active ingredients, others enhance and support the work of those active ingredients, some are nutritive, still others buffer compounds that might act harshly if isolated, and so on. All of these chemicals act in subtly different ways, in concert with each other, to create the effect we want.

For this reason, most traditional herbalists consider the strength of herbal medicine to be in the whole herb. Whole herbs are usually more effective and tend to be safer due to the presence of all their complementary constituents.

This benefit of herbs is another drug downfall. While drugs are very useful for relieving symptoms and are necessary at times, the broader action of herbs is superior for restoring underlying health. The conventional approach of isolating an active ingredient from a plant (as, for example, aspirin was first isolated from constituents of meadowsweet) creates dramatic, narrowly focused activity that is much more likely to produce side effects and to be ultimately less effective.

Drugs generally employ a single isolated substance to cause a single specific effect. These single actions produced by drugs are usually very severe. There is nothing else built into the drug to control or compensate for the force of its single action. Drugs often instigate other symptoms that may be as or more unpleasant as the symptom for which the drug is being taken (such as vomiting produced by a painkiller). The singular action of drugs can also upset the balance of the body so gravely as to set the stage for other illness later on. The propensity for yeast overgrowth after the use of antibiotics is an example. By simply trying to smooth out the bubble in one isolated spot, another bubble pops up somewhere else. Another metaphor is the seesaw: Drugs quickly drive body processes so far up or down in one direction that the other end of the seesaw rises or drops and then must be dealt with.

Herbs are generally balanced by nature, and when using an herb in its whole form, side effects are almost never an issue. Many traditional herbalists believe that there is an innate ecological wisdom in the way a given plant is composed, having evolved to contain that unique and specific combination of components. Perhaps the perfection created by nature could not be replicated in the laboratory.

In addition to the fact that the whole plant base includes compounds that may mitigate any deleterious effects of active ingredients, an herb is usually made up of a lower percentage of the active ingredient than is a drug. Herbs are by nature more dilute, thanks to the presence of inert plant material as well as less-active or inactive constituents.

Herbs Restore Health to the Whole, Not Relief to the Part

Herbs are traditionally used in the context of natural medicine, which seeks to correct the underlying pathology. This usually involves healing action on the interconnected systems and organs of the whole body, with the ultimate goal being to restore health and equilibrium. Drugs are usually made to alleviate symptoms, which are usually only telltale markers of some other trouble.

It's important to note also that this difference is not only a function of the differences between herb chemistry and drug chemistry, but of *the philosophies and intent with which they are used.* It *is* possible to use herbs only to treat a symptom and not the pathological process or imbalance that's triggering the symptom. It's just not often that you will find a natural health practitioner who is interested in using herbs only in that way. That mind-set is unique to conventional medicine.

Generally, practitioners who use herbs are not concerned merely with quieting symptoms. Such use may be part of treatment initially for immediate relief, but herbs and other therapies will be used simultaneously to restore the body's proper function. In herbal medicine, it is always preferable to eliminate the symptom by eliminating its cause. It is also preferable to activate the body's own functioning, rather than to *replace* a function. For example, in natural/herbal medicine it is preferable to stimulate the body to return to normal hormonal production and regulation, where in conventional medicine it is acceptable simply to replace hormones that are missing or insufficient.

Thus herbs not only by their own nature offer innumerable ways to eliminate underlying causes of disease and symptoms for a wide range of conditions, but their custodians by nature are practitioners who are inclined to direct their use specifically toward healing the whole.

Furthermore, herbs are health enhancers, while drugs are treatments. Drugs are not designed to restore balance or enhance the whole body in any way. They cannot be expected to do so because drugs themselves are not balanced. They are only taken as treatment when you are sick, never when you are well.

Drugs developed out of a model that is focused on disease treatment, usually at a point where people are already very sick. If the doctor always sees the patient after he or she is very broken, the doctor will need and demand only tools that fix what is very broken.

Herbs can be used as "treatment," but they are also used effectively to boost health further. In fact, herbs shine in this area. Many herbs are useful even when you are well. They work with the body, not just against disease, so they are the best way to get well and stay well.

Drugs Are Easier—Or Are They?

The main advantage of drugs is convenience. If you have a headache, you can take two ibuprofen tablets and the headache goes away fast. Brewing up two cups of willow bark tea is more inconvenient. Herbs usually do take longer to work than drugs, and often require more effort and responsibility than taking prescribed pills.

But there are costs and payoffs to everything. There are definite costs associated with the convenience of drugs, both in terms of physical health and dollars. Drugs are not only exorbitantly expensive to buy, they also create further costs down the road because of the way they work (or don't). That's because they frequently ignore the problem underlying the symptoms; thus the real problem may persist, get worse, and require more treatment. Drugs may also suppress the disease on the surface by pushing it inward, resulting in more serious illness that is even harder to control.

In addition, drugs may create new problems in their wake (from side effects, to rebound effects, to new diseases borne of new imbalances or weaknesses). More treatment of one kind or another is then required to fix these new problems. Dr. Howard Posner from Philadelphia notes in the PBS documentary *The Medicine Garden* that it's not uncommon to see patients given second- and third-line drugs to treat the side effects of the first drugs. Michael Terra, in his book *The Way of Herbs*, calls it "increased attempts to beat the system into submission." When increasingly powerful interventions are used to treat these "satellite" problems, a never-ending vicious cycle ensues that is bad for the patient *and* the cost of health care.

By making the host weak and favoring survival of the fittest microorganisms, drugs can also influence the evolution of disease, affecting not just your health but that of society. The "hot issue" of antibiotic-resistant bacteria is just one example. The problem is predictable by common sense, yet trillions of dollars in industries are built on the dismissal of this logic. Whether you're treating bacteria, cancer, fleas, or garden insects, if you douse it all with harsh chemicals you will kill all but the hardiest bacteria, cancer cells, fleas, or aphids. You also weaken the human, pet, or garden. Then the surviving fittest—those hardy pathogens, cells, or insects—can proliferate with less resistance from the compromised host.

Anything that weakens you in any way is ultimately antithetic to healing. Disease and degeneration befall the weak host, whose mechanisms of repair and healing or resistance are depressed or defective. With that in mind, any substance or method used to provide relief is undesirable if it weakens the host. So what if it kills the pathogens today if it renders you too feeble to fend off attacks tomorrow?

It is in your interest to use medicines that boost your own healing mechanisms. Herbs are so effective, cost-efficient, nontoxic, and noninvasive that the personal effort required is worth it. And the kind of commitment that is cultivated by their use leads to enhanced health, prevention, and attitudes that promote health in the first place.

ARE ALL HERBS SAFE?

Most are, but not all. It is possible to do harm with herbs; there is no question about that. Herbalists and doctors alike have used the adage "The dose makes the poison." There are a handful of herbs that are naturally so powerful that they could be harmful if misused. These herbs are identified throughout the book, where relevant. It's important to distinguish the majority (very mild herbs that are therapeutic only in large doses) from the small minority (potent herbs that must be used sparingly). Knowledge of traditional uses is key.

Herbs could also be harmful if used improperly, without information, to treat something for which they are not really effective, thereby allowing a condition to worsen under the illusion that it is being treated. However, this would not really be the herb's fault; it would be the fault of an uninformed person using something unwisely and not heeding the body's messages. That's an education problem, something that certainly needs to be addressed (and which this book is intended to help resolve).

Nevertheless, it must be emphasized that most herbs, because they are so balanced and dilute and because the active ingredients are spread over such a broad spectrum of action, are safe for almost anyone to use. A number of herbs, like some foods, can be taken in as much of a quantity as you can tolerate because no matter how much you take, they will only help you. Herb toxicity is much more rare than drug toxicity (although, ironically, herb toxicity gets far more attention).

If you went into a herb store and randomly grabbed a few bottles of herbs off the shelf and swallowed them all down, chances are great that you'd be just fine. Certainly you shouldn't be doing that, but it's likely that just about anything you'd ever find in a herb store would not hurt you. If you did swallow the contents of a random bottle of herbal supplements, you might have diarrhea or feel a bit queasy, but in most cases that would be the extent of the damage. (For example, a woman who recently attempted suicide by taking a bottle of valerian root experienced muscle tremors and fatigue lasting one day, with medical tests revealing no liver toxicity or other abnormalities.[5]) You can surely imagine the kinds of things that would happen if you did that with a random bottle of pharmaceutical drugs.

Drug side effects are a serious issue. Drug reactions outnumber herb reactions worldwide by more than 99 to 1.[6] In the public broadcasting radio documentary *The Medicine Garden*, produced by David Freudberg, Freudberg reports that:

- There are 10 million cases of negative drug reactions *every year*, according to the consumer advocacy organization Public Citizen.
- Of those, 600,000 result in hospitalization *every year*.
- Worldwide, other countries that use herbal medicine (especially in Europe) have excellent adverse-reaction reporting systems, and herbs account for *less than 1 percent* of negative reactions. Pharmaceuticals account for virtually all negative reactions to remedies worldwide.[7]

These findings are consistent with the clinical experience of most herbalists, naturopaths, and other natural health practitioners—including Karta Purkh, his colleagues, and those interviewed in this documentary. Consistently, those consulted reported that 1 to 2 percent of all individuals experience *mild* reactions.[8]

In *The Medicine Garden*, Robert Temple, who evaluates drugs for the FDA, says that's hard to swallow. In typical clinical studies of drugs, he says, it's common to see 25 to 30 percent of subjects having adverse reactions. "It's inconceivable that plant-derived materials are not associated with the same kinds of side effects," he charges. But he's looking at drugs. He evaluates drugs. Drugs are single substances that produce a single effect. Herbs are not concentrated and isolated. It's like comparing massage to major surgery: What's inconceivable is that they *would* have the same side effects.

Dr. Andrew Weil, M.D., has relied on botanicals for the last fifteen years personally and in his practice, and estimates that for every prescription drug he prescribes, he recommends forty to fifty botanicals. He says this has never produced a single adverse reaction. A couple of rashes, a couple of upset stomachs—in which case the patient was told to discontinue use. This, he says, is utterly insignificant compared to what you see with drugs. Relative to the use of pharmaceuticals, there's no contest. The risks of drug toxicity are significant, both in numbers of reactions and kinds of reactions—"which include death and permanent disability," he said in *The Medicine Garden*. He also said he is very upset at the widespread prescription of steroid drugs for trivial conditions.

Paul Bergner, editor of the journal *Medical Herbalism*, recently pointed out:

> Approximately 8% of all hospital admissions in the U.S. are due to adverse reactions to synthetic drugs. That's a minimum of 2,000,000. At least 100,000 people a year die from them. That's just in the U.S., and that's a conservative estimate. That means at least three times as many people are killed in the U.S. by pharmaceutical drugs as are killed by drunken drivers. Thousands die each year from supposedly "safe" over-the-counter remedies. Deaths or hospitalizations due to herbs are so rare that they're hard to find. The U.S. National Poison Control Centers does not even have a category in their database for adverse reactions to medicinal herbs.

Herb safety issues, including myths, are discussed further in Chapter 24, "Urban Myths and Sidewalk Talk," pages 472–495.

ARE DRUGS EVER BETTER THAN HERBS?

For most conditions, only as a last resort. While sometimes drugs are unavoidable, such instances are invariably at the latter stages of a condition that has been allowed to progress. And natural healing is much more sophisticated, effective, and powerful than most people think it is. Herbal medicine is not a "cute fantasy" or "nice hobby"—it's serious, worthy medicine, and the rest of the world knows it.

Herbs can treat just about any health problem you can come up with, from acute issues to long-term chronic conditions to tricky, challenging puzzles. Karta Purkh says, "Unless someone has a genetic disorder, such as Down's syndrome, I feel virtually any ailment can be cured naturally with herbal medicine. Some, certainly, are more challenging than others, and some will require a variety of interventions."

Often, herbal medicine (and other natural alternatives) offers options for healing that conventional methods cannot. Since the average doctor at this time simply doesn't learn much about natural alternatives, the conventional prognosis for your condition may be pessimistic. Such pessimism, which can certainly interfere with healing, is of great concern to many natural healing authorities.

Drugs have without question saved lives, and sometimes they are necessary. You should use the most appropriate treatment in your individual situation. It's just that herbs and other mild natural treatments often are very appropriate, yet drugs are used instead because of lack of knowledge, understanding, and respect for herbs. This often amounts to the use of a wrecking ball when all that's needed is a love tap.

Furthermore, the kind of situation in which drugs really are more appropriate can frequently be avoided in the first place. The kind of zero-hour emergency that makes high-tech methods necessary can often be prevented with herbs as well as lifestyle choices. Generally, you don't have to get to the crisis point where the "big guns" are absolutely necessary. But even when total prevention is not achieved, early-stage problems can be handled using gentle, mild methods, far in advance of the need for desperate save-the-day measures.

Before you use a sledgehammer, see if a gentle nudge won't do the trick. Or, as Dr. Andrew Weil bluntly puts it: "If you are faced with the prospect of taking drugs to treat a health problem, you will want to know if there are any natural agents you may use instead."[9]

IS THERE ANYTHING HERBS CAN'T DO?

Yes. Herbs cannot directly treat serious trauma or mechanical injury. For example, herbs cannot suture wounds, set broken bones, or relieve pressure on the brain from a skull fracture. Conventional medicine is extremely skillful and successful at treating trauma and serious injury. (However, herbs can speed healing and reduce discomfort in numerous ways as an adjunct to trauma treatment or after surgery—to reduce bruising, promote tissue regeneration, slow bleeding, and so on. We will discuss later how to use them in these situations.)

Other than that, herbs have a fantastic range of health-care uses. They can help you feel good, look good, and live better as well as longer. They can relieve pain, not only by dulling your sense of it but by eliminating its cause. They can take the lead in or assist in the healing of most diseases. And unlike drugs and surgery, *they can help strengthen the body so that it is less likely to succumb to illness in the first place.* They are the most versatile medicines available because they can alter the "bad" *and* promote the "good." They can have a direct effect on a problem now, or they can create global changes in the entire body and all its systems, for a long-lasting effect on present and future problems.

Even diseases that we would not recommend you try to treat yourself or with an herbalist are, in fact, treated herbally in other parts of the world, where thousands of years of practice have made herbal medicine an extremely sophisticated science. Michael Weiner, Ph.D., notes that in China, even acute appendicitis is treated herbally—with about 20,000 reported cases reflecting an overall nonsurgical cure rate of 90 percent. "This is only one example of a philosophical difference which enables one school of practice to effectively employ herbs for a condition which the other generally considers to be strictly in the surgeon's realm," Weiner notes.[10]

PHARMACOGNOSY

When herbs are studied or taught by traditional healers, it is with all the larger context of the entire traditional healing system in which herbal medicine matured, a healing system that is holistic in its approach to the body, health, and life. In those systems, herbs are used in the context of a person's entire life, and complemented by other aspects of the lifestyle. Many American herbalists study herbal medicine within this perspective, and they are considered traditional herbalists.

However, there is another way that herbs are studied in the West, from within the context of conventional scientific medicine, called pharmacognosy—the botanical cousin of pharmacology. In pharmacognosy, the scientific principles of the West are applied to herbal medicine. All substances are analyzed and broken down by their components, which are studied for their individual effects. This is usually done in the absence of the context that gives herbal medicine its rich dimensions. The herbs are plucked out of the healing system of origin, leaving behind all of the accompanying wisdom, observation, and intuition that made them most useful, understandable, and safe in their native culture.

Orthodox scientists like this approach to herbs, and even insist upon it, saying that is the only "scientific" way to approach any kind of medicine. Thus herbs are treated like drugs in an attempt to wedge them into more familiar concepts and filter them through the current scientific paradigm, so that they can be understood in terms of modern scientific thought.

But since herbs are not drugs they often don't fit very well into the present scientific model, and they suffer in the interpretation. The structurally oriented thinking of Western science doesn't necessarily lead to useful explanations of herbs (or other healing systems or modalities), which are viewed functionally in other cultures; and reductive methods of analysis don't necessarily spotlight herbs' greatest potentials. When science tries to mix apples and oranges in this way, the apple sometimes gets illegitimized for its failure to fit in the same box as the orange.

Scientists frequently complain that they cannot understand herbs or see any benefit to them, but that is because they have insisted on taking home a new toy, chucking the instruction book, and taking it apart until it cannot be put back together again. For example, they try to make an herb kill a pathogen in a petri dish when that's not the way it works; the herb may instead effect global changes in the host that make the host an unfavorable environment for that pathogen. Scientifically, such an herb might be pronounced "ineffective."

Pharmacognosists frequently view herbs merely as diluted drugs. That is not what herbal medicine "merely" is. It is a way of life and incorporates a panoramic set of views about health and the body. Pharmacognosists may insist that medicinal herbs are not foods or nutritional supplements, because anything used to treat disease or improve health must conform to the definition of the word *drug*. Pharmacognosists also typically see no difference between natural and synthetic substances.

Unfortunately, though we'd like to hope otherwise, classifying herbs as "drugs" may be the only way herbs will ever get studied, taught, and covered by insurance in this country. However, classifying herbs this way wouldn't change the biochemical facts: No matter what name you give it, a whole herb and a concentrated drug are two very different things. At any rate, pharmacognosy does not equal herbal medicine. Pharmacognosy is the pharmacological analysis of herbs.

SETTING THE SEMANTICS STRAIGHT

One last issue to clarify is definitions of terms used frequently to distinguish different kinds of medicine. The phrases used in this regard are sometimes questionable, sometimes used interchangeably when they are not interchangeable, and often mean different things to different people.

To help clear up this confusion, below we provide a glossary of terms that defines what we mean when we use them. It may also help you sort out what others are referring to, or at least alert you to the possibility of misuse or multiple meanings.

Conventional medicine—The most common term used to describe the medicine that has evolved in the West over the past 100 years or so. Synonyms for this term as we use them include **allopathic** medicine, **standard** medicine, and **orthodox** medicine. (While it is sometimes called **Western** medicine, this is not entirely accurate because Europe can be considered "the West," yet is very sophisticated and advanced in its use of herbal and other natural medicine.)

Alternative medicine—A broad field that encompasses all of the natural and holistic therapies not recognized as "conventional," as well as a host of controversial treatments and therapies that are not necessarily natural or holistic. We don't use this phrase much, except when quoting others, because it can be confusing and misleading.

Holistic medicine—While considered by some to be a broad subset of "alternative medicine," other practitioners feel that true holistic medicine encompasses anything and everything that works for the whole patient—alternative or conventional, whether natural or synthetic. By the latter definition, **natural** medicine is not an interchangeable phrase, even though it is often used as such. Natural medicine refers specifically to the use of natural and nontoxic substances as well as preventive lifestyle measures to promote health, and is the most accurate term to describe herbal medicine. Many natural health practitioners feel that the "whole" in "holistic" refers to the whole person, not necessarily to the whole range of medical options available, and point out that many aspects of conventional medicine do not treat the whole patient. Most agree that holistic medicine does emphasize addressing the whole body and life of a person, both in sickness and in health. Our perspective is that all health problems should be treated holistically—considering the whole person *and* considering all options from all fields—but that very often, natural medicine is the most appropriate avenue.

Traditional medicine—The traditional, often ancient healing systems of specific cultures, such as Chinese medicine, Ayurveda from India, Tibetan medicine, or Native American healing. These are essentially holistic healing systems associated with the cultures that have refined them.

Herbal medicine—the art and science of using plants, foods, and spices to heal and maintain health. Much of what we know about herbs originally came from records of their well-developed use in traditional medicine. An herbalist may be trained specifically in herbal medicine by itself, or may be a health professional such as medical doctor, naturopath, osteopath, homeopath, physician's assistant, or nurse practitioner who studied herbal medicine.

Naturopathic medicine—Naturopathic medicine, or naturopathy, is based on a combination of modern medicine and traditional healing philosophies and techniques. Naturopathic physicians (NDs) are general health practitioners trained as specialists in natural medicine. They are licensed physicians (in Washington state and eleven other states, as of September 1996), but are not licensed to prescribe drugs. Their training emphasizes natural and holistic approaches.

Naturopaths may choose to specialize in an area of interest to them, so some may use herbs extensively in their practices, while others use homeopathy or favor nutritional therapies. Some naturopaths may be herbalists, but this is not necessarily the case. Still, botanical medicine is usually part of naturopathic therapy, and NDs are the only health-care professionals licensed specifically to treat using medicinal herbs, and the only physicians who are expressly trained to do so.

Homeopathic medicine—Homeopathy is a system of medicine whose fundamental approach to the patient is holistic, but whose healing methods are highly specific. Medicines may be made from plants, animal substances, or chemicals and are diluted according to a precise process until very little of the original substance remains. Although homeopathy sometimes uses plant substances and herbalists may sometimes recommend homeopathic medicines as part of a treatment plan, *homeopathy and herbal medicine are not the same thing.* Homeopathy is a very complex and unique system that we do not cover in this book.

Integrative medicine—This phrase was coined by Dr. Andrew Weil, M.D., to communicate the essence of his approach: combining the best ideas and practices from around the world and from different systems, both those we call conventional and those we call alternative. Sometimes this type of approach is also referred to as **complementary** medicine.

GETTING STARTED

In many areas of health education, there is a lack of acknowledgment or respect for the idea of "starting where you are"—introducing things slowly so you don't get overwhelmed, and allowing that doing something imperfectly is better than not doing it at all. Most beginning herb users do not want to worry about whether yarrow that was grown on the east slope of a shady hillside is better than that grown on a sunny pasture with a southern exposure. (For some herbs that can matter, but if you're not there yet, it doesn't mean you can't get great benefits from herbs. Most herb users never get that sophisticated, and the actual benefits of doing so can be marginal.)

Conversely, we believe it is important to go beyond the utterly simplistic. At this point, almost anyone on the street can tell you to take echinacea for a cold. Hundreds of women's magazine articles are now featuring little herbal how-tos and tidbits (without context, in a try-this-for-that fashion).

There are 500,000 species of botanicals in use on earth that have effective and safe medicinal uses. Among them, there is almost certainly something you can use to get your body to do its job. You don't have to suffer and live with your health problems. You can get well—naturally. Let's get started.

2

History of Ayurveda, Ancient Healing Wisdom

M ost other countries, in both the West and the East, are ahead of America in understanding and using herbal medicine. But the East is the origin of most of what is known today about herbal medicine, thanks to several larger, conceptual systems we often call Eastern healing.

When we talk about Eastern healing, we generally mean healing systems of Asia—from India, China, Japan, Tibet, and southeast Asia. Each of these regions has developed distinctive concepts about health and healing, but all share some fundamental common ground that we recognize as Eastern healing for its distinct differences from what is known as Western medicine.

What is now frequently called holistic healing really descended from Eastern thought about healing. The chief philosophies that make medicine holistic—understanding, observing, treating and maintaining the whole body and the whole person, rather than an ailing or broken part; an emphasis on increasing health and healing rather than decreasing disease and symptoms—are essential ideas that originated in the East.

Eastern healing systems, of course, are based on much more than just a general focus on health and the whole person. Each system is based on observations and beliefs about the human body and what creates wellness as well as disease. These observations and beliefs provide direction regarding ways to eat, sleep, exercise, and manage the influences of various environments, both internal and external, as well as what herbs to take. They provide tangible tools and frameworks for applying what you learn.

It is easiest to understand and apply concepts in context, rather than abstractly. Therefore, we believe that it will be valuable, as you begin learning how to integrate healing herbs into your life, to have at least a rudimentary understanding of one of the systems that has yielded so much of what we know about herbs today. Connecting herbal recommendations to their sources and influences, and seeing the beliefs about health and the body that surround those recommendations, give perspective to what you are trying to do.

In the interest of providing this context, we considered offering a chapter on one of any number of Eastern healing systems. The choice came down to two, Ayurveda (from India) and traditional Chinese medicine (TCM). These are the two oldest and most sophisticated healing systems on record. There are crucial bottom-line philosophic similarities shared by these two systems; there are also some functional and practical differences.

We chose Ayurveda for a number of reasons. First, quite simply, it is the one that we know the most about. Karta Purkh in particular owes much of his education as well as personal health to the specifics of Ayurvedic healing. He has studied for many years under Yogi Bhajan, a master of Ayurveda and yoga, so much of his experience with Ayurveda comes not only from historical record but from the direct tutelage of one of India's premier authorities on the subject. In turn, having studied with Karta Purkh, my knowledge of herbs and Eastern healing favors Ayurveda.

Secondly, the purpose of providing this background is to give you some structure for dealing with your body using the kind of thinking that is common to Eastern healing—an orderly guided tour out of the conventional mode of thought about the body and disease. With the goal of enhanced understanding and insight, the simpler system makes a better foundation. While both TCM and Ayurveda have their complexities (and both Ayurvedic and Chinese herbs are widely recommended and discussed throughout this book), TCM as a system of thought is less easily broken down into a "first-timer's guide to Eastern healing." It is less easily condensed and, we feel, carries more risk of being confusing at this stage of your journey. But we do encourage you to learn more about TCM if your interest is piqued. There are several excellent books on this extremely powerful system, and they are listed in "Recommended Reading" on page 517.

As a layperson I have found Ayurveda to be the most digestible and most easily translated introduction to Eastern healing thought and practice, but it too has its intricacies. Of course, there are a number of books wholly on the subject of Ayurveda; some of these are also listed in "Recommended Reading" on page 517. What follows is a relatively brief distillation of a 7,000-year-old healing system that has at its core a sophisticated, extensive, and profoundly valuable herbal science.

BACKGROUND ON AYURVEDA

Ayurveda is the oldest continually practiced healing system on the planet. There are written records going back 5,000 years and an oral tradition going back thousands of years before that.

Ayurveda has probably been most popularized in the west by Dr. Deepak Chopra and to a lesser degree by a few other authors. Still, it's not very well understood in America. The practice of Ayurvedic medicine here lags behind acupuncture, for example, probably by about ten years. In the previous decade, the idea that long needles could unblock or reconnect invisible energy traveling along meridians throughout the body, bring about dramatic healing, or replace anesthesia would elicit unprintable comments from many doctors. Now, even though acupuncture is still not completely understood or explainable in conventional scientific terms, it is accepted because it's undeniably effective. There are now a great many acupuncturists practicing in the United States, and the treatment is covered by most insurance.

Mind, body, and spirit are inextricably entwined in Ayurveda and other Eastern traditions of health care. Ayurveda and yoga are sister practices, two sides of the same coin. Ayurveda is the physical, health, and medical side of the philosophies and guiding principles by which Ayurvedists live. Yoga is the science of spiritual development. Karta Purkh's mentor and teacher is a traditionally trained master both of Ayurvedic medicine and of yoga.

Ayurveda literally means "the science of life" (*Ayur* = Life, *Veda* = Science). Ayurveda looks to create a balance among body, mind, emotion, spirit, and environment. It places emphasis on the ability of the human body to heal itself, with the *assistance and support* of a variety of nontoxic therapies. Ayurveda offers the layperson a framework for understanding the body and how to best support its quest for balance.

Ancient Ayurvedists observed and experimented with how people could best live to be as happy and healthy as possible. Over many generations of patient, careful observation and systematic exploration, they recorded in encyclopedic writings what they found worked and did not work about every aspect of living. The culture at this time was extremely stable, affording the opportunity to observe the same people closely over very long periods of time—in extended families over generations, for example. There are libraries in India filled with 5,000 years' worth of written records and information in thousands of volumes.

Many of the health and medical "discoveries" being heralded today as breakthroughs by scientists were long ago observed and documented by the Ayurvedists. Modern science is now acknowledging the efficacy of more healing foods, nutrients, and herbs by the day—most of which were already proven in the eyes of the Ayurvedists to be useful and effective.

With the British takeover of India in the 1850s, Ayurvedic medical education was suppressed. Ayurveda could not be taken from the people, however, since it was so much a part of the way they lived and cared for themselves. So it continued on as a grassroots, people-based folk-healing legacy. After independence was regained in the late 1940s, the medical schools bounced back quickly.

Ayurvedic medicine is the origin of most healing systems on the planet today; all Asian medical systems evolved from the core of Ayurveda. Even acupuncture, largely thought to be a Chinese modality, may have originated from Ayurveda; archaeological digs in northern India have unearthed accurate acupuncture maps.

Ancient Ayurvedists were wanderers and traveled widely, sharing their knowledge of health and medicine. After Ayurvedic medicine was well developed in India, these scholars and practitioners traveled to gain and share knowledge—up over the Himalayas to Mongolia, China, and Tibet, then down through Japan and southeast Asia, and eventually as far as Greece.

Different cultures came to emphasize different aspects of the system of Ayurveda and interpreted it in their own ways, individualizing some aspects considerably. Different cultures employ different sets of herbs (usually those native to their own lands). And this is good: We have something to learn from each culture and the way they use natural medicines for healing and prevention. That is why this book, or for that matter herbal medicine at large, is in no way limited to the specifics of core Ayurvedic medicine. And you don't need to understand every interpretation of Ayurveda developed by every culture worldwide to benefit from all of it. But Ayurveda was the foundation for natural healing in the global sense, so it's a good foundation for your own natural healing in the personal sense.

AYURVEDIC USE OF HERBS

Ayurvedists have relied on herbs as the absolute centerpiece of the health-care system, successfully, for thousands of years. Therefore they have a lot to teach us about how to use herbs most effectively to restore and maintain health.

The Ayurvedic view of herbal medicine always considers the application of herbal and nutritional supplements in light of all other factors of a person's lifestyle. Herbs are used holistically along with an emphasis on diet, exercise, and stress management.

Categories of Herbs

Ayurveda classifies herbs into six main categories of action. Based on their main chemical components, they can be recognized by six characteristic *tastes*—sweet, sour, salty, pungent, bitter, and astringent.

In addition, herbs in Ayurveda are recognized by *energetics*: as warming or cooling, and as drying or "wet" (not necessarily literally "wet," as in dripping, but in that they tend to be juicier or moister, and also send the body in that direction). The tastes, through their action, drive the energetics—they produce hot or cold energy, dry or moist energy. Later in the chapter we will detail the energies produced by each of the tastes.

The specifics of herbal therapy in Ayurveda are driven by a given individual's need to increase or decrease these energies in his or her body in order to heal, or to stay well. Excess heat is controlled by cooling herbs; excess oiliness or moisture by drying herbs, and so on. Herbs may be chosen because they are cooling and drying, or warming and drying, or because they are warming and moistening. It all depends on the condition being addressed, and the general body type.

Each taste tends to produce a certain type of energy, although there are exceptions (for example, pungent herbs are generally heating, but mint is an exception—it is pungent and cooling). In turn, the energetics of herbs tend to push body processes in a certain direction. "Cold" herbs tend to reduce, slow, and dry. That can mean slowing the metabolism or digestion, reducing inflammation, or treating fever, as just a few examples. "Hot" herbs tend to increase, speed up, and expand. For example, they may promote circulation, increase appetite, stimulate glandular secretions, shorten the menstrual cycle, or raise metabolism or body temperature.

Herbs (and foods) can also have more than one taste. Pineapple is sour and sweet; green beans are sweet and astringent; onion is pungent and sweet. Rosemary is sour, astringent, *and* sweet.

Sweet-tasting plants' active compounds are often macronutrients—carbohydrates, fats, or amino acids (proteins). These herbs are builders, promoting tissue mass and health. Sweet-tasting plants form the bulk of all traditional diets around the globe. Most grains and nuts are predominantly sweet. Most general, long-term, nourishing tonics are sweet. One reason for that may be a certain type of long-chain carbohydrate, called polysaccharide, which research shows is a common denominator among many immunostimulant tonics. Sweet herbs and foods are generally cooling and wet.

Herbs with a sour taste produce their action through organic acids. This group of herbs tends to cleanse the body of toxins and promote digestion. Acidic herbs tend to be high in vitamin content, such as vitamin C in lemons. Citrus peels are, in fact, used herbally to promote digestion and stimulate appetite. Sour herbs are generally warming and wet.

Salts are mineral compounds that help the body retain fluids and improve digestion and bowel action. Salty herbs control gas and coughs. Kelp is an example of a salty herb. Salty herbs are generally warming and wet.

Herbs with "bite," or pungent herbs, usually contain volatile oils—ginger, for example. Black pepper is an excellent pungent herb, and is used in Ayurvedic therapy as a digestive tonic and blood purifier. Other pungent herbs found in the well-known umbellifer (carrot) family include dill, fennel, coriander, caraway, cumin, and anise, which are all excellent digestive and antiflatulence (carminative) remedies. The "herbs of life," as Yogi

Bhajan terms them, include pungent marjoram, rosemary, oregano, and thyme. Pungent herbs are generally warming and drying.

Bitter herbal preparations usually contain alkaloids and glycosides as components. These medicines are cleansing and can remove toxins from the blood. Many pharmaceutical drugs that have been created from herbs come from this bitter category, such as digitalis from foxglove. The king of the bitter herbs is turmeric (the herb that gives the yellow color to curry). Turmeric has wide use in Ayurveda, as we will discuss. Bitter herbs are usually cooling and drying.

Astringency, the taste produced by the presence of chemical constituents called tannins, is characteristic of those herbs that are used for tissue contraction and fluid absorption, such as in the treatment of diarrhea, hemorrhage, or excessive urination. For example, the astringent (tightening, drawing) leaves of strawberry, raspberry, and blackberry are used as tonics for the mucous membrane of the digestive tract, the uterus, and the kidneys. Astringent herbs are typically cooling and drying.

If we understand the basic tastes and energetics of herbs, we can begin to see the logic in how they work. You can become more instinctive about matching herbs to conditions. For "hot" diseases such as those involving inflammation, cool bitter herbs are best. For oozy, leaky conditions, astringents are often recommended. For cold conditions (such as arthritic stiffness or depressed, slow glandular function), warming herbs are used. You can begin to understand why some herbs can stop bleeding or bring down a fever. Traditional cultures using these herbs have observed such effects empirically over a long history of use.

AYURVEDIC BODY TYPES

To choose which herbs are right for you, you can match herbal tastes and energetics not only to a specific condition but to your characteristic mind-body qualities. The system of Ayurvedic medicine offers guideposts that let you distinguish the most appropriate herbs for the job by matching their properties with *your* properties.

One of the most pragmatic and functional aspects of Ayurveda is its fairly detailed, well-defined system of body typing. This provides a logical, consistent, and credible basis for making decisions and taking actions regarding your health, healing, prevention, and treatment. It lets you narrow down your options from among the vast and sometimes overwhelming array of choices among herbs and related healing substances. It lets you predict your most likely weaknesses, imbalances, and potential health problems, and determine how you can adjust your lifestyle to head off problems at the pass, before they even arise.

The Doshas

The unique system of Ayurvedic body types is based on the definition of three *doshas,* or energetic tendencies. These "master forces" of health are responsible for maintaining balance in the daily and long-term health of the individual. Disease is defined in Ayurveda as an imbalance of the doshas.

The doshas are characterized by temperature, moisture, weight, and texture. These qualities are related to the functions, systems, or qualities that each dosha governs in the body.

The *kapha* (earth) dosha maintains structure, solidity, growth, and lubrication in the body, forming connective and musculoskeletal tissue as well as mucus and other secretions. It is wet/oily, cold, heavy, slow, and stable, and promotes those qualities in the body. The *pitta* (fire) dosha maintains digestive and glandular secretions, body heat, and metabolism, including digestive enzymes and bile. It is wet and oily, hot, light, and intense. *Vata* (air) dosha maintains movement in the body, such as respiration and joint mobility. It is dry, cold, light, and irregular.

Primary Dosha Characteristics

Vata (AIR)	*Pitta* (FIRE)	*Kapha* (EARTH)
DRY	Oily	Oily
Cold	*HOT*	Cold
Light	Light	*HEAVY*
Irregular	Intense	Stable

In the Ayurvedic school of thought, everything happening in your body at any moment is a result of the doshas, and everything you do and don't do affects their balance. All three doshas are ebbing or flowing in every body (and in the environment around us) at any given time.

In a person, the dosha most likely to overpower and dominate defines that person's "constitution," or body type. Thus, the doshas—*kapha* (earth), *pitta* (fire), and *vata* (air)—not only represent and describe specific characteristics or "leanings" that can occur in anyone or anything, they also define the body types that most manifest those doshas.

For example, *pitta* refers to a specific kind of energy (hot, wet, light, and intense) and a set of trends or symptoms influenced by that energy. It is descriptive: Body processes can be *pitta*; weather can be *pitta*; food can be *pitta*.

But additionally, *pitta* is a body type—the fire type, one whose body is most likely to manifest *pitta*-type strengths and weaknesses. The *pitta* body type will be most likely to overemphasize *pitta* (fire) trends and tendencies, and to be affected by *pitta* food, weather, and so on.

Doshas are, in this sense, like faults—they represent the ways that a particular body type tends to go out of balance. Doshas can go out of whack in the body at any given time. Foods, stresses, exposures, and other things in our environment can overstimulate a particular dosha and make it overactive.

The body type is a good predictor of which dosha is most likely to try to overpower the other two and dominate. You can think of the doshas as the three legs of a stool; the body type is characterized by which leg wants to get longer than the others and tip the stool. The job of the other two is then to stretch out and help the stool regain balance. Sometimes we need to help that process along with food, herbs, or lifestyle adjustments.

Keeping this in mind, the fundamental concerns when looking at health from a Ayurvedic point of view are:

- How balanced the doshas are—or not—in relationship to one another currently (the short-term concern), and
- What our constitution, defined by our primary dosha, will tend to do over the rest of our lives (the long-term concern).

One of the things that makes this system of understanding your body so valuable is that it is an excellent predictor of how your body will behave. When you can predict with great accuracy the types of diseases to which you are most prone, you can act in advance to stave them off. It lets you fine-tune the basics of healthy lifestyle. By understanding the long-term likelihood for your body to go out of balance in a very particular way, you can live accordingly to manage it.

Determining Your Type

The Ayurvedists believe that the constitution is determined by heredity. Regardless of how it is determined, characteristics of a particular constitution are already evident in infancy.

There are a number of different body types, because not all bodies manifest the tendencies of one primary dosha. There are dual-dosha types and even a tri-dosha type in which all three—*vata, pitta,* and *kapha*—are about equally strong. Thus it is possible to be:

Single type	Combo types
Vata (air)	*Vata-pitta* (air-fire)
Pitta (fire)	*Pitta-kapha* (fire-earth)
Kapha (earth)	*Vata-kapha* (air-earth)
	Tri-dosha (equal parts of each tendency)

There is no "best" body type to be. Each has its advantages and disadvantages. The single-dosha body types tend to have fewer but more serious and in-depth health problems. Dual-dosha types and the tri-dosha type will tend to have a wider variety of less severe issues. The tri-dosha type is least likely to become seriously imbalanced (because all three doshas are vying for equal dominance) but can be trickier to treat when it does, because anything you do to one dosha throws the other two out of whack. Treating tri-dosha usually requires very mild, slow nudges rather than aggressive activity.

The constitution reflects not only tendencies of the body but also tendencies of the mind—personality characteristics. The fire type tends to be passionate, colorful, argumentative, competitive, decisive, and convincing—fiery! The air type tends to be creative, nervous, restless, disorganized (think airy, ethereal, "spacey"). The earth type is prone to be—what else?—down-to-earth: conservative, loyal, slow, calm, and steady.

THE BODY-TYPE TEST

Determining your constitution may involve a little sleuthing. Most Americans have all three doshas totally wacky by adulthood. This is largely due to the way we live and care for ourselves (or don't).

Children who grow up in an environment of awareness regarding these elements and influences, and whose lives from birth are adjusted to complement their constitutions, will consistently display classic signs of their types throughout life. However, for many Americans, trying to identify what dosha primarily drives their health is puzzling because so much of what *seems* primary and innate is actually the result of imbalance. In a culture marked by unhealthy eating, smoking, drinking, drug abuse, and a sedentary lifestyle, this is not surprising. The test that follows will help you to determine your constitution.

Some people will find that their answers clearly fall into line within one dosha. There are forty-six questions, and if more than two-thirds, or thirty, of your answers fall in one column, that's a good indication of a single-dosha constitution. For example, when I take the test I have a whopping thirty-nine out of forty-six *pitta* (fire) answers, with two *kapha* (earth) and five *vata* (air) answers.

If your answers are almost evenly divided among the three columns, you are most likely the tri-dosha type. If you have twenty-five, fifteen, and six (or something similar), then you are a dual dosha, with the two dominant ones representing your constitution. For instance, twenty-five *vata* (air) answers and fifteen *pitta* (fire) answers would suggest a *vata-pitta* (air-fire).

Answering Truthfully

If you have trouble deciding on answers for some of the questions, either about your body or your personality, it may be because time, modern environments, and habits have distorted or concealed your true constitution. Your constitution represents tendencies that include gifts and potential, but a lifestyle that abuses your body may mean that potential is never realized and the gifts get buried. Tendencies are just that—natural inclinations, not fixed, immovable features. They can be masked by other developments over time.

A classic example of this is a *pitta* (fire) type, normally a naturally muscular and medium-to-lean body type, who may have a great deal of fat piled on top of his or her essentially medium-sized frame, and whose muscles may be poorly developed despite *pittas'* natural tendency to be very developed. We would call such a person a *pitta* (fire) type with excess *kapha* (earth). The imbalance screens the fundamental dosha.

Most Americans require some work just to get back to exhibiting the normal tendencies of the primary dosha. Karta Purkh notes, "Usually, at first, you have to deal with things as you find them, scraping away layer by layer till you hit bedrock—the bottom-line dosha that determines the constitution. Once you reach that point, you can work on yourself constitutionally for the rest of your life—as people in other cultures do from the very beginning."

If a particular aspect of your dosha is not clear, it can help to think back to what you were like as a child. Ask your parents or friends, if you cannot remember. How did you compare to other kids? If you were strong, muscular, and fiery until your twenties, then spent the next thirty years in a sitting job eating burgers for lunch every day, you may look and feel and act like a *kapha* (earth type), but you probably are actually a *pitta* (fire type), like the example above. If you were quick, light, dreamy, and creative as a child, it's a good bet you're *vata* (air type)— even if you feel your creativity is now quashed by sixteen-hour workdays with three kids at home. Your child self may provide clues to the true constitution underneath.

Occasionally, you might find that the opposite is true. For example, I am a *pitta* (fire type) who was heavily weighted with excess *kapha* (earth) all through childhood. I was slow and thick like *kapha* (predictable, in retrospect, since my diet favored sweets and fats, both energetically "heavy" and aggravating of *kapha*). If you look only at what I was like back then, you might say I was an earth type. In fact, that was a case of poor habits leading to a body and symptoms that concealed my real constitution. After I began caring for myself appropriately and brought my body into balance, my true nature emerged. (For this reason, it's best to think back to when you were *very* young. When I was two, I was very "fire type"; I was about six when the sugar and fat began to take their toll visibly.)

An even better way to choose the best answers is to think about what you revert to under stress. You may be able to modify certain physical and mental aspects of yourself, but when the going gets tough, chances are you snap back into certain behaviors and succumb to certain types of illnesses. Those "default programs" point you toward your constitution. For example, you may have taught yourself to be assertive, but under pressure you may still become quiet and reticent. You may have learned to be calm, relax, and let others take the lead, but under strain you may revert back to taking control, being intense and critical.

Keep in mind when choosing answers that you are looking for the description that is most like you and most uniquely you. Of course we are all, at some time or another, all of those things listed in all three columns. The question is, Which one is so exceedingly you that about two-thirds of the population is less so?

One friend was studying the quiz and complaining about the "Mental" column: "But I'm all those things, sometimes. Sometimes I'm restless and curious, sometimes I'm sharp and irritable, sometimes I'm placid and receptive." True; so am I. But if I ask myself, "Which of those am I *more than most other people I know?*" I have to admit it's sharp and irritable. Almost everyone is aggressive, intense, and rebellious sometimes. But when I look at everyone around me, I have to admit that I'm more that way than most other people.

I explained to my friend that while she may manifest all of those states at some point, what she's like most of the time from my point of view—and especially in a pinch—is placid and receptive. Certainly I can be open and mellow, and she can be intense and strong-willed. But in a heated debate, I will become more fiery and she will become more reasoned. That's where the answers lie.

Finally, ask other people about their experience of you if you are uncertain. In my friend's case, I was clear about which of her many qualities dominate, even when she wasn't. Another way of asking this question of yourself is, "What am I famous for?" What qualities do people admire about you over and over, and what do you get teased about?

Take the following quiz by choosing the most appropriate description (either from the *vata*, *pitta* or *kapha* column) for each quality or process listed. Choose only one answer for each line. At the end, total up the number of answers in each column. If you are uncertain about which answer is best or truest for you, or about how to interpret your score, refer back to the discussion of determining your body type on pages 44–45.

Constitutions Test

	VATA (Air)	PITTA (Fire)	KAPHA (Earth)
General Nature, Personality, Habits/Interests	Variable, frail, artistic, restless, nonconformist, indecisive, quick, changeable; moving, traveling, stories, dance	Intense, aggressive, athletic, leader, critical, rebellious, visionary, persistent, purposeful; goal-setting, politics, drama	Solid, smooth, slow, strong, stable, steady; water, sailing, business, family
Mental	Fluctuating, restless, curious	High intelligence, sharp, irritable	Well-considered conclusions, placid, receptive
Positive Emotions/Traits	Creative, artistic, multifaceted	Productive, determined, perceptive	Loyal, calm, content
Negative Emotions/Traits	Anxiety, fear, insecurity, restlessness; "spacey"	Jealous, judgmental, greedy, irritable, aggressive	Depression, greed, detachment, apathy
Spiritual Attitude	Changeable, unsteady, rebellious	Determined, fanatic, leader	Steady, loyal, conservative
Spending Habits	Quick, impulsive	Methodical, moderate	Slow, saves
Speech	Chaotic, continuous, quick; talkative	Cutting, incisive, argumentative, convincing	Slow, melodious, defined, reticent
Sleep	Insomnia, erratic	Sound, short	Prolonged, deep, heavy, excessive; difficulty waking

	VATA (Air)	PITTA (Fire)	KAPHA (Earth)
Dreams	Many dreams— remembers; flying, jumping, running, tall things, nightmares	Fiery, passionate, color, conflict	Water, romance; few dreams— doesn't remember
Memory	Short good, long poor (generally poor)	Sharp, clear	Slow, prolonged
Physical Stamina	Low, poor, start and stop quickly	Moderate, heat intolerance	Good stamina, inertia, slow to start, constant, good endurance
Body Temperature	Very Cold	Warm or Hot	Moderately Cold
Body Tissue Moisture (skin, hair, membranes, etc.)	Dry	Oily (moist/wet)	Oily (moist/wet)
Frame	Slender, tall or short; veins, bones, tendons visible	Medium; muscles defined	Thick, large, stout; little definition; prone to obesity
Body Fat	Low	Moderate/medium	Heavy, obesity tendency
Head	Small, wobbly	Moderate size	Large, steady
Forehead	Small	Folds, lines	Large

Constitutions Test (continued)

	VATA (Air)	PITTA (Fire)	KAPHA (Earth)
Eyebrows	Thin, small, irregular	Fine, moderate	Thick, bushy
Eyelashes	Dry, firm, small	Fine, thin, small	Large, oily, thick
Eyes	Active, dry, brown, black, small, squinting, shifting gaze	Medium, penetrating, piercing; green, gray, yellow	Big, wide, prominent, blue, thick, oily eyelids, wet (tears)
Nose	Small, crooked, dry skin and nostrils	Medium size	Thick, firm, oily skin, moist nostrils
Lips	Thin, dark, dry, unsteady, small	Moderate, red, soft	Thick, large, oily, firm, smooth
Teeth	Protruded, crooked, cracked	Moderate size	Large, white
Gums	Thin, dry, receding	Soft, pink, bleed	Soft, pink, moist
Shoulders	Flat, small	Moderate	Broad, thick, oily skin
Chest	Narrow, poorly developed	Moderate	Broad, well developed
Arms	Small, thin	Moderate	Large, thick, long, developed, full
Hands	Thin, small, dry, rough, cracked, veins, prominent knuckles	Medium, warm, pink	Large, thick, moist or oily, cool, wide
Calves	Hard, small	Soft, loose	Round, full

	VATA (Air)	PITTA (Fire)	KAPHA (Earth)
Feet	Thin, small, dry, rough, cracked	Moderate, soft, pink	Large, thick, full
Skin	Rough, dry, cool, dark, thin, cracked, visible veins	Moist, pink, red, yellow/olive; moles, freckles; rashes, acne; warm, soft, oily; perspires	Thick, oily, cool, pale
Nails	Small, thin, dry, rough, brittle, fragile	Moderate, soft, pink	Thick, large, smooth, white
Hair	Dry, kinky, brown, black	Soft, oily, fine; scant, early baldness, blond, gray, red, light brown	Thick, oily, wavy; dark or light
Joints	Thin, dry, "crackly"	Medium, soft, loose	Thick, move smoothly
Appetite	Variable, low	Sharp, large	Regular, steady
Digestion	Irregular, gas	Rapid, hot, acid	Smooth, efficient
Urine	Scant, difficult, concentrated, gray	Profuse, burning, stinging, yellow, red	White, milky, cold, profuse
Feces	Hard, dry, small, gas	Loose, diarrhea, oily, burning	Moderate, solid, mucus, thick, regular, heavy, slow
Sweat, Body Odor	Little	Profuse, hot, strong smell	Moderate, cold, pleasant smell

Constitutions Test (continued)

	VATA (Air)	PITTA (Fire)	KAPHA (Earth)
Voice	Weak, hoarse	High pitch, sharp, strained	Deep, pleasant, clear tone
Menstruation	Irregular, missed periods, scant, dark, cramps	Regular, profuse bleeding, bright red blood, PMS, moderate cramps	Easy, regular, light blood, edema (water retention)
Sexual	Erratic, desire strong, low energy, low fertility	Moderate, passionate, dominating	Strong, sensual, low but constant libido, energy good, stamina, devoted, high fertility
Sensitivity (dislikes)	Fear of cold, wind, dryness	Dislike of heat, sun, fire	Fear of cold, damp, likes wind, sun
Disease Resistance	Poor, weak immunity	Medium, infections	Strong immunity
Disease Tendencies	PAIN, headaches, arthritis, nerve, joints, constipation	INFLAMMATION, fever, infection, skin, hemorrhoids, high blood pressure, ulcer, liver conditions	MUCUS, respiratory, kidney, sinus, edema, tumor, cholesterol, excessive growth/secretion
Medication Reaction	Quick, low dosage, side effects, nerve reactions	Medium, aspirin sensitivity	Slow, high dose
TOTAL NUMBER OF ANSWERS	_____	_____	_____

This quiz was compiled from many different sources and translations of traditional Ayurvedic texts, as well as the teachings of Yogi Bhajan. Similar charts appear in other books about Ayurveda, including the excellent *The Yoga of Herbs* by Drs. David Frawley and Vasant Lad.

VATA OR ECTOMORPH?

Three Western classifications of body shape and build that are acknowledged by some health, sports, and fitness professionals (though not widely accepted in American medicine) often correspond at least to some degree with the Ayurvedic constitutions. The Ayurvedic types address a much wider range of characteristics, and with much greater depth. The Western versions are used primarily in the context of physical fitness. However, this is another way of giving yourself some clues if you're stuck.

The ectomorphic body is naturally "thin" (though that doesn't guarantee it will be lean), usually tall, gangly or lanky, with long, slender bone structure. *Vatas* (air types) are most often ectomorphs.

The mesomorph is the "medium"—usually of medium height or shorter, builds muscle easily and loses fat easily, tends to be well defined and have a moderately sized frame. (A bodybuilding joke says that the mesomorph is the one who builds more muscle than you do just by spotting you as *you* lift weights!) When the mesomorph gains fat, it is usually in the hips and thighs. *Pittas* (fire types) are most often mesomorphs.

The endomorph has the greatest tendency to be "heavyset"—though this does not mean that he or she is destined to be fat; just that this type is going to be the first to show it in the absence of healthy eating. (It's not as if the other types won't also pay the price for a bad diet; it just may take longer for the bill to arrive. And a poorly-cared-for mesomorph can be fatter than a well-cared-for endomorph.) The endomorph has a large frame and tends to gain fat around the belly. *Kaphas* (earth types) are usually endomorphs.

Obviously, there are blends with these types, just as there are with the Ayurvedic constitutions. A mesomorph-ectomorph might be smaller-boned, leaner, lighter, and more delicate; a mesomorph-endomorph will tend to carry a little more fat and be bigger, taller, and stronger.

DOSHAS REFLECT WHAT'S DEEP INSIDE

Finally, it's important to keep in mind that the dosha concept refers primarily to energies *within* the body. They are hallmarks of body processes. We tend to associate "warm" and "cold" with our superficial external responses to temperature, but the doshas are not necessarily concerned with those. A fire type may not literally feel hot on the outside all the time; what makes them *pitta* is that their internal processes are hotter and faster than those of some two-thirds of the population. My husband, who is *vata* (air type), may feel warmer than I on a cold winter day, even though I am *pitta* (fire). But I am still more likely to heat up faster in hot weather; I enjoy heat more and I am more affected by it. I have hotter digestion and tend toward burning and inflammatory conditions. He is more likely than I am to have cold, dry joints and stiffness. How warm or cold we *feel* may be irrelevant.

REAL PEOPLE PROTOTYPES

To put a face on this perspective, here are three examples of the main constitutional body types in whom you might see yourself—or other people you know.

Kapha (Earth Type)

KARL

Age:	42
Height:	6'0"
Weight:	210 pounds
Hair:	Light brown, oily and wavy
Eyes:	Blue
Skin:	Pale, oily
Build:	Large and thick, "big-boned," always battling bulge around the middle

DISEASE HISTORY:
Sinusitis, pneumonia, bronchitis, hay fever, colds, kidney infection, cysts on back, hand, nose

Athletic:	Football lineman in high school
Sleep:	Sound sleeper; loves to sleep in when he can
Love life:	Didn't date much; married twenty years
Residence:	Lived in the same city all his life
Work:	Long hours as a computer analyst (been at company for fifteen years)

Friends say: Reliable and stable, but stubborn
Children: Four
Sex: Once a week, slow to rouse, long stamina once he gets
               started
Recreation: Family picnics and canoeing
Food: Loves greasy, salty meals and snacks, especially Mexican
               food, pizza, and potato chips
Car: Family station wagon
Money: Modest investments for kids' college

Describes his life as happy. "I guess I'm a little boring," he says, grinning.

Pitta (Fire Type)

SUSAN
Age: 36
Height: 5'6"
Weight: 140 pounds
Hair: Bright red, curly
Eyes: Green, wears glasses
Skin: Fair, burns easily, many freckles
Build: Compact and muscular
Other: Heavy perspiration and strong body odor

DISEASE HISTORY:
Canker sores, PMS, ulcer, gastritis, adult acne, assorted rashes

Athletic: Competitive runner
Sleep: Doesn't need much; goes to bed late, gets up fairly early
Love life: Many boyfriends
               First marriage five years; many fights
               Second marriage two years so far; passionately in love
Residence: Three different cities since entered workforce
Work: Regional office manager, promoted several times, obsessed
               with work
Friends say: Very intelligent, motivated, and passionate, but has a
               quick temper, tends to be controlling
Children: None (two miscarriages); ambivalent about taking the time

Sex:	Three to four times per week; many orgasms; fast, hot, and sweaty
Recreation:	Gourmet cooking, hiking, skiing, theater
Food:	Likes spicy food, especially Thai and Chinese; also Italian (lives for garlic!)
Car:	Shiny red sport utility vehicle
Money:	Has some savings, but enjoys indulging in vacations, new sports gear, and home improvements when her bonus checks are good

Describes her life as exciting, meaningful, but hectic; always wishing for more time.

Vata (Air Type)

TERRI

Age:	46
Height:	5'9"
Weight:	122 pounds
Hair:	Short, brittle, dry, straight
Eyes:	Brown
Skin:	Chapped, with corns and calluses
Build:	Lanky, bony
Other:	Always cold, loves the sun
	Loves excitement and adventure, but gets exhausted easily

DISEASE HISTORY:
Amenorrhea (ceased menstruation) several times, chronic constipation, headaches, insomnia, anxiety, fatigue; already has beginnings of osteoarthritis in a few joints
Already menopausal (started at 44); has hot flashes, emotional swings, vaginal dryness

Athletic:	Walks
Sleep:	Doesn't fall asleep or stay asleep easily; often uses sedating substances
Love life:	Dates several people at one time, never married, few serious relationships

Residence: Five different cities since graduated from college, plus
                lived in Europe for a while
Work: Art director for ad agency; very innovative and imaginative,
                often late to work; only a few productive hours per day
Friends say: Very artistic but unreliable, "space case"
Children: Never pregnant
Sex: Every night if possible, many positions, fantasies; orgasmic
                only half the time
Recreation: Painting, reading, music, travel, animals, classes in exotic
                subjects, creative writing
Food: Loves sweets; often skips meals and heads straight for dessert
Car: Ten-year-old Jaguar
Money: Always broke. "It just flows through my fingers."

Describes her life as "a roller-coaster—I never know what will happen next."

Keep in mind that if you are a combination type you will be a blend of these profiles, identifying with characteristics from two (or three, in the case of tri-dosha). Even if you are one type all the way, obviously you will not be *exactly* like one of these people. For example, I am a classic fire type, but while I do share most of "Susan's" characteristics, I have dark hair, eyes, and skin, and I identify more with "Terri" in terms of recreation, sleep, and taste for sweets. (And as it happens, among my own constitution-quiz answers, the few that don't fall in the *pitta*/fire column are on the *vata*/air side.) These prototypes are all based on real people, but we chose the most dramatic examples we could to underscore and help you recognize the types more easily.

WORKING WITH YOUR CONSTITUTION

Once you have a pretty good idea of where you stand in terms of your dominant dosha, you can begin to recognize and even predict some of your health issues (most people are amazed at how neatly their most nagging problems and concerns fit with their body types). Then you can begin to apply herbal healing specifics with a more discerning perspective, choosing some tonics or remedies over others because of their appropriateness for your particular type of body.

With Ayurveda, you use foods, teas, herbs, and nutrient substances to enhance your gifts—those aspects of your constitution that are advantages. You also accommodate or address your potential difficulties. At any given time, you might eat, supplement, or incorporate other lifestyle adjustments to:

- Address a specific, current issue of balance
- Enhance the benefits of your type
- Ease and soothe the negative tendencies of your type, in order to stave off health problems in the future

When you have one single dosha that is obviously dominant, your ideal health maintenance scheme is concentrated on suppressing that one dosha, which will lean toward overpowering the others, creating imbalance if not controlled.

For example, if you are *vata* (air-type) constitution, then *vata* energy wants to get stronger or "bigger" than the other two; your *vata* tendencies will cause certain conditions or vulnerabilities to flare up or show themselves. The way you eat, exercise, supplement, and live should be angled toward keeping *vata* under control. An air-type person's best herbs and foods are thus actually described as "anti-*vata*," strange as that may sound! It's not against *you*; it's against an aspect of you that's likely to get too large and unruly, and cause trouble.

For example, to treat excess *vata* (air), herbs can be used to decrease *vata*, and to boost and strengthen *pitta* (fire) and *kapha* (earth). Balance is achieved by suppressing or calming the dominant dosha and by strengthening the other two doshas, in effect raising their profiles.

In a tri-dosha person, all three doshas are trying to dominate, vying for the number-one position. This means fewer problems because there is inherent balance in all three reaching for equal status. However, when there is a problem, balancing this body type can be challenging; the strategy is like a tightrope balancing act. If you try to warm and lubricate *vata*, you may aggravate the fire and wetness of *pitta* and the wetness of *kapha*. If you try to cool *pitta*, you will aggravate the cold of *vata* and *kapha*. Tridoshas generally need to use very mild, slow remedies so as not to create sudden increases or decreases in any one dosha.

Healing by Constitution

Ayurveda deals with disease not as isolated and unpredictable symptoms, but rather as a function of predictable imbalance among the doshas. It is not something mysterious that strikes without provocation or warning. In Ayurvedic herbal medicine, you certainly address symptoms if they exist, but once surface issues are handled, you work long term with your true constitution to maintain health.

In a system like this, symptoms translate into patterns. The herbalist, especially with experience and background in Ayurveda or Chinese medicine, looks at acne, cysts, and exhaustion, and suspects liver congestion. He or she does not recommend acne medication, stimulants, and surgery. Some temporary-relief botanicals might be appropriate, but the real and permanent relief comes from rooting out the cause. By looking at the whole picture and identifying a common root, you can avoid whacking indiscriminately at all the branches. (This might be noted as one of the key differences between "treatment" and "healing.")

Moreover, in Ayurveda we may look at a person with four or five different conditions that seem unrelated in the modern conventional model, and attribute them all to imbalances typical of, say, a fire-type constitution. In that framework, the symptoms or diseases make sense, and the person can be treated constitutionally, rather than for five different conditions with five individual treatments.

Flexible Treatment for Doshas in Flux

Your needs will change as your lifestyle influences the state of the doshas. To begin with, you may be dealing with symptoms of a constitution very much out of balance, and the symptoms you are experiencing may not be symptoms that are normally associated with your constitution.

Therefore, it is important to understand that food and herbs are first addressed *at the dosha you're currently working on.* When treating specific problems, choose herbs that are directed at the dosha *of your condition,* not necessarily your body type. For example, "treating *pitta*" (fire) doesn't always mean treating a fire-constitution person. It may mean treating a *pitta* condition, a condition or imbalance of heat or fire, in *any* person.

The fact is that any person may exhibit symptoms at any time in his or her life that are not typical of the core body type, and this reflects imbalance or illness. It's less typical, but fire types do get respiratory mucus conditions (*kapha* must be treated or reduced). *Kapha* (earth types) do experience rough, hoarse, dry symptoms when *vata* (air, cold and dry) is aggravated and must be reduced. A *kapha* person with a fever or inflammation (a condition of excess heat) will need an "anti-*pitta*" remedy (something that cools and dries by increasing *vata* or cold, dry energy).

When I began using herbal medicine, I had excess *kapha* (earth)—I was cold all the time and dampness affected me terribly, even though I am inherently a fire-type constitution. The use of warming herbs and foods (anti-*kapha*) instantly dealt with the symptom of being cold; over a much longer period, working at a deeper level, the use of herbs boosted and nourished all systems, dealing with the sources of imbalance. After a point, I no longer needed to use lots of warming herbs and foods just to stay warm; I *was* warm.

Once I reached the point of balance, I had to learn to be careful not to go too far in the other direction. With excess *kapha* it was good for me to eat massive amounts of garlic, onions, and hot spices, even though this is normally not advised for fire types. Now I have to curb my intake of these foods, for my natural tendency is to get internally overheated. Warming foods, herbs, and spices can cause diseases of heat.

And indeed, when I overdo *pitta*-enhancing foods, and/or when I fuel *pitta*-aggravating activity and mental stress (anger, intensity, competition, argument or debate, pressure, hurrying) for prolonged periods, I tend to develop inflammatory skin conditions.

When the body is essentially healthy, occasional imbalances usually reflect the innate constitution. The strengths and weaknesses associated with your constitution reflect clearly in your health experiences. I am continually amazed at how succinctly the constitutions predict dysfunction. All the "skinny," *vata* (air-type) people I know tend to have joint problems, arthritis, aches, and stiffness. As a fire type, the most serious illness I have had in the last eight years is shingles, a disease of heat (blistering!) and skin inflammation and an eruption of intense stress. Vintage fire type! The *kapha* (earth-type) people I know all have the most mucus problems— colds, flus, sinus, and allergy issues.

Using the System to Polish, Not Punish

The objective of the body typing is not to pigeonhole yourself or label yourself into a corner, or use the indications for each body type to regiment yourself rigidly into a spartan, joyless existence. That would be the antithesis of what we're after, both physically and spiritually. The point is to note your issues (or potential ones) and live your life accordingly, with awareness, as much as possible.

What I have always said about basic fueling also applies to eating, supplementing, and otherwise living in a manner fitting for your constitution: It is not necessary to be perfect. In fact, striving too hard for perfection can be adverse to health if it makes you miserable or discouraged, or if it means you're following a "program" instead of listening to your body and being flexible about how you respond to it. What is important is knowing what works best and being consistent—not pristine or compulsive—about working in an informed manner with what you've got.

The bodies we are given may prevent us from making drastic, fundamental changes in how we are built, but that doesn't mean we can't have the best possible body for our type. Any type can be lean, healthy, and fit. Your basic constitution can be molded to a large degree by a basically poor lifestyle or a basically good one.

GETTING TO KNOW WHAT'S GOOD FOR YOU, AND WHEN

The charts and tables on the next few pages are designed to give insight into what enhances and aggravates each of the doshas and constitutions, and to illustrate how certain choices of foods, herbs, and even environments can upset or restore balance.

We hope the knowledge of your constitutional type remains with you as you learn about herbs, foods, and nutrients for health. When you have the option of using any of several herbs with an affinity for a particular condition, you can factor your constitution into your choice, choosing cooling, warming, drying, heavy, or moist herbs according to your constitutional needs. You can refer back to this chapter to see if foods or herbs recommended for a specific issue are particularly good for you, or are best avoided.

(If the best solution for an acute condition happens to be incompatible with your constitution, it may be okay to use it short term; just be cautious and watch for signs that it is aggravating you. In most cases, however, there are enough options so that you can choose a remedy that also complements your type.)

Choosing foods and herbs by tastes and energetics is certainly a concept that may take some getting used to. Other cultures teach these distinctions to their children at a very young age. People of Vedic cultures learn their constitutional strengths and weaknesses by the time they are about seven years old, and live accordingly so that their "disease potential" is never realized (or is at least minimized). The grandparents are often the patriarchal and matriarchal figures that do a great deal of the cooking and prepare the tonics and remedies. In the United States we are generally very divorced from such awareness. Many people give little thought to choosing between cereal or a doughnut for breakfast, let alone something as subtle as whether a cooling or warming, bitter or astringent food is best for their bodies.

(Some of these charts are adapted in part from other works on Ayurveda [by Vasant Lad, David Frawley, Robert Svoboda—see "Recommended Reading"]—as well as the teachings of Yogi Bhajan.)

COMMON HEALTH SYMPTOMS OF THE DOSHAS

	Vata	*Pitta*	*Kapha*
Primary:	Pain (generally) Pain (cutting, pricking)	Inflammation Pain (burning)	Pus Pain (dull)
Other:	Cracking (skin) Dryness (skin, joints, stool) Stiffness Tension Immobility Hoarseness Bloating Crackling joints	Redness (eyes, skin, membrane) Blisters Green Color (nasal mucus, pus) Yellow Color (urine, stool, skin)	Phlegm Mucus Itching Heaviness Coldness Greasiness Pale skin Sweet taste (in mouth, on skin) Drowsiness Indigestion Edema Obesity

Remember, the tastes (of herbs and foods) drive the energetics. The following chart details how:

Tastes and Energetics

SWEET	Cold	Wet	Heavy
SOUR	Hot	Wet	Light
SALTY	Hot	Wet	Heavy
PUNGENT	Hot	Dry	Light
BITTER	Cold	Dry	Light
ASTRINGENT	Cold	Dry	Heavy

Sweet herbs include cardamom and fennel.
Sour herbs include hawthorn berry.
Salty herbs include kelp.
Pungent herbs include cayenne and pipali.
Bitter herbs include turmeric, goldenseal, and barberry.
Astringent herbs include rosemary and aloe.

Sweet foods include milk, rice, honey, wheat
  (usually macronutrients are sweet).
Sour foods include yogurt, sour cream, lemon, vinegar, gooseberries.
Salty foods include sea vegetables, some fish (and of course,
  anything salted).
Pungent foods include garlic, ginger, cayenne, horseradish.
Bitter foods include eggplant, kale, collard greens, bittermelon,
  unsweetened cocoa.
Astringent foods include pomegranate, unripe banana, cranberries.

Therapeutic Tastes for Doshas

Most Therapeutic Tastes	Best	Second Best	Third Best
VATA (Air)	Salty	Sour	Sweet
PITTA (Fire)	Bitter	Sweet	Astringent
KAPHA (Earth)	Pungent	Bitter	Astringent

The rationale for the therapeutic tastes is as follows:

The best things to treat the dosha are those which are most
opposite (thus decreasing or controlling it).
The tastes that match the dosha will increase it to excess.

Vata (air) is cold, dry, and light.
Salty is best for *vata* because it is hot, wet, and heavy.
Sour is good for *vata* because it is hot and wet.
Sweet is good for *vata* because it is wet and heavy.
   Bitter is the worst for vata; *it is cold, dry, and light*
   Astringent is second worst for vata; *it is cold and dry.*

Pitta (fire) is hot, wet, and light.
Bitter is best for *pitta* because it is cold (the most cooling of all the
   tastes) and dry.
Sweet is good for *pitta* because it is cold and heavy.
Astringent is good for *pitta* because it is cold, dry, and heavy.
   Sour is the worst for pitta; *it is hot, wet, and light.*
   Pungent is second worst for pitta; *it is hot and light.*

Kapha (earth) is cool, wet, and heavy.
Pungent is best for *kapha* because it is hot, dry, and light.
Bitter is good for *kapha* because it is cold and light.
Astringent is good for *kapha* because it is dry.
   Sweet is the worst for kapha; *it is cold, wet, and heavy.*
   Salty is second worst for kapha; *it is wet and heavy.*

FOOD FOR DOSHAS

The food charts that follow list foods that are best and worst for each
of the doshas.

Consider yourself warned: People often look at this list and say
"What? All of the foods I'm supposed to avoid are my favorites!" Classic
Ayurveda says you're likely to be attracted to what balances your dosha,
but Karta Purkh suggests that contemporary experience is just the opposite, especially when translating across other cultures. Perhaps historically

in India, upbringing was such that people developed a taste for what healed them. In modern times, people seem to be attracted to—and even addicted to—what aggravates us. Thus the hot and fiery *pitta* (fire type) is drawn to spicy foods, the *kapha* (earth type) is drawn to grease and salt, the *vata* (air type) tends to forget completely to eat, and so on.

It's hard sometimes to persuade people to try for balance because we tend to want to go for what's familiar, comfortable, and fuels the characteristics for which we get praise or affirmation. We may think of our dosha as giving us our "edge"—the *pitta* likes being hot and fierce; *vata* likes floating along in the clouds; *kapha* likes feeling steady and solid.

But being balanced doesn't mean you lose your fundamental characteristics. You're just *less* of it—less enough to be healthier and more stable. If *vata* warms up and gets moist, he or she will still be drier than the other two-thirds of the population—just not fifteen times drier. And so on.

So the purpose of eating this way is not to torture yourself. It is to feel better, to prevent disease and discomfort by nurturing balance. It doesn't mean never eating those foods that tend to aggravate your constitution (just as a low-fat diet doesn't mean *never* eating foods that are high in fat). That would be unrealistic, and unnecessary besides. What it means is that you are aware and conscious, and can emphasize other foods as much as possible while eating the "avoid" foods more sparingly. (That's why we say "favor" and "avoid" rather than "always" and "never.")

It also means that you have another way to pay attention to your health, and another way to make connections and draw conclusions about what kind of signals your body is giving you. And it allows you to respond appropriately. For example, as a *pitta* (fire type) it's predictable that I absolutely adore garlic and onions. I'm aware that they're potential troublemakers for me, and I know that if I'm experiencing *pitta*-type problems (i.e., *pitta* is aggravated or running rampant) it works to avoid them completely for a while.

Moreover, if I were to eat an exceptionally garlicky meal and subsequently experience skin breakouts or heartburn, I would have some way to connect my actions to my condition, and could add correction. Someone without these distinctions might simply begin to medicate themselves, popping antacids or stronger drugs that push the body further out of balance, while continuing to eat the aggravating foods. This is how minor troubles turn into major ones.

SOME NOTES ABOUT USING THE CHARTS

These "foods to favor" and "foods to avoid" for each dosha are based on the traditions of the Ayurvedic constitutional diets, which are historically taught and used in Indian culture. The lists have been modified over the years to reflect dietary idiosyncrasies of American culture and the results of these diets in a Western setting. Observations by Karta Purkh and other herbalists and natural health practitioners have confirmed most of the ancient Ayurvedic wisdom about which foods control or aggravate the doshas, but have also added some contemporary insights.

You will note that the foods are divided into categories and that meat is not among the categories. This is primarily because the core of this list comes from the observations and experiences of the people of India, who mainly consume a vegetarian diet. There are many reasons to limit or avoid meat, and since we do encourage a grain-based diet generally for best health, we present the body-type food suggestions through the filter of traditional Ayurveda. Thus we have not attempted to "rate" meat for the body types.

These are general guidelines based on general observations. For most people, most of them will be accurate, but there are always exceptions. These should be used as *one* point of reference for devising your healthiest and most enjoyable diet. There are obviously other factors in a healthy diet, which are discussed at other points in this book and in other books. Individual requirements also vary—for example, you may dislike, be allergic or sensitive to, or unable to obtain foods in the "favor" column.

Likewise, the degree to which you manifest a particular dosha determines how aggravating the "avoid" foods for that type will be. (I didn't have to pay much attention to the "avoid" foods for *pitta* until I entered the *pitta*/fire phase of life, thus bolstering my already hot and fiery tendencies; alas, suddenly I found garlic aggravating!) And combination body types may be less aggravated than single body types by foods that stimulate even the primary doshas—for example, *vata-pitta* types may find *vata*'s "avoid" foods to be less aggravating than "pure" *vata* types.

Once again, if you're not presently reflecting your core constitution, treat the dosha that is currently dominant, not the innate constitution. (Before I reached my current state of health and was imbalanced toward excess *kapha*, I had to eat as if I were *kapha*—to warm up. A cooling *pitta* diet would not have been appropriate at that time.)

All of this means that the point is not to follow this zealously and without question, but to use its input along with other input to note what works best for you.

Another important point: Relativity is everything. Strawberries, bananas, and peaches are on the "avoid" list for *pitta* because they are mildly heating compared to other fruits; realistically, however, this is not going to present a major problem if you are not burning up with *pitta* and not consuming pounds of it daily. It's a technicality: Those fruits are warming compared to grapes and pears, but they would rate a .01 on a scale where chilies were a 10.

If you pay attention, you will begin to be able to "sense" what foods will truly aggravate you and which ones will complement or balance. This will happen especially as you become more attuned to the Asian concept of food and herb energetics and tastes. The deeper your awareness of a food's warming tendency, drying ability, or "oiliness," etc., and the better you understand your body type, the more you will become conscious of, say, the effect of a hot, spicy food if you are a hot type, or the effect of wet, slimy food if you are already cold and wet, or the effect of crumbly, dry food if you are an air type.

Likewise, if you are experiencing symptoms or conditions and are having trouble pinpointing the cause, see if you can note common dosha characteristics both in your health condition and your environment. Try keeping a record of foods, activities, stresses, seasons, and other influences, and their energetic properties. For example, one *pitta* friend who is entering midlife couldn't understand why she was suddenly having rashes. She didn't think she'd been eating much hot stuff, but when pressed realized she'd been using garlic and hot sauce liberally in her soups. To her, the rash seemed mysterious; to me, given the *pitta* influence of hot food on her already *pitta* constitution—as she entered the "hottest" phase of life—skin inflammation was predictable. The other two constitutions can have the same type of experience. Pay attention to the influences of the doshas in your diet and environment.

Earth Type *(Kapha)*

	FAVOR	AVOID
Grains	Amaranth, barley, buckwheat, corn, millet, quinoa, rye	Oats, rice, wheat
Fruits	Apples, apricots, berries, cherries, cranberries, peaches, pears, raisins, strawberries	Avocados, bananas, coconut, dates, grapefruit, grapes, melons, oranges, plums; **sweet and sour fruits**
Vegetables	Asparagus, beets, bell peppers, broccoli, brussels sprouts, cabbage, carrots, cauliflower, celery, corn, eggplant, garlic, green beans, leeks, lettuce, onions, parsley, peas, potatoes, radish, spinach, turnips; **raw, pungent and bitter vegetables**	Artichoke, cucumber, olives, pumpkin, tomatoes, starchy squash; **sweet and juicy vegetables**
Beans/Legumes	Aduki beans, black beans, black-eyed peas, garbanzo beans, lima beans, navy beans, pinto beans, split peas	Mung beans, kidney beans, lentils, soybeans, cold soy milk
Nuts/Seeds		All nuts; sesame seeds
Dairy	Ghee (clarified butter), goat's milk *(small amounts)*	Butter, buttermilk, cheese, cow's milk, ice cream, sour cream, yogurt
Beverages	Apple juice, carob drinks, carrot juice, mixed vegetable juice, soy milk *if spiced and warm*	

	FAVOR	AVOID
Spices/Condiments	Ajwain, allspice, anise, asafoetida, basil, bay leaf, black pepper, caraway, cardamom, cayenne, cinnamon, cloves, coriander, cumin, dill, fennel, fenugreek, garlic, ginger, horseradish, marjoram, mint, mustard seeds, nutmeg, onion, oregano, paprika, parsley, peppermint, poppy seed, rosemary, saffron, sage, star anise, tarragon, thyme, turmeric, vanilla	Soy sauce, tamari
Sweeteners	Honey, fruit juice sweeteners (apple and pear)	Fructose, maple syrup, molasses, Sucanat, white sugar

Fire Type *(Pitta)*

	FAVOR	AVOID
Grains	Barley, oats, rice, wheat	Amaranth, buckwheat, corn, millet, rye
Fruits	Apples, apricots, avocado, berries, coconut, dates, figs, grapes, pears, plums, raisins, watermelon; **sweet fruits**	Bananas (unless ripe), cranberries, grapefruit, lemons, peaches, straw-berries; **sour fruits**
Vegetables	Artichoke, asparagus, bell pepper, broccoli, brussels sprouts, cabbage, cauli-flower, cucumber, celery, green beans, leafy greens, lettuce, olives, parsley, peas, potatoes, squash, watercress; **sweet and bitter vegetables**	Beets, carrots, eggplant, garlic, horseradish, onions, pumpkin, radish, spinach, tomatoes; **pungent vegetables**
Beans/Legumes	Aduki beans, black beans, black-eyed peas, garbanzo beans, kidney beans, lentils, lima beans, mung beans, navy beans, pinto beans, soy beans, split peas, tempeh, tofu, white beans	
Nuts/Seeds	Coconut; psyllium, pump-kin and sunflower seeds	All nuts; sesame seeds
Dairy	Cottage cheese, ghee (clarified butter), cow's milk, goat's milk, most mild, soft cheeses	Buttermilk, hard cheeses, feta cheese, sour cream, yogurt

	FAVOR	AVOID
Beverages	Apple juice, coconut milk, goat milk, grape juice, soy milk	**Alcohol, coffee, caffeine drinks,** cranberry juice, grapefruit juice, lemonade, orange juice, tomato juice
Spices/Condiments	Basil (fresh), black pepper, caraway, cardamom, cilantro, coriander, cumin, dill, fennel, mint, parsley, peppermint, turmeric, vanilla, wintergreen	Ajwain, allspice, anise, asafoetida, basil (dried), bay leaf, caraway, cayenne, cloves, fenugreek, garlic, ginger, horseradish, marjoram, mustard seeds, nutmeg, oregano, paprika, rosemary, saffron, sage, savory, star anise, tarragon, thyme; soy sauce, tamari
Sweeteners	Barley malt, brown rice syrup, fructose, fruit juice concentrate, maple syrup	Honey, molasses

Air Type *(Vata)*

	FAVOR	AVOID
Grains	Amaranth, oats, wheat, rice	Cold/dry/puffed cereals, barley, buckwheat, corn, millet, quinoa, rye
Fruits	Apricots, avocado, bananas, berries, cherries, coconut, dates, grapefruit, grapes, lemons, limes, oranges, pears, peaches, pineapple, plums, rhubarb, strawberries; **sweet fruits**	Apples, cranberries, dried fruit, pears, prunes, watermelon
Vegetables	Artichoke, asparagus, beets, carrots, cucumber, green beans, leeks, mustard greens, olives, onions, pumpkin, radish, rutabaga, sweet potato, squash, watercress, **cooked vegetables**	Broccoli, brussels sprouts, cabbage, cauliflower, celery, corn, eggplant, leafy greens, lettuce, mushrooms, peas, peppers, potatoes (white), spinach, tomatoes, turnips; **frozen, dried, or raw vegetables**
Beans/Legumes	Aduki beans, mung beans, soy cheese, soy milk, tofu	All large, dense beans
Nuts/Seeds	Almonds, brazil nuts, cashews, coconut, filberts, macadamia nuts, pecans, pine nuts, pistachios, walnuts	
Dairy	All dairy, in moderation	

	FAVOR	AVOID
Beverages	Apricot juice, carrot juice, hot dairy drinks, grape juice, grapefruit juice, orange juice, pineapple juice, soy milk *if spiced and hot*	Apple juice, coffee and caffeine drinks, cranberry juice
Spices/Condiments	Ajwain, allspice, anise, asafoetida, basil, bay leaf, black pepper, caraway, cardamom, cinnamon, cloves, coriander, cumin, dill, fennel, fenugreek, garlic, ginger, horseradish, marjoram, mint, mustard seeds, nutmeg, oregano, paprika, parsley, peppermint, rosemary, saffron, sage, savory, star anise, tarragon, thyme, turmeric, vanilla, wintergreen	
Sweeteners	Fructose, fruit juice sweeteners, honey, maple syrup, molasses	White sugar

Note: Tri-dosha types don't have to avoid any foods; provided that they are not experiencing imbalances, they can eat moderately from all food lists.

Note: Sweeteners are listed with the caveat that we mean "permitted in small amounts." We do not encourage anyone, regardless of body type, actually to "emphasize" any sweetener in the diet. Sweeteners listed in the "favor" columns are the ones *less* likely than others to inflame or unbalance that particular dosha/type. However, less (or none) of any added sweetener is preferable. Generally, *pitta* (fire) does better with sweets than the other two (since sweet is cooling, and *pitta*'s fast metabolism burns reasonable amounts of sugar quickly). *Kapha,* which is the dosha that favors excess growth, does not need the added "building" property of sweet, and is the most aggravated by it. All types should avoid refined white sugar and corn syrup. Heavily processed foods are not healthy or nutritious for anyone.

DOSHA CYCLES

The doshas don't fluctuate and battle for center stage only inside our bodies; their dance is evident in the environment around us. In the cycles of the seasons and the length of a lifetime, *vata, pitta,* and *kapha* take turns "driving the bus." It's helpful to know how the dosha that dominates a particular season or stage of life can affect you, so you can adjust as much as possible using factors that are within your control.

Seasons

The dosha of the season will vary depending on locale. For example, summer is the unhealthiest season in most places around the world because of the heat and humidity, but in Seattle it's the healthiest because it's about the only time we get to dry up at all. Seattle is a very *kapha* climate—cold and wet. It aggravates *kapha* (earth types) more than the other constitutions.

If you really want to fine-tune, you can adjust herbal therapies and foods according to the season's dosha. This is especially important when you already have too much of the prevailing dosha of the season. *Kapha* (earth) types who want to thrive through winter in Seattle need to pay extra attention to warming and drying strategies. Likewise, *pitta* (fire-type) constitutions will do better during hot, humid weather if they emphasize cooling and drying. *Vata* (air) types in the desert should intervene with moistening foods and herbs.

Life Cycle

The same goes for life cycles: *Vata* types will be most prone to disease and discomfort during the "air time" of life; *pitta* types will be most susceptible to illness and injury during the "fire time," and *kapha* types will be most vulnerable during the "earth phase" of life.

The already intense *pitta* (fire-type) constitution, for instance, may experience the height of inflammation in the "heat" of young adulthood and midlife, and should adapt health care accordingly.

Remember, these are tendencies; managing them is entirely possible.

Early—Earth/*Kapha*

Through puberty, *kapha* is strongest it will ever be in life. *Kapha* constitutions are especially aggravated during this exceptionally *kapha* time. For example, Karta Purkh is *kapha* and had serious respiratory illnesses throughout childhood, including pneumonia.

Adult—Fire/*Pitta*

Raging hormones, intensity, out there trying to "make it." Inflammatory diseases, ulcers, hemorrhoids are classic *pitta*/midlife conditions.

Old Age—Air/*Vata*

Cool down, dry out. This is the hardest life phase for already cool/dry *vatas*. Tendencies are toward dryness, "crackly" joints, and fatigue. Arthritis, gas, and constipation are common.

3

Perspectives on Research

In our culture, science determines the belief system. So we work within that high-tech system to prove how powerful these low-tech, ancient interventions can be.

—Dean Ornish, M.D.
Author of *Dr. Dean Ornish's Program for Reversing Heart Disease*,
in *Healing and the Mind* with Bill Moyers

If I have a patient with newly diagnosed high blood pressure, and I recommend 10 sessions of biofeedback training for the person to relax his or her sympathetic nervous system, the chances are that the patient will have to pay for that out-of-pocket. But if I write a prescription for antihypertensive drugs for the rest of the person's life, the insurance company pays happily. That should not be. . . . But how do you convince executives of insurance companies to do what is in their own self-interest? These people say they do not have the data to show them that an intervention such as biofeedback is both effective and cost-effective. Why don't they have the data? Because most of the people who do research in this country, the people who have the money, facilities, and inclination to conduct research, are not interested in studying these things. They are not interested because they have come out of an educational system that portrayed such interventions as weak, unimportant, and uninteresting— not the real "meat" of science.

—Andrew Weil, M.D.
Alternative & Complementary Therapies, September/October 1995,
"The Body's Healing Systems: The Future of Medical Education"

There is an art and a science to herbal medicine, and in our culture, there is a great deal of emphasis on the science. Even those of us who are not trained professionally in science are brought up to seek "truth" and evidence from within scientific parameters, and even to feel foolish if we choose to rely on anything outside those parameters. Within medicine and elsewhere in our culture, this is changing, but slowly.

The framework provided by science has value—and it also has flaws and biases that should be recognized. Healthy skepticism about what is not "scientific" is encouraged in this culture. Perhaps, to even things out, we should have an equally healthy skepticism about science itself as well.

Research is a very complex business. Economics, politics, timing, and many factors vulnerable to human fallibility play into whether something is researched or not, as well as whether the research is effective and appropriate for the subject. There's not some monolithic unanimity about research. That's not "bad"—it's just important to take into account. The research industry has the right to have an agenda; you just need to be aware that it may not be *your* agenda.

We don't suggest that you reject all scientific information; we just suggest that you not reflexively reject everything that cannot be fit into one particular scientific model—and that you stay open to the possibility of other valid models.

STANDARDS OF PROOF

Modern research is verifying almost daily the efficacy of herbs and related natural substances. Therefore, some of what you read in this book is backed by "scientific verification" as established by the standards of conventional science. Whenever that is the case, it is indicated. Other herbs may receive this type of verification soon, or there may be preliminary data, but there is nothing yet considered substantial by the standards of orthodox science. Some of the information provided is based on what is considered anecdotal evidence, clinical (based on the authors' experience and that of colleagues, or on clinical studies) evidence, historical accounts, or "folk wisdom."

Sometimes "all" we have is thousands or millions of people over hundreds or thousands of years, and the reasonable conclusions of other cultures' practitioners over that time regarding the traditional use of the herbs. In those cultures, that is the standard of proof. Not every culture honors or requires the same standards created by our scientists. In herbalism, historical and traditional use is highly respected and valued.

An herbalist works with botanicals based on everything from traditional to empirical to controlled scientific evidence. Any presentation of herbs with any scope will reflect that. However, nothing recommended in this book is untested; it's just that some of it has not (yet) been tested to one particular standard: that of conventional science. Nothing we recommend has only been used by one or two, or even fifty or one hundred people. Everything we discuss, even if not "scientifically proven" by some standards, is based on historical use over very long periods of time by thousands of people, and more often by many millions of people.

For my own personal use, I made the decision some time ago that if something nontoxic (such as a food or spice I might eat all the time anyway) is preventive or healing for even one or two other people, it can't hurt to try it (especially if the reasoning for its effectiveness makes sense to me). Certainly if ethnic healers observed it working consistently for a particular purpose over thousands of years, there is all the more reason to try it. I respect that wisdom and believe it is relevant; it more than suffices as evidence for me. If that wisdom was subsequently passed on to an American herbalist, who observes the same patterns repeating themselves in his or her own practice, that strengthens the position further still. If I myself experience the expected result, that clinches it. If a U.S. scientist reproduces that effect in a lab setting, that's nice, but not necessary for my healing.

Tom Wolfe, owner of Smile Herb Shop in College Park, Maryland, and a professional member of the American Herbalist Guild, developed the following 1-to-5 rating system for use in his store to help consumers understand the varying levels of health evidence supporting different botanicals. He proposes that the industry as a whole adopt a similar standard.

1. Anecdotal Proof: Observations not known to be tradition
2. Empirical Proof: Observations accepted as traditional practice
3. Open Clinical Trials: Clinical observation by trained practitioners
4. Placebo-Controlled Clinical Trials: Scientifically valid studies
5. Peer Consensus: Including groups such as the American Herbalist Guild (and, hopefully someday, the Food and Drug Administration and American Medical Association)[1]

As you read, explore, and discover, you will have to choose for yourself what your standard of proof will be. In the meantime, pursue the facts behind any statement that "no evidence exists" to support use of an herb. It may actually mean "no evidence from double-blind placebo-controlled studies exists yet" but millions of people all over the world have used the herb efficaciously for centuries. To some people—perhaps to you—that *is* evidence.

IF A STUDY WASN'T SEEN BY YOUR DOCTOR, DOES THAT MEAN IT DOESN'T EXIST?

A doctor once said to me, "No case study showing cancer can be cured by natural means exists because I've never seen it and no one has ever seen it."

This is not true, nor is it true of AIDS, arthritis, or any number of other conditions about which the same comment has been made. What is striking about the comment is not whether it addresses cancer or colds, but rather the egocentrism involved: "If I didn't see it, it doesn't exist." Is it possible for any one doctor to encounter all research and case studies on all subjects?

This is a common misperception under which many doctors seem to labor—that if a study existed, it would have magically shown up on their desks. Unfortunately, their patients may believe it: "If it was any good, my doctor would have heard about it." Sad to say, this simply is not true. There are economic interests in limiting support for natural options. Says Jane Heimlich in her book *What Your Doctor Won't Tell You,* "Your doctor may never know about many helpful new treatments because it's the policy of the American Medical Association to promote profitability of the medical industry, not healthy diets, vitamins, and inexpensive new treatments."

My friend Kaaren Nichols, M.D., has observed how difficult it is to obtain information about studies conducted on alternative methods in medicine. "You have to actively search for such studies," she explains, "and many physicians assume that if the studies are not in the medical journals they read, the research has not been done." If a doctor says, "Well, I've never seen a study on that," it can mean that either a study wasn't done because the companies who fund studies weren't interested in it because it's not patentable, or there have been lots of studies done but the doctor has never seen them.

Medical journals can also refuse to publish studies, further weakening the argument that "if there were studies, I would have seen them in the reputable journals." Writing about the lack of focus on healing in medicine, Dr. Larry Dossey, M.D., in *Healing Words* states, "Medical journals have generally refused, until recently, to publish studies on healing."

For example, almost 300 studies contributing to the premise that mental efforts can affect living organisms at a distance have been ignored or rejected by most scientists, says Dossey. Over 100 of these exhibit the most stringent criteria of "good science" and show that prayer is indeed capable of causing significant changes in living beings, from one-celled organisms to humans. Dossey at first assumed that this enormous body of scientific proof would be common knowledge among scientifically trained physicians, just because it existed. Says Dossey, "I came to realize the truth of what many historians of science have described: A body of knowledge that does not fit with the prevailing ideas can be ignored as if it does not exist, no matter how scientifically valid it may be. Scientists, including physicians, can have blind spots in their vision."[2]

Even if a study does not exist, that does not mean there wouldn't be evidence if studies were done. Lack of studies is not proof that something is ineffective.

How do studies get done? The Catch-22 is that you first need evidence that there is some validity to the hypothesis. If political winds are not blowing in your favor, this can trip you up. In Bill Moyers' *Healing and the Mind*, Dr. Dean Ornish of *Reversing Heart Disease* fame was discussing his efforts to get funding for his original study, which did eventually show that heart disease can be reversed through lifestyle intervention. He told Moyers

> When I first began planning this study, we had a great deal of difficulty getting funding from the National Institutes of Health or the American Heart Association or major foundations. . . . [T]hey said, "It is impossible to reverse heart disease. And even if you could, you would have to use drugs, and a year is not long enough, and no one can change their lifestyle anyway and stick with it." . . . I would respond, "Well, let's find out. That is what science is all about." . . . [T]hey would answer back, "No, we know it can't be done, so we won't even bother."

That is what anyone who hopes to research something outside the existing paradigm is up against. Thus one lesson is that when someone states "there is no research" supporting something (assuming for the moment that the statement is correct), it doesn't mean that fifty studies were done and no favorable evidence turned up. It may mean that no one was willing to fund the study. Obviously, that wouldn't necessarily mean the study was not worth funding.

Finally, there is the issue of what constitutes a "good" study. We must keep in mind that criteria for "good science" arose from scientific opinion. What medicine reveres as "the scientific method," which is often presented as being beyond reproach, arbitrarily assigns a particular standard of truth. As Larry Dossey wryly points out in *Healing Words*, "We invented the scientific method; it did not descend from on high."

When all is said and done, scientific "proof" is simply a matter of replicating a certain result, a certain number of times, in a certain way—until a group of people in the field feel it is consistently and adequately proven.

THE MYTH OF OBJECTIVITY

In all proving processes there are "unknowables." There are variables that are not considered relevant to the outcome at the time, but which may later turn out to affect the outcome very much indeed. In any research experiment, one has to decide which variables will be controlled and which won't. All variables cannot be controlled. And the choices about what will be controlled are made by human beings, based on human experience, intelligence, and instincts—and necessarily, also human error and biases. Most scientists today, for example, would not try to control for the variable of someone praying for the subjects—yet there is a substantial and growing body of evidence that prayer is a variable.

Dr. Larry Dossey's best-selling book *Healing Words* offers evidence of nonlocal events—thought or mind activity of one person affecting the result in another being, whether in a healing or an experiment, a person or a microorganism. If a person's thoughts, emotions, beliefs, and attitudes can affect outcomes, then we have to question seriously the supposedly airtight "objectivity" of the gold-standard double-blind placebo study.

Enlightened thinkers have long acknowledged and drawn attention to the role of beliefs and expectations in shaping outcomes. Research itself continues to support this. It is increasingly difficult to pretend that researchers can divorce their views and preconceptions from the activity and result of a study. Double-blind controls attempt to eliminate the possibility of unaccounted-for physical influences, but they don't account for the state of mind of the experimenter and how that might factor into the outcome.

Scientists naturally resist the idea that their thoughts and expectations can creep into the carefully constructed double-blind study and "throw" it. This has enormous implications for the practice of science, research, and the medicine that is based so thoroughly on that research. No scientist wants his or her objectivity challenged.

From an alternative-medicine point of view, researchers' influence on outcomes is a major concern, given the attitudes and prejudices demonstrated by some conventional scientists. If expectations, beliefs, and agendas can influence outcomes, there are certainly people you might not want conducting experiments on the efficacy of alternatives. One can only imagine what they are hoping to find—or not find. What if researchers want to find a (profitable) new drug safe and effective? What if they privately are convinced that ginger cannot be anti-inflammatory? And so it goes.

The spring 1996 *Noetic Sciences Review* reports recent findings that add to the growing body of evidence for the effect of "experimenter expectations." Several researchers are preparing for publication a study supporting the hypothesis that "consciousness can interact directly with the physical world, that experimenters cannot be seen as detached from the object of their studies, and that beliefs and expectations make a difference, even under conditions in which the results cannot be explained by ordinary sensory interactions."

In this experiment, a pair of researchers conducted a collaborative study of a process in which one believed strongly and the other was a skeptic. They drew from the same volunteers, used the same equipment in the same lab, and used the same randomization procedure. Their results were totally different: The skeptic found no effect on volunteers from the procedure, while the believer found significant effects.

This is just one study representing many. If you are interested in how nonlocal consciousness affects research and, more importantly, healing, we strongly recommend Larry Dossey's wonderful book *Healing Words*. In the meantime, it certainly seems wise to suspend total, abject belief in "the scientific method." The myth of impassive, robotically objective scientists is just that—a myth.

ANECDOTAL EVIDENCE

"One report means nothing. It's not scientifically or mathematically sound. You just can't draw conclusions from one person."—Anonymous Doctor

During my last sinus infection (in 1990), I took echinacea and goldenseal, and the infection cleared up on its own without antibiotics. I never got another one. What does that tell you?

To the hard-core conventional scientist, this story tells you nothing. The most hard-line will agree with the doctor quoted above and say that you cannot and must not draw any conclusions from this event.

However, such an approach is not only closed-minded and impossibly theoretical, it's also impractical. How can one ignore the evidence of one's own senses? What is the value in that, and is it even possible to do? If you take antibiotics for infections all your life and they don't work very well, and the infections always come back (and you get other infections as a result of the antibiotics)—and then you try an herb and the infection goes away and never comes back—you're going to have a hard time convincing me to ignore this data because it is "unstable."

Moreover, the argument against drawing conclusions would be somewhat more understandable if I said that I took ground-up paper towels mixed with sawdust and brown sugar, put it in capsules, and it made my sinus infection go away, even though no one had ever tried it before and there wasn't a single other anecdote that corroborated mine. However, when you use a treatment that millions of people have used before you, all around the world, and you duplicate the result produced historically by those people—what is unstable about that?

It's the very antithesis of true health and health care to insist that results we see and feel with our own senses are worthless, that we need scientists from laboratories to tell us whether something works for us or not. If you want to give me a walloping, crushingly powerful drug that is likely to have serious side effects, then absolutely test it like crazy first. But don't tell me we have to test an ordinary, harmless food like eggplant before I am "allowed" to say that eating it had an impact on my health—especially not when it was recommended to me in the first place because the same effect I experienced had been observed around the world by healers and patients.

The fact is that even after the most rigorous trials, we still cannot say with certainty that a result was produced by what we think produced it. Even someone taking the most rigorously tested drug in history cannot *prove* that relief was produced by the drug. It may have been the drug, but we'll never really know. Even scientists don't ever have absolute evidence.

TAKING BACK YOUR POWER: HOW SCIENCE STUNTS SELF-WISDOM

Part of what "quackbusters" (people who consider themselves arbiters of truth who "save" the consumer from "charlatans") don't like is people without "proper training" making evaluations or suggestions. That includes "self-treating"—learning and applying knowledge on your own.

Leaving the issue of trained alternative-medicine practitioners aside for a moment, what does that say about you and me? It says we are unable, or should be unable, to listen to our own bodies and have enough basic information to keep them well, and to heal them when they are not well. It says we are not qualified to do that. We must go to The Experts, do what they say, and not question them. This leaves you helpless to draw your own conclusions or make decisions about yourself. It usurps your power, deflates your esteem, and devalues common sense.

There is definitely a middle ground in this issue. We certainly don't think we should perform surgery on ourselves. We don't think we should self-medicate for months or years when we're not getting any better. We believe in going to an expert when that expertise is needed to get the job done. I seek the assistance of doctors as well as accountants, insurance agents, and car-repair specialists when appropriate.

We do not, however, believe that as laypeople you are unable to make many everyday decisions about your health. You *can* do that, both preventively and to heal much of what goes awry.

The term *folk remedy* is sometimes used so disparagingly by doctors and scientists that some herbalists don't like to further its use. The word *folk* may be used by design, to make a remedy sound less effective or authoritative. But there is something that we feel ought to be honored about folk remedies. In one sense, the concept means people using everyday things, on their own, to get well and stay well. What is so implausible about people taking care of themselves, after all? Folk remedies are taught to people by other people. It's people-based medicine. There is value to that.

The question you might ask yourself is, If substances have been used successfully by other cultures for hundreds or even thousands of years, is that good enough for me or not? Are you going to wait for the person in the white lab coat to tell you, ten years from now, that it looks promising but "more research is needed"? Or that it worked in a test tube (even though it's already worked for millions of people over five centuries)?

It's okay for you to trust and respect yourself—your instincts, your beliefs, your results. In fact, such self-awareness and trust in your instincts is absolutely necessary for outstanding personal health as well as for the success of any health-care system. If the burden of responsibility is always shouldered by the doctor alone, health care will never budge from the stuck place that it's in. It's not healthy for the doctor or for patients. It's a dysfunctional relationship.

THE MEANING OF THE MECHANISM

Another argument sometimes leveled at natural therapies and preventions is that they are inferior if we can't identify the mechanism of action. I asked one doctor what he would do if he had a choice between eating an ordinary food like eggplant every day to cure a condition, and it would be effective without knowing exactly why it worked, or taking a pharmaceutical drug for which we know the exact mechanism of action, but which had six serious toxic side effects. He said he would choose the drug.

That's an extremely hard line to take, and not everyone takes it. It is, unfortunately, an example of the lengths of unreasonability to which some orthodox thinkers will go to justify wholesale rejection of any natural therapy. However, most studies attempt to ascertain empirical effectiveness, not necessarily the mechanism—and the empirical evidence, not the mechanism, is the standard of proof. This means that often, even for drugs, effectiveness is "proven" to satisfaction before the mechanism is necessarily identified.

Thus the mechanism argument is very flawed if it is used to try to discredit herbal medicine. The mechanism of action for aspirin, for example, was not known until recently; now scientists think we know, but every month we gain still more understanding. Indeed, says the *University of California at Berkeley Wellness Letter*, "until recently, the way aspirin works has been poorly understood."[3] That didn't stop people from manufacturing or taking it. It also didn't stop it from working, regardless of the reason. Aspirin was used freely to relieve headaches for 100 years before we knew the mechanism.

And despite poor understanding of the mechanism, we've never seen or heard anyone calling aspirin an "unproven remedy" that we would be "irresponsible" to recommend. Why is that? And why should whole-plant, food, and spice remedies—which in the vast majority of cases are milder and more harmless than a drug like aspirin—be held to a more stringent standard of proof than that? Especially in the case of a food or spice, there can be no harm in it even if it doesn't work.

Larry Dossey writes in *Healing Words*, "To acknowledge that we don't know how something works is not a particularly damaging confession in medicine. No one knew how penicillin worked (or that it even existed) when Fleming made his famous observation that the growth of bacteria was inhibited by fungi. If the scientific community had used ignorance of the process as a justification for rejecting his discovery, the introduction of life-saving antibiotics would have been delayed. . . . As history shows, full explanations frequently come later." It is more important to know *that* it works than *how* it works.

Science is a moving target. "Knowledge" is constantly being overturned by new evidence that gives rise to newer, even more plausible theories. It is probably dubious ever to say "We have proven how this works," or to claim that as the sole edge of superiority over something else that may work just as well. Not only does it imply that something besides effectiveness is the issue (which should not be), but it implies total confidence that at no time in the future might we discover that we were wrong about the mechanism.

It is also easier to isolate the mechanism of action for man-made pharmaceuticals than whole plants or foods. With drugs, you generally have an isolated individual chemical whose action is easy to trace in the body. It can take ages to isolate and assess all of the hundreds, even thousands, of potentially active compounds in a whole plant. Some modify others, some are acting through different pathways, some support the action of more active compounds. (And if it has a very long history of effectiveness in populations, and is nontoxic, why go through all that? To satisfy whom?)

In addition to it being easier to study the mechanisms of man-made pharmaceuticals, it may be more urgent to do so. I am personally more concerned and rigorous about understanding what a concentrated pharmaceutical drug is doing inside me and why than I am about eggplant (or cinnamon, astragalus, carrots, soybeans, nettles, or chilies). Something we weren't necessarily meant to eat, something that does not exist in nature, something that is lacking all of its parts or is made more concentrated than it was naturally created to be, something people have never consumed before—*that* I worry about. *That* I would require detailed information about before taking.

Oddly enough, we notice that many people feel just the opposite. Rather than demand details about drugs or invasive therapies, those are meekly accepted while herbs are fretted over. This double standard is in effect in science, medicine, and the insurance industry as well as the lay public. Witness Dr. Dean Ornish's struggle to find funding to study his lifestyle program and, even now, to have insurance companies cover it— even though those same insurance companies will spend $12 billion annually on bypass surgeries, at $30,000 to $40,000 apiece, half of which will need to be redone within 5 years, and another $4 billion annually on angioplasties at $10,000 each, almost 40 percent of which need to be redone in 4 to 6 months.[4]

As for the public, I have met many people who will swallow drug pills without asking what they are or what they're for, but will eye you suspiciously for taking echinacea (or ask nine thousand questions about it before they dare take ten drops of tincture). There's absolutely nothing wrong with asking questions, but why not apply the same standard to conventional medicine? One must wonder how we got so twisted around, so that highly manipulated synthetic substances became so implicitly trustworthy, while whole plants and foods are routinely subjected to affrontive interrogation.

Laypeople with whom I have had discussions about herbs have

demanded, "Well, *why* did the parsley work?" or "*How* did the nutmeg do that?" Sometimes I know, because that kind of information is available about many herbs. But sometimes I don't have an answer. And to me, that's okay. Also, I could fire back, "Well, do you know why the doctor gave you a cortisone shot? Do you know what it's doing to your joint? Do you know how the antibiotic works? Do you know the components of the antihistamines you're taking and what they are doing to you?" In my experience, people generally don't. Drugs are innocent until proven guilty and herbs are guilty until proven innocent. This is ironic, since drugs on the whole have a much greater power to harm. To draw on an analogy we used earlier, it's like questioning the therapeutic massage while blithely submitting to major surgery.

PLACEBOS

One of the things that make scientists uncomfortable about not knowing the mechanism driving a result is the possibility that the result is due to the "placebo effect." Medicine has long acknowledged the effectiveness of placebos—technically innocuous substances and procedures—in producing healing results. But the words that have been used for such practices—*sham, quackery,* and so on—reveal the general view that such use is disdained, for all the results it might produce. "Placebo" is often negatively associated with "fake" or "fraud" when it is suspected of being used purposefully.

When someone claims that an herb's success must have been due to the placebo effect, this is generally meant to suggest that nothing about the herb itself was effective. Such statements are typically made by someone who is not knowledgeable about the herb or about herbs in general. Anyone who makes a modicum of effort to look for evidence that specific herbs produce specific outcomes will find it, in many forms—including, in many cases, the forms recognized by orthodox science. In most cases, among those herbs for which we don't know the exact mechanism, there is enough historical evidence of repeatable outcomes to reasonably rule out "mere" placebo effect. An unclear mechanism does not automatically make an herb a placebo.

Note, however, that if in an individual case an herb has a placebo effect, that too says something powerful about healing. For example, if I found myself healed after using a substance and in some way was able to determine absolutely that it was a placebo effect, I would still think something remarkable had happened. Moreover, I would still be healed.

Placebos, when they work, illustrate the power of belief in the medicine itself. The generally understood fact about placebo is that in any given group of 100 sick people, if every one is given a harmless, useless inert pill, about one-third will nearly always get well. In other words, the illness actually disappears as a response to having been given a medicine and believing that the medicine will help. Renowned physician and women's health specialist Christiane Northrup, M.D., author of *Women's Bodies, Women's Wisdom*, asks a great question: How many more of the patients in this type of placebo situation might get well if the power of suggestion were actively, consciously supported? What if half, or three-quarters, or all would get well?[5]

While the notion of conscious support for the placebo effect is distasteful, even horrifying, to many physicians and scientists (the whole point of double-blind random studies is to control the placebo effect away), there is a burgeoning field of medicine that supports these views. It's called psychoneuroimmunology, or mind/body medicine.

Given all of the evidence, it is absurd to suggest that most herbs are placebos. "Anyone who considers herbalism quackery or herbs at best placebo medicine is simply demonstrating their ignorance," says David Hoffman in *The Elements of Herbalism*. But clearly, neither are placebos totally undesirable. And if someone were to actually wish to offer a potential placebo intentionally to a patient, the typically innocuous herb makes a better choice than the typically harmful drug. Antibiotics, routinely prescribed for viral illnesses against which they are useless, are an example of "placebos" for demanding patients—and they do great harm when used in this way.

THE WISDOM OF HEALERS AROUND THE WORLD

Many scientists insist that we must "rigorously test" every plant and food before it can be recommended to the American public, even if it has been used effectively and safely in other cultures for hundreds or thousands of years. It's not good enough that healers in China or India have been working with the substance for all of recorded history; that's not "scientific." This mistrust says something about the American scientific view of the healing arts and sciences of other cultures.

As a result of this disregard for the wisdom of the world's healers, an enormous body of valuable information is dismissed. "We've become so totally infatuated with our brand of objectivity that it has hidden from our view much of the wisdom of the rest of the world," observes Dr. Larry Dossey.[6]

Other cultures don't test things the way we do; therefore, some herbs they use are considered untested. But they are not untested; they are simply not tested to the standards *we* have adopted. By some standards, they are very well tested and clearly effective. Says David Eisenberg, M.D., internist at Beth Israel Hospital in Boston, in *Healing and the Mind* with Bill Moyers, "The Chinese weren't interested in chemistry as we know it. They didn't have organic chemists to isolate the active ingredients. They had people who observed whether whole herbs helped with certain problems."

Never mind historical tradition; even controlled studies are often suspect if conducted in other countries. It is thought that only Americans know how to do "good science." For example, European studies showing that garlic lowers cholesterol had to be repeated at Yale at heaven knows what cost before the outcome was considered acceptable.

Centuries or millennia of use is also a good safety record. People simply would have stopped taking certain remedies a long time ago if they were harming them. Healers in China and India don't want to hurt people, either. And as Daniel B. Mowrey, Ph.D., noted in *Let's Live*, December 1995, "The goal of research is to establish centuries of data in a relatively short time." Those centuries of data are not inferior; rather, they are the desirable goal that research tries to emulate. To me, it seems more relevant if a substance has been used for 3,000 years by an observant culture than if it underwent six months of clinical trials at a modern university.

In their own cultures, traditional healers have earned the respect and trust of their communities because they produce results. The people who have mastered the healing arts of their cultures use experience and intuition when dealing with herbs and people's bodies, often based on concepts that cannot always be explained in conventional medical terms. They are trained intensively in subtleties that American doctors are not, just as the reverse is true.

Unfortunately, the thinking in much of science is that we are too sophisticated to bother with concepts that don't provide hard physical data. If we can't grasp an approach or philosophy involved in another culture's medicine, there is a tendency to dismiss it as being lacking, rather than to question what may be lacking in our own capacity for comprehension (or to cultivate an expanded comprehension). There is unwillingness to bend in the direction of others' standards, demanding instead that they conform to ours. We assume that the inability of apples and oranges to blend is somehow due to the inherent inferiority of the apple.

When considering herbs that are based "only" on the observations of the healers of other cultures, remember that most of what is now backed by scientific research was originally only recommended by healers in other cultures. In fact, that's how those herbs came to be studied; scientists took note of their traditional reputations and began testing them.

PROBLEMS WITH JUDGING HERBS
BY DRUG STANDARDS

What *is* the incentive to take a food or spice that has anecdotally and clinically worked around the globe for hundreds or thousands of years, and spend lots of money to understand its mechanism and ferret out the active parts of it? The incentive is not efficacy, because when the whole herb works, it works whether or not we understand it completely.

The incentive is economic. Economic forces have enormous bearing on what is funded, researched, marketed, and endorsed by authorities. Why does our medical system favor standardized pharmaceutical drugs? Because standardized pharmaceuticals can be patented. Isolating a compound and making it into a pill can be patented. Eggplant cannot be patented. Cinnamon cannot be patented. Plant roots or tree barks cannot be one company's sole "discovery" or monopoly, nor can a company charge a fortune for something that is readily available around the world.

At the core of the changeover 100 years ago from botanical medicine to pharmaceutical medicine is capitalism. As we detail in Chapter 1, "Herbs: The Original Medicine," those with influence could foresee clearly that there would be very little money in botanical medicine, but an endless wealth of opportunity for those who could isolate, patent, and synthetically reproduce the purified active components of botanicals. To do that costs enormous amounts of money, and the investment is recovered only by charging enormous amounts of money.

Thus the herb industry is faced with a Catch-22: It is continually charged with not having researched its products enough and not having enough "evidence" of their effectiveness, but there is no economic incentive (or even adequate compensation) for researching something that is cheaply available to everyone.

How can an herb company afford to invest the exorbitant sums demanded by the kind of research conventional science respects, when they will never be able to make it back in product sales? A company that wildcrafts, packages, and markets a plant can never patent that plant; it is no one's sole property. Should herb companies, just out of the goodness of their hearts, study the plants they market—while drug companies extract an ingredient, copy it, magnify its potency 100 times, add a bunch of other stuff to it, and sell it as a unique product to which no one else can lay claim? Drug companies routinely justify the exorbitant sums charged for pharmaceuticals by pointing to their huge research investments. How would an herb company make back that huge investment? By charging $100 for a bottle of garlic pills when we can go to the grocery store and buy three bulbs for a dollar?

James A. Duke, Ph.D., one of the foremost authorities on botanical medicine in the country, whose experience includes twenty-five years of government service with the U. S. Department of Agriculture (USDA) as a botanist and medicinal plant researcher, noted in *HerbalGram,* "What drug company wants to invest $231 million to prove an herb like feverfew, which you and I could grow at home, can prevent migraine? How would they get their $231 million back if we raised homegrown feverfew and self-medicated, and how much would they lose in sales of remedial migraine medications if this herb prevented 70 percent of migraine headaches?"[7]

The consumer loses if herbs are judged based on the inability to produce evidence that parallels that which is required for a drug. A consumer may forgo use of an herb or food that is completely nontoxic, extremely inexpensive, and very effective because he or she has been convinced that "not enough evidence exists to support its use."

Let's look at some examples. Treatment with saw palmetto berry, in Europe considered a proven remedy for enlarged prostate, costs only 40 cents a day, compared to the pharmaceutical drug finasteride, at about

$1.75 a day. Similarly, cholestyramine, a cholesterol-lowering drug, costs nearly $4 a day more than garlic tablets, which have been shown to lower serum cholesterol and trigylcerides (and have other heart-healthy effects).[8]

Who benefits more from the herb and who benefits more from the drug? Would you rather spend 40 cents a day than $1.75 a day? And which is better for making a cost-effective health-care system? On the other hand, which is better for the drug company that makes finasteride? Are they happy about you taking saw palmetto berry?

Duke suggests:

> Ask your congressperson: "Who benefits most from preventive medicine: the consumer, the government, the medical establishment, or the pharmaceutical industry?" Clearly, the doctors and pharmaceutical industry stand to lose, if preventive medicine prevails. Then why is 90 percent of government funds targeted for curative medicines? . . . As it stands today, the FDA prohibits the sale of herbal alternatives, if there are any preventive or curative messages implied. The FDA tolerates tobacco while prohibiting the sale of licorice or lobelia to help people stop tobacco, or antioxidant teas or even carrots to prevent lung cancer or willow bark to prevent heart attack. The FDA tolerates the sale of alcohol while prohibiting the sale of evening primrose to curb the alcohol habit, or milk thistle seed or dandelion flowers to prevent cirrhosis, or antioxidant teas to prevent oral, kidney, or liver cancer. They tell us that without scientific proof of efficacy, these herbs cannot be sold with health messages. Are they helping the American consumer or the pharmaceutical industry?[9]

Duke suggests that the burden of proof be put not on herb companies, but rather "on the agency which confiscates an inexpensive, longstanding, and empirically proven botanical, while favoring the exorbitant synthetics and expensive, unproven, or unnecessary interventions . . . [that] cause thousands of deaths a year. . . ." He further suggests requiring "legislation that would require a pharmaceutical firm, in any new synthetic drug trial, to compare its new drug, not only with a placebo, but also with one or two of the better herbal alternatives. If the drug company finds, as I predict it will in many cases, that the herbal alternative is nearly as safe and efficacious as their synthetic option, they could be granted marketing rights to both the herbal and the synthetic alternative."[10]

Dr. Larry Dossey also points out that "healing has laws that appear to differ from those of other sciences. Scientists insist that all phenomena obey the same laws, and that they consequently should be expected to jump through the same hoops experimentally. . . . The assumption is that healing should be expected to work like drugs or irradiation, which are given in standard doses."[11]

When herbs are expected to work like drugs, one-size-fits-all research concepts may conceal the real value of the substance. The prevailing "doctrine of specific cause" also affects natural medicine research adversely when scientists trained to see medicine only in terms of killing external threats are assigned to evaluate herbs or nutrients. When garlic, astragalus, or vitamin C fail to directly destroy pathogens or cancer cells in a petri dish, scientists abandon study of those agents, saying they are ineffective.[12] The most sophisticated minds may miss the simplest concepts: that those substances make *us* more effective at doing the killing.

"MORE RESEARCH IS NEEDED": IT'S NEVER ENOUGH

A doctor who wishes to remain anonymous said that we are the greatest system in the world because we test everything. But does that really make us great? We're not convinced that the idolatry of research is a criterion for a "great" medical system. Again, there is no doubt it has value, but not to the exclusion of everything else.

A phenomenon you may have noticed is that researchers decide we need to do research, so they do research. And then they do more research. And more research. And more research. And after all that, often the only conclusion they offer is "more research is needed."

Play a game with yourself for one month. Clip every newspaper magazine article that reports on research findings but concludes, "More research is needed." Write down every time this is said on radio or TV news. Tally it up at the end of the month. Once you start playing this game, you'll never stop seeing and hearing that phrase echoing throughout your news.

It's not that "more research is needed" is untrue; we agree that even the most exacting and extensive research doesn't necessarily "prove" anything and should be taken with a grain of salt. What's interesting about it is that research is so revered, even though it's never definitive and the researchers themselves almost always say, in effect, "We're still not sure." It's also amazing how endlessly something can be researched based on that conclusion.

As of this writing, Dean Ornish's "Reversal Program" still has yet to get the nod from large insurance companies like Cigna, Aetna, and Prudential, even though Ornish has solid scientific documentation and the therapy is far cheaper than bypass surgery. "The therapy shows promise, they say, but further studies are needed."[13]

From the venerable *New York Times*, here's one of my favorites of all time: "The latest development, scientists say, is good news tinged with great uncertainty."[14] Doesn't that say it all?

CRUNCHING THE NUMBERS

I've heard it said time and time again: "We need to study alternatives in a rigorous manner. You need numbers behind things."

Do we always need numbers behind things? Maybe we do and maybe we don't. We hope that we have at least provoked some thought about that.

But supposing we do want "numbers." How do we get them? We need dollars—and the respect that brings dollars. Can we get that respect without first having research? It's like that old conundrum of needing experience to get a job, but needing a job to get experience. It's easy to get locked out.

Things are improving—marginally and slowly. In 1992, the National Institutes of Health established its Office of Alternative Medicine (OAM), thus conferring somewhat increased respectability on holistic healing. In 1994, two new alternative medical journals were launched: *Alternative Therapies in Health and Medicine* and *Alternative & Complementary Therapies*, both targeted at conventional physicians.[15]

The NIH is encouraging exploration of alternative medicine but, says Dr. Andrew Weil flatly, "They are too small. They don't have enough money."[16] Doctor, researcher, and author Jeffrey Bland, Ph.D., puts it succinctly: "The National Institutes of Health allocate billions of dollars annually on research into and treatment of disease. Less than 1 percent of the budget is spent on anything related to functional health."[17]

The NIH's Office of Alternative Medicine (OAM) has established eight new specialty centers across the country that will investigate and explore alternative medical therapies with "scientific rigor." Safety, cost-effectiveness, and efficacy of various therapies—for conditions ranging from AIDS to pain to allergy to cancer—will be studied. The grants total $850,000 over three years for the eight centers. The OAM also awarded a handful of smaller grants of $20,000 to $30,000 each.

While it's exciting that the NIH is funding some research of natural medicine, it's also interesting to note the still relatively paltry sums being devoted to this area. A $30,000 grant is considered mere pocket change in the research world. The Office of Alternative Medicine's budget represents a fraction of the overall funding power of the NIH. The OAM's budget in 1995 was $5.4 million—an increase of $1.1 million over 1994. The overall NIH budget is about $10 *billion*. Not even a full $1 million was doled out for those eight centers to share over three years.

This must be considered before complaining about how little research there is on natural medicine. First of all, in the world scope—taking into account all of the scientific research done in other countries, even if you don't count the clinical and anecdotal data kept over thousands of years in an "unorthodox" manner by other cultures—it's not true that there is little research. But in the United States the amount of research done on natural medicine is very small compared to the amount of research we have on drugs. This is the predictable result of $5 million in funding compared to $10 billion. And just five years ago there was zero money in the coffers for study of alternative medicine at all. The OAM didn't even exist.

CLOSING WORDS

I found this text on the Internet, written by naturopath Sharol Tilgner, N.D., reprinted here with her permission. We think it sums up very well:

> In the U.S. as well as other industrialized countries, scientists are
> looked upon by some with the same awe and reverence one would give
> to a priest or shaman. There is often no questioning the researchers'

authority, how the information was obtained, or if there is an ulterior motive behind their research. . . . I am appalled at how easily our society is willing to blindly follow the word of scientists. . . . The research lab is a contrived situation and far-removed from everyday life. Many factors can cause the research to be unrealistic when compared with the daily life of a human, including: environment, preparation of plant material, method of administration, varying idiosyncratic reactions between the patient and plant interaction, energetic qualities of the plant not being accounted for, plant constituents not having the same action as the whole plant, research is often on animals, not humans. . . . Ulterior motives are possible in the researcher as well as the financial backers of the research. . . . Contradictions can be found between one researcher and her experiments and other researchers. . . . The important thing to keep in mind when reading research articles is to use the information as a building block to understand the larger picture. . . . Do not let it become the whole picture, and always question the motives behind the research.

4

Immune System 101

The man is not sick because he has an illness;
he has an illness because he is sick.

—Proverb quoted in *Between Heaven and Earth,*
A Guide to Chinese Medicine,
by Harriet Beinfeld and Efrem Korngold

Natural medicine emphasizes prevention, and your body's own powers in the area of prevention are chiefly storehoused throughout your immune system. So it's smart medicine to understand how this vitally important system works—and how to work with it.

We both have long believed that an understanding and appreciation of your body inspires and empowers you to care for it appropriately, much more so than if someone simply gives you a laundry list of how-tos for doing so and tells you that you "should." In the case of the immune system, there's lots to appreciate, so let's take a step back and learn about the marvelous systems our body has in place to keep us healthy. I find that I feel stronger, healthier, and more invincible just knowing how my immune system works, and how sophisticated and powerful it is! Not only does that make me all the more motivated and pleased to do things to maintain and support it; I think that's a bit of mind-body medicine that works on my behalf. Besides, it's difficult to heal, nourish, or nurture something that's a total mystery to you.

MORE THAN THE SUM OF ITS PARTS

The immune system is not a system in the same way that the other systems of the body are; it is not merely a physical set of connecting tubes or glands. It's really a concept as well as a system. There is so much of your body involved in immune function, and immune function is so closely linked to proper functioning of other systems, that it is hard to set it apart as a stand-alone system. Chinese doctors first referred to the immune system as "defensive energy" about 2,000 years ago.[1] This offers some apt imagery.

There are discrete cells and organs that are part of the immune system, however. Some organs serve the immune system exclusively; some have other jobs as well. By varying estimates, one-fourth to one-half of cells in the body are exclusively dedicated to immune function. This makes it the largest system of the body—and with good reason. The immune system has a tremendously crucial and mammoth job to do.

Crudely put, the immune system is designed to get what's not "us" out of us. Every cell has some immune function in terms of keeping outsiders out, to prevent things that are not supposed to be in that cell from getting in. The entire apparatus keeps an ever-present vigil and is prepared—ideally—to coordinate an effective search-and-destroy mission whenever it recognizes a threat.

Our ability to withstand infectious disease, cut short the development of abnormalities, and be cleansed of toxins is dependent upon the health of this system. To a great degree, when you talk about the strength of the immune system, you're talking about your body's level of total health. They are mutually dependent.

A variety of organs and cells supervises, replenishes, and integrates the immune process. Let's take a look at the sophisticated crew that works so diligently to keep you healthy.

Immune-specific organs are the *thymus* (a ductless gland situated near the throat) and *spleen* (a large lymphatic organ in the upper left part of the abdomen). Some health practitioners hold that the tonsils are also immune organs. The thymus manufactures cells and produces hormones that coordinate immune activity. Low blood levels of these hormones are associated with depressed immunity and increased susceptibility to infection.

In the spleen, bacteria are engulfed and destroyed. Worn-out red blood cells and platelets are processed and eliminated here as well. The spleen also acts as a blood reservoir.

The kidneys, liver, and intestines—busy multitasking organs that they are—are involved in immune system tasks as well, even though they do other jobs. The liver, especially, plays a pivotal role. This organ is our main toxin filter and also produces most of the body's lymph. In addition, it eliminates "used" cells.

Elements we sometimes don't think of as being part of the immune system include the skin and mucous membranes, such as those in the digestive system, nose, mouth, and throat, which act as the body's first line of defense for filtering out interlopers. Many an invader has been stopped in its tracks right here, before it can make any further inroads into your body.

The lymphatic system is an extensive network of vessels that runs parallel to the blood vessels and stores, filters, circulates, and eliminates waste. It is like the body's sewer system, and there is a "sewer pipe" to every cell in the body. In fact, the lymphatic system is about four times as large as the circulatory venous system.

Lymph fluid allows the flow of waste materials through the vessels. It flows in one direction—toward the heart. No single muscle pumps it, in the way that the heart pumps blood through the circulatory system. To some degree, all of your muscle power pumps the lymph system. (This could be why regular moderate exercise appears to increase immunity. The regular movement of your muscular system keeps the lymphatic system moving. Massage can do this, too.)

The lymph system is a one-way drain from cells out of the body. The fluid dumps into the blood, and the waste is then filtered by the kidneys, the large intestine and the liver. Lymph nodes are storehouses, congregated in areas where a lot of lymph vessels intersect. These "way station" reservoirs provide a temporary collecting point so that your body doesn't get completely overwhelmed as toxins or dead invaders—such as viruses engulfed by immune cells—are produced or collected. As "filters" they can swell up when they get too full of solid matter, such as when there is so much overload that they can't keep up with the flow. The nodes themselves can also become infected.

White blood cells are manufactured in the bone marrow and thymus and, when mature, are distributed throughout the cells of your body. The five kinds of white cells—lymphocytes, phagocytes, basophils, neutrophils, and eosinophils—can differentiate themselves into further "subtypes" that have specialty jobs.

Phagocytes can differentiate as monocytes, macrophages, or granulocytes. *Monocytes* can expand to become *macrophages* once they enter tissue fluid. These important cells then either attach themselves to tissue or circulate freely to act as the primary detectives of foreigners. Then they chemically alert other cells to do the necessary killing. They are also "microbe gobblers," and help to clean up the waste left behind after the "riot" and filter out accumulated "trash" in lymph nodes.

Basophils are produced in response to allergen exposure. They release a protein called histamine. Histamine is supposed to protect you from valid threats, but may be produced inappropriately, creating an unneeded reaction, when an overactive immune system begins to perceive normally innocuous substances as threats. The over-the-counter *anti*histamines you take to suppress an allergic reaction are actually squelching this immune response. (They are not dealing with the source of imbalance that allows for the inappropriate reaction.)

Neutrophils are the white blood cells called upon when the macrophages first detect invaders. They are free-roaming cells that find and attack bacteria and viruses.

Eosinophils are the toxic-waste cleanup crew. They are specially designated to deal with chemical contamination as opposed to pathogenic infection. Inflammation (which we perceive as discomfort and often reflexively try to suppress) is actually an immune-system response, an attempt to flush toxins through increased heat, blood supply, mucus production, or skin outbreaks.

Lymphocytes are produced by the thymus gland or in lymph nodes. They are transformed into T cells (or T lymphocytes) or B cells.

T cells may be one of two kinds: helper T cells or killer T cells. Helpers are the efficient communicators who take note of invaders and send the message that defense is needed. The killer T cells then perform their elimination task, latching onto the invader and literally poisoning it.

The helper-Ts communicate with hormonal messengers (called messenger molecules or cytokines), including interferon and interleukin. These two substances have been studied for their possible use against cancer and AIDS, even though as purified drugs they are extremely toxic when used in "therapeutic" doses. Another immune-stimulating messenger is tumor necrosis factor.

Natural killer (NK) cells specialize in destruction of foreign cells such as virus or cancer. NK cells recognize and destroy precancerous cells before they can get out of control and become cancer. According to Lara Pizzorno, M.A., the average human being produces 300 cancer cells every day.[2] As long as your immune system is functioning properly, this is no cause for alarm.

NK cells are special because they're "freelancers." They don't need to be activated by messages from other cells. They can directly recognize and eradicate the foes.

B cells circulate in the blood and manufacture antibodies. Antibodies are proteins that recognize and latch onto antigens, the proteins that mark the surface of invaders. B cells may snuff out the invaders themselves, or they may call in white blood cells to do the job.

Suppressor T cells keep the squad from getting too zealous or over-protective. They help ensure that the system takes a balanced and appropriate approach to resisting invasion. An overactive immune system can take the form of allergies or autoimmune disease (in which the immune system loses track of what's "you" and what isn't, and systematically attacks the body's own tissue, as in the case of rheumatoid arthritis or lupus).

Now, isn't that incredible? I find it fascinating that all this work is going on in my body, all the time. It also makes me feel mighty, given how much effort is being expended by so much of my body to keep me well. I feel safe with these "protection police" on duty.

On the other hand, I recognize that being out there "on the street" night and day can leave even the best cops somewhat vulnerable. And given the size of the job at hand (a job that never ends, as long as I live), it occurs to me that a force like this can use all the help and nourishment it can get—to keep from getting tired and worn out, confused, depleted, and starved, or just plain overwhelmed. Besides, I'm so appreciative of all the work being done on my behalf that I want to help.

As it happens, there's a lot we can do to enhance these amazing safe-guards. We can live and care for ourselves in such a way that we do not place undue, added stress on our bodies, creating no more challenges than are necessary. We can also supplement with herbs that are specifically designed to help those safeguards deal more efficiently with the challenges that do come along. I've been doing just that for a long time—both "living lightly" for least impact and burden on the system, and using herbs for added support—and the results are wonderful. Millions of people are doing the same, with excellent results.

Let's now take a look at exactly how we can create the most favorable environment for enhanced immune functioning—and thus the most favorable environment for great health.

5

Prevention 101:
Immune-Boosting Basics

N atural healing excels at prevention. That's not to say it isn't a valuable answer for many existing health conditions; we will deal later with common health concerns and how to treat their symptoms and causes herbally. But ultimately, it's not desirable to get to the point where you need treatments. Herbal medicine can be part of a preventive way of living—along with good food and exercise, and pure water and air—that helps you get to the point where you won't have to "treat" yourself. Then you can spend your energies building and enhancing. Let's look at the ways in which the immune system assists with prevention of disease—and how you can assist the immune system.

EACH CELL TO ITS OWN JOB

Immune cells begin their lives as cells called stem cells. At this point they are generic cells. The body can potentially create any type of red or white blood cell out of them, as needed. Mature immune cells can be divided into two types: memory cells and effector cells. These cells offer different types of immunity.

Memory cells are the kind that remember specific invaders—bugs, toxins, or other compounds—to which they are exposed, and can recall and alert the system if and when they ever meet again. They "make enemies" with specific invaders. Vaccines are designed to affect these cells to create lasting immunity (theoretically). This kind of immunity is called *humoral immunity.*

Memory cells recognize antigens, or identifying proteins, on the surface of foreign cells. The immune system's response to these protein "markers" is the antibody. Antibodies are also proteins, and they can be made to match the antigen. They have the ability either to destroy the marked invader or to signal for its execution by white blood cells made for that job.

Effector cells, on the other hand, are jack-of-all-trade cells. They are not disease specific, but rather take action against all foreigners, not just specific ones they have "memorized." The kind of immunity offered by effector cells is called *cell-mediated immunity.*

Herbs that support, strengthen, or enhance components of the immune system are immunostimulants—general immune system stimulators. They increase cell-mediated immunity, the general level of immune-system activity. There are herbs that can directly kill, or poison, certain kinds of pathogens, and/or have affinity for certain parts of the body, such as the lung or liver. (None has yet been found to act against only one specific disease or "remember" an antigen.) But herbs that increase general immunity are the most valued herbs in traditional healing systems because when general immune functions become stronger and more efficient, you are generally more resistant to almost everything.

This is in contrast to conventional medicine's emphasis on disease-specific therapies that directly kill invaders, acting independently of your own functioning. As a result, there are very few drugs that can combat viral infection (since viruses must be killed by the activity of your own immune system). Those that attempt it (such as AZT for AIDS) are extreme and not very effective.

IT'S NOT THEM; IT'S US

Challenges to our immune system are numerous and constant, especially in our culture, for many reasons. Our lifestyles on the whole tend not to be the most immune supportive in the world. The typical American diet is high in fat, sugar, and processed food and low in fresh food, fiber, and nutritional variety. And let's not forget the low-grade long-term starvation we call dieting—reportedly half of all Americans are abusing themselves in this way at any given time. There's the stress and tension of the average American workday—the hours, the boss, the commute—as well as family and trying to do it all, have it all, and be it all. There are environmental stresses—air and water pollution, chemicals, toxins. When we do get sick, heavy-artillery drugs suppress our immune response and cause imbalances as they eliminate symptoms.

The fact is, germs are always there. We don't really "catch" things—everyone lives in a soup of thousands of bacteria species and viruses. Imagine trying to control all of *them!*

Disease is most often a function of host resistance (or lack thereof, as the case may be). Microbes are opportunists. They get a foothold when they have an opening, when the host (you) is weak. In that sense, it's not so much the bugs that make us sick. We're sick already, sick in the sense of being weak.

So the key is to remain as impenetrable as possible. Then the bugs will fail in their efforts to infect you. If you nurture your own internal resistance instead of attacking the external bugs, you don't have to worry so much about trying to control everything else in the outside environment. Instead of worrying about "antibiotic-resistant strains of bugs," you can become a bug-resistant strain of human!

GENERAL IMMUNE FITNESS BASICS

Clearly, there are things in life that sap your immune system's vigor and capacity. There are also things that give your immune system a break, or even actively nurture it. So in the simplest sense, the strategy for strengthening the system is to increase the positive influences in your life as much as possible, and reduce the negative ones as much as possible.

As an overview, what this would mean is reducing mental stress, consumption of simple sugar, alcohol, saturated and certain other harmful fats, and cutting out smoking and drug use. It would mean increasing your intake of whole grains, legumes, fresh fruits and vegetables; getting plenty of fresh, clean water, rest, relaxation, and quality sleep; doing moderate exercise; and experiencing as much genuine joy, happiness, and self-expression as you can manage.

Certainly that's a lot of things to do, and it may seem overwhelming if all of those areas need work right now. But the nice thing about this concept of reducing the negative and increasing the positive is that it's a process. You can feel good about every step you take. One negative influence removed from your life makes a difference—there's no getting around that. It's simply one less burden on your immune system. One addition on the plus side gives greater mass to your health power. Do what you can, and appreciate yourself for the changes you make.

Following are some general recommendations in each lifestyle area for supporting your immune system.

Food and Diet

A Foundation for Healing: Some Words about Diet

The more your body already reflects a commitment to health through basic care, the more that herbs can help you accomplish. Herbal healing works best on a clean and strong foundation.

It should not be surprising that what we eat has the power both to harm and to heal. Food runs virtually every body operation in some way. The food we take in is all that our bodies have to work with to perform the millions of tasks they do during every second we are alive. Every one of our 60 trillion cells depends on what goes into our mouths and stomachs. It may be a worn cliché to say "We are what we eat," but it's absolutely true. Because of this, the efficiency of your body's operations depends on whether the food you take in is appropriate for the job.

And in addition to some foods being more appropriate than others to provide fuel for energy, some foods definitely enhance functioning and even block, repair, or reverse damage and disease. Research, especially since the late 1980s, is exploding with information about food that can take us beyond simply being well-fed and -fueled (though that is a basic priority). Food can boost immunity—or it can blunt it.

Basic Healthy Eating

Every year, the average American consumes 100 pounds of refined sugar, 55 pounds of fats, and 300 cans of soda pop, among other things.[1] It is simply not possible to build optimum health using these kinds of materials. If you want better-than-average health and immunity, you need to take better than average care of yourself. That starts with diet.

For maximum immune benefit: Your diet should generally be natural, unprocessed, and whole. Don't stress yourself by eating a lot of what you don't need and/or not enough of what you do need. Get enough fuel often enough: 50 to 65 percent complex carb, 20 to 30 percent protein, and 15 to 30 percent fat. Eat a wide variety of foods.

- Eat plenty of fresh fruits and vegetables—at least three of each a day.
- Limit refined carbohydrates, saturated fats, hydrogenated and partially hydrogenated fats (including margarine), and foods with stimulants, drugs, hormones, and chemicals.
- Try to eat as few animal products, especially meats, as possible.
- Organically grown is better whenever possible—it's worth the cost not to consume chemicals whose effects no one really knows. Dr. Andrew Weil says in *Spontaneous Healing,* "I cannot emphasize too strongly that residues of toxic chemicals in foods we eat are major health hazards, affecting us in ways that current medical science and governmental policy often fail to recognize. . . . Do not believe people who try to allay your concerns about toxic exposures. This is a real threat, and you must learn to take protective measures."
- Don't starve yourself. Dieting not only doesn't work, it makes you sick. If you consistently destroy body proteins to manufacture glucose to maintain blood sugar, then immunity will decline.
- Avoid white sugar. White sugar is one of the most insidious immune suppressors in the American diet. Some people who are counting fat grams like crazy continue to consume sugar by the pound. Research shows that sugar does suppress immune function. One study found that 100 grams of glucose, sucrose, fructose, or honey significantly impaired the ability of subjects' white blood cells to engulf and destroy bacteria.[2] Another study shows suppressive effects starting 30 minutes after consumption and lasting more than five hours.[3] Whole-grain complex carbs don't appear to have the same effect. Sugar has even been observed in vitro—under the microscope—to be destructive to cells.

Sugar and other refined foods also raise trigylcerides (blood fats) as well as blood sugar.

When I eat sweets, I choose those sweetened with Fruitsource (made from grapes and rice) or barley malt or rice syrup. Failing that, I choose honey, molasses, maple syrup, fruit juices. These are sweeter, so less can be used; they also at least have a marginal amount of nutrient value, whereas white sugar has absolutely none. Processed white sugar gives me a headache that no other sweetener does; I assume my body is trying to tell me something.

Fine-tuning

In addition to good basic fueling, my diet includes antioxidant foods and healthful oils, and is almost 100 percent organic and vegetarian. People who know this about me often ask me why I did not detail these issues in *BodyFueling®*; in fact, I encouraged people not to worry about those issues initially and to focus instead on handling the "macro."

BodyFueling® was designed in part to avoid the "recommendation overwhelm" that many people experience when trying to make positive health and lifestyle changes. If people who have been doing nothing "right" at all for three or five decades suddenly want to do some good things for themselves, giving them twenty-five recommendations and claiming that all are equally important can send them off the deep end.

Also, there is such a lack of information, awareness, and understanding about the most basic needs of the body that I found it much more productive to get people started doing five or so of the most crucial, bottom-line things and enjoying the great benefits of those changes. People making just those changes—eating enough, eating often enough, eating the right proportions of macronutrients, exercising fueled, and eliminating fats and sugars—would see huge improvements in health and fitness, even if they did eat nonorganic food and didn't take vitamins or herbs.

BodyFueling® is a foundation. It gets people to the place where they can say, "Okay, what next?" Now we can talk about vitamins, minerals, phytonutrients, antioxidants, herbs, Ayurvedic or Chinese body-type diets, organics, and a host of other enhancing issues that do indeed build on the basics. Now we can deal with which foods, in the massive smorgasbord of foods that might fuel you, are optimal for your specific constitution and specific lifestyle, or which foods in that range of choices contain anti-aging or cancer-fighting phytonutrients.

Very Specific Diets

One could adopt any number of specialized dietary guidelines beyond these fairly basic recommendations. You can eat foods that enhance your Ayurvedic body type and avoid those that aggravate your body type's tendencies and conditions. You can eat foods that balance yin and yang, as befits the seasons or the time of day. You can follow a strict macrobiotic diet.

There are books that detail thoroughly these and other types of eating, and you may wish to try them now or at some time in the future. Some of the books that cover such diets in detail are included in our bibliography. But the purpose of this book is to help you integrate into your life some of the most useful and basic principles of herbal medicine and related natural healing traditions. It is to help you, as a layperson, understand these ways of thinking and doing things—and to be able to apply them without feeling you have to become a totally different person overnight.

Vegetarianism

There is no space in this book to discuss at length the many health and environmental strikes that have mounted against animal products—especially meat—in the past decade or two. However, it is hard to ignore vegetarianism completely in any discussion of healthy diet. Reduction in intake of meat and meat products seems to result in better health in just about every conceivable area.

Vegetarian women are less than one-fourth as likely as meat-eaters to get breast cancer. Vegetarian men have a 46 percent lower chance of suffering a heart attack than men who eat meat. Vegetarian diets help prevent or treat strokes, osteoporosis, kidney stones, cancers, diabetes, hypoglycemia, rheumatoid arthritis, ulcers, obesity, hernias, gallstones, high blood pressure, asthma, and many other diseases (countries with more meat consumption have more of those diseases). Meat consumption is now being linked to many negative "symptoms" of aging, including senility and Alzheimer's. And vegetarians do live longer: The greater the meat consumption, the greater the death rate from all causes combined.

The great majority of meats add more fat to our diets than is healthy, and it's the worst kind of fat for our bodies to deal with. Other health issues have been raised regarding meat, from the hormones and antibiotics injected routinely into the animals, to the possibility that they might eat contaminated or chemically treated feed, and even the possibility of "aggressive energy" produced in those who consume meat filled with adrenaline from animals in extreme fear states just prior to slaughter.

Then there are the environmental concerns: Producing one hamburger uses enough fossil fuel to drive a small car 20 miles and enough water for 187 showers. More than half of all water and most of the grain used in the United States goes to raising animals for our meals. Between 1960 and 1985, nearly 40 percent of all Central American rain forests were destroyed to make cheap grazing land for cows later eaten by North Americans and Europeans.

Despite all of that, we do not intend this to be an admonishment of nonvegetarians and we do not insist that everyone in the world become a vegetarian (as if we could, anyway!). All we suggest is that you consider these issues on an ongoing basis and keep reevaluating your choices. Healthy eating—healthy *anything*—does not have to mean making one definitive decision about something for the rest of your life. The perception that it does mean just that keeps many people from making any movement at all, because such a commitment is almost impossible to swallow.

Karta Purkh and his family are lacto-vegetarian (eat some dairy products, no eggs), and I am about 98 percent lacto-ovo vegetarian—a few free-range eggs a month, a few organic dairy products a week, and fish a few times a year.

I want to be clear, however, that for me this is a relatively recent development; it has taken place over the last three or four years. When I began "fueling" in 1990, I was eating poultry daily, sometimes more than once a day (although even then I hadn't eaten red meat for almost ten years). I didn't try to force myself to stop eating something I liked. Meat was eliminated from my diet very slowly and gradually.

I say *it was eliminated*, and not *I eliminated it*, because it happened almost without intent, of its own accord. I didn't wake up one day and say, "I am now a vegetarian." I didn't make a single conscious decision. It happened naturally as I added more and more other foods into my diet and slowly lost my taste for meats. As many vegetarians do, I found that I thrive without any meat in my diet.

Some health practitioners actually feel that there are people who are healthier with meat than without (based on various theories about blood type, body types, and evolutionary adaptations). However, others counter that even the person who experiences minor health discomforts on a meatless diet (dry skin, cravings, or constipation, for example) might be able to achieve balance in other ways—using herbs, for example—rather than by including meat. The need for meat by some people may be genuine, but it's equally plausible that the meat is masking or crutching some other deficiency that could be met even more healthfully.

Certainly, diets should be individualized to some degree. And we agree that *excess* consumption of animal protein represents the core problem. But this book is about taking your health to the next level. And when you get to the point of fine-tuning, then at least a reduction in meat consumption may be worth considering. While many people can do well with a moderate meat-eating diet (assuming the meat is healthfully prepared and other healthy habits are in place), there is simply a well established correlation between diets high in animal protein and disease.

Diet as Medicine

An exciting branch of recent research has identified biologically active substances in foods—plant foods, including fruits, vegetables, legumes, and grains—that have health-enhancing or possibly curative abilities. Often these are the very substances that also give the food its color, flavor, or smell. These substances are being called *phytochemicals* (*phyto-* being from the Greek word for "plant"), or *phytonutrients*, or sometimes *nutraceuticals* or *foodaceuticals*. The idea behind these terms is that food can be medicinal as well as nutritious.

To explain the difference between a food being nutritious and medicinal, let's look at an example. Citrus fruits have long been considered to be nutritious in the traditional sense of the word, in part because they are high in vitamin C. Vitamin C is a nutrient that we need to stay healthy, and there are minimums established so that we do not become deficient in that nutrient. Citrus fruit also has carbohydrate value, carbohydrate being a macronutrient (like protein and fat), as opposed to a micronutrient (like vitamins and minerals). Carbohydrate has nutritional value—it's fuel that runs our bodies.

Recently, citrus foods have been discovered also to contain a compound called limonene, which is not a nutrient like a vitamin or mineral and does not provide fuel. It does, however, appear to boost cancer-fighting ability by increasing proliferation of certain enzymes and enhancing killer cell activity. Limonene may be medicinal. Dr. Andrew Weil offers some other good terms: *natural therapeutic agents* and *natural preventive agents*. Regardless of the word you use, the implication is clear: Some foods contain valuable compounds and substances that, distinct from their nutritional value, pack an enormous preventive wallop and may also promote healing of existing illness.

Phytochemicals can be said to have pharmacologic actions—predictable activity that can be isolated and defined as pushing a body process in one direction or another. But, being natural constituents of foods rather than concentrated synthetics, they provide their helpful activity without the downside of possible toxic injury or unpleasant side effects—and in most cases, with the bonuses of nutritious fuel and a tasty experience along the way.

This type of substance is being discovered in a wide range of foods we already value nutritionally, and it's exciting to know that these foods can provide additional health-enhancing and disease-fighting benefits not previously known or understood. Literally hundreds of these substances are currently being investigated.

Best Phytonutrient Bets

Here is a summary of the information available as of this writing on the most researched phytonutrients. Including as many of the following foods in your diet as you can will let you reap significant anti-cancer, anti-aging, and other benefits.

> Soy—*Isoflavones* in soybeans appear to protect against cancer. *Genistein* is the isoflavone getting the most attention currently, and appears to fight cancer in several ways. As a phytoestrogen (plant estrogen), genistein can plug up receptors for the real thing—putting the brakes on some cancers, including breast cancer, that are stimulated by estrogen. One study showed that a soy-based diet increases the menstrual cycle by about two days, and a longer menstrual cycle means less exposure to estrogen. This may be one reason (though there are undoubtedly others) that Japanese women have one-fifth the breast-cancer rate of American women.[4] Genistein may also reduce menopausal symptoms and prevent osteoporosis.

Other Beans—The soybean is emerging as a phytochemical winner, as shown above, but kidney beans, chickpeas, and lentils have *saponins* (a type of compound also found in many medicinal herbs), which may slow cancer-cell production and spreading.

Tomatoes—*Lycopene* (a carotenoid, in the same family as beta-carotene, among others) is an antioxidant, so it protects against cell damage. It is linked to reduced growth of colon and bladder cancer cells in mice, may reduce risk of prostate cancer and prostate disease, and may also lower risk of cardiovascular disease. *P-coumaric acid* stops the production of cancer-causing nitrosamines. *Coumarins* are also anti-inflammatory.

Citrus—*Limonene:* A substance that increases production of cancer-cell-breakdown-and-disposal enzymes thought to break down carcinogens and stimulate cancer-killing immune cells. The vitamin C and soluble fiber are good for you, too. *Glucarase* inactivates carcinogens and eliminates them.[5] Lycopene, mentioned earlier, is also found in red grapefruit.

Orange Vegetables and Fruits—Squash, sweet potatoes, carrots, mangoes, pumpkins, and cantaloupes get their color from carotenes, the antioxidant chemicals found in these foods. *Alpha-carotene* increases vitamin A activity, slows lung-cancer cell growth in mice, and boosts general immunity. *Beta-carotene* is an antioxidant that has been linked to decreased risk of many types of cancer as well as generally improved immunity. (Other carotenes in other foods that may be equally or even more valuable: *lycopene, lutein, zeaxanthin,* and *cryptoxanthin.*)

Crucifers—*Indoles* in crucifers (broccoli, Brussels sprouts, cabbage, and other cruciferous vegetables) affect estrogen metabolism by increasing enzymes that weaken cancer-promoting estrogens. Animal studies show that this slows cancer growth. Indoles may also assist in toxin elimination and increase general immunity. *Sulforaphanes:* Another crucifer chemical. Animal studies show it inhibits breast-cancer tumor growth; also assists cancer-fighting enzymes in removing carcinogens from cells.

Grapes—*Ellagic acid* blocks the body's production of cancer-helper enzymes. In mice, an extract of Concord grapes was as effective as the cancer drug methotrexate in slowing tumor growth.[6] Turnips are another source of ellagic acid.

Garlic and Onions—*Allyl sulfide (allicin)* Garlic and onions are discussed in detail elsewhere in this book of their dozens of benefits, but decreased risk of stomach and colon cancer, lower LDL cholesterol, and reduced blood clotting are among allicin's benefits. It also may encourage the production of gluthathione S-transferase, an enzyme that helps rid the body of carcinogens.

Berries—*Polyphenols* are found in red grapes and red wine, strawberries and blueberries (also artichokes and yams). They may flush carcinogenic toxins and lower risk of heart disease. They include *flavonoids*, which are compounds linked to dozens of health-protective benefits: They interfere with carcinogenic hormones, fight cell damage from oxidation, strengthen blood vessels, decrease capillary permeability, protect skin integrity, and are anti-inflammatory and good for the eyes. *P-coumaric acid* (see tomatoes) is also found in strawberries.

Flaxseed—*Lignans* are antioxidant polyphenols, and flaxseed contains lignan precursors. Lignans may help prevent some estrogen-related cancers by binding to estrogen receptors in breast tissue and interfering with estrogen's cancer-promoting activity there. Flaxseed is also a good source of healthful omega-3 fatty acids. (The seeds can be used ground up and sprinkled on food, or the oil can be used.)

Leafy Greens—*Lutein* in spinach, mustard, turnip, and collard greens, as well as yellow squash, are carotenoid antioxidants that appear to protect against some cancers, slow degenerative eye disease, and increase immunity. Dark, leafy greens also contain indoles (see crucifers).

The above fruits and vegetables are probably best eaten fresh and raw (except for beans, obviously) but are also probably just as effective lightly cooked (steamed is best) as well. A few, such as the sulforaphanes in crucifers, are reported to be enhanced by light steaming or microwaving. Don't overcook vegetables, since phytochemicals may be destroyed in the process just as some vitamins and minerals are. Juicing is a good way to concentrate nutrients, so it's probably a good way to concentrate phytochemicals as well. Canned and frozen fruits and vegetables are probably better than none at all.

Isn't it interesting how everything comes full circle? The same foods that have been recommended for so many other reasons—their nutrients in the classic sense, their low fat content, their fiber, their displacement of unhealthy foods—are also the foods being found to contain these health-promoting substances. Coincidence? Note also that no one has yet turned up any potent health-enhancing phytochemicals in steak, milk, or Twinkies.

At any rate, now you have yet another reason to emphasize plant foods in your diet. Not only are these foods nutritious in the traditional sense, they also have specific disease-fighting properties. There appear to be numerous reasons why people whose diets consist mainly of these foods have less of the diseases Americans struggle with the most.

There is yet another good reason for that long-held recommendation to eat a wide variety of foods: Phytochemicals may be synergistic. The more of these different foods you eat, the more of the "phytochemical smorgasbord" you will benefit from, and the more chance you have of combining them in ways that may later be found to enhance the actions of individual substances.

How Do Phytochemicals Work?

The exact mechanism of action is not yet known for every single phytochemical identified to date. However, there are many observations and theories about them. Most of the compounds with some confirmed activity are anticancer (preventing or fixing cell malignancy through various mechanisms), heart protective, anti-aging or antioxidant (blocking or repairing oxidative damage to cells), or anti-inflammatory.

Some of the cancer-preventive and -healing compounds seem to be quite sophisticated and wide-ranging in their actions. They may block the formation of malignancy, cut off the blood supply to malignant cells, boost production of cancer-flushing enzymes, or counteract carcinogens (cancer-forming or -triggering toxins) themselves, either by detoxifying or preventing them from establishing on target organs. They may also support our own repair mechanisms.

Phytochemicals with *antioxidant* capabilities are of special interest. Antioxidants are substances (usually chemicals or nutrients in foods and herbs) that can protect our cells from damage by counteracting a body process that is similar to oxidation (like rusting). Oxidative damage represents the dominant theory today for what causes aging.

Antioxidants have the ability to neutralize free radicals, which are highly reactive and unstable molecules that cause cellular damage. These destructive molecules may bond with and alter molecules, damage cells and tissues, and feed carcinogens. All of our cells are exposed to these toxic, destructive molecular bits, which are the by-products of external stresses and exposures as well as normal internal processes. They are constantly on the loose in our bodies. By some estimates, each of the 60 trillion cells in our bodies suffers 10,000 free-radical "hits" daily.[7]

You can appreciate how sophisticated and powerful our bodies are to repair that much damage routinely. When our repair mechanisms don't keep up, however, we run into trouble. Many scientists now believe that the havoc wreaked by free radicals is a factor in cancer and numerous other diseases, as well as much of the damage we attribute to "getting older." The oxidation of LDL ("bad") cholesterol is also partly to blame for atherosclerosis.

Fortunately, there are ways to assuage the ravages of these toxic molecular saboteurs. One is prevention. Free-radical damage is accelerated by environmental factors, many of which are in our control. These include diet, emotional stress, smoking, drinking, exposure to excessive sunlight, and exposure to industrial processes, ozones, radiation, nitrates, exhaust, and other chemicals and pollutants.

Another way to fight free radicals is with regular intake of antioxidant-rich herbs and foods. These appear to help our bodies resist, retard, or defuse the effects of exposures we cannot prevent. They can also help our repair mechanisms fix the DNA damage. In addition to phytochemical compounds in herbs and foods, some common nutrients also show free-radical-quenching or other antioxidant activity. These include vitamins A, C, and E, the mineral selenium, and the amino acid glutathione.

Food versus Pills

As phytonutrients show up on our shelves as synthetic pills, there are some things to think about before you dismiss carrots and reach for capsules.

As with herbs, there is the question of whether the phytochemicals are effective by themselves, or whether other components in the food or plant are required for their function, or at least to enhance the primary component's activity. Many phytochemicals, like active compounds in herbs, may be synergistic with other compounds. No one is sure yet exactly how this happens, or which ones work together. Quite simply, isolated extracts in a pill may not work as well as the whole food.

This was underscored when a couple of much-ballyhooed studies showed slightly higher rates of lung cancer among smokers taking beta-carotene supplements than among those who didn't take them. There were problems with these studies, though, and they don't represent the average person eating beta-carotene-rich fruits and vegetables, or taking moderate amounts of antioxidant supplements.

What's crucial to note (and what much of the media and public missed, unfortunately) is that:

1. Beta-carotene was used in isolation from the other carotenoid compounds that accompany it in foods.
2. Synthetic beta-carotene was used, and there are molecular differences between natural and synthetic that influence how the body uses beta-carotene. The atomic structure of the natural form makes it a more potent antioxidant, according to several other studies.[8]
3. The studies were not controlled for other lifestyle risk factors, such as drinking alcohol in addition to smoking.
4. Hundreds of studies have already shown that eating high amounts of fruits and vegetables, including carotenoid-rich ones, reduces cancer risks (and decreases risk of oral leukoplakia in smokers, a precancerous change in the mucous membrane of the mouth).
5. Even these studies showed lower cancer in *non*smokers taking the supplements; only smokers had increased cancer. (It should never surprise us when smokers get cancer, no matter what else they are doing. No supplement is a substitute for quitting smoking.)

Make no mistake—the bottom line is still that people who eat more fruits and veggies have the least cancer. It may not be the beta-carotene in those fruits and veggies that provides the whole effect. (The decision to study it alone came from the single-isolated-ingredient paradigm we have discussed.) Or beta-carotene may need other compounds in the food as co-factors. Or beta-carotene isolated (or synthetic) may interfere with the activity or absorption of more powerful, not-yet-studied carotenoids or other compounds.

You may just have to eat the whole food. That's certainly how other cultures have historically used foods for health and healing, rather than seeking "anticancer compound designer pills"—a pursuit that is peculiar to our health-care thinking and, in our opinion, not the path that truly leads to wellness. Looking for all answers to be contained in a 325-milligram tablet is looking for health in all the wrong places.

Natural Health magazine, in its March/April 1996 article "Reinventing the Vegetable," quoted many health professionals who support the varied whole-foods approach over the magic-pill fantasy and criticize the obsession with single nutrients. Paul A. Lachance, Ph.D., professor of nutrition and food science at Rutgers University, said, "There's a real complexity to this chemistry, and a danger in trying to get all of these chemicals out of a handful of pills. The issue is one of perspective, and the fact is, you've got to eat your veggies."

Finally, it is interesting to note that many of the foods being studied, and in which potent phytochemicals have already been identified, already have a long history as remedies in other cultures. This is just one of many examples of how science is actually playing catch-up with an existing body of knowledge. Sometimes substances already considered effective in other cultures based on observation are presented as a new discovery, when in fact their benefits have simply been made newly credible.

Exercise

Exercise definitely affects immunity, and that effect can be positive or negative. Too much can depress your immune function, while the "right amount" can definitely enhance it.

Naturally, there is no definitive consensus yet regarding the exact amount of exercise that will cause the immune system to go on hiatus or cause it to shore up its forces. However, the general consensus of most research on exercise and immunity suggests that a "long, hard workout"— anything much more than an hour for most people—puts certain immune cells on vacation for six to nine hours, leaving you open and vulnerable to cold and flu viruses and other pathogens. Heavy training of more than an hour a day seems to bring a diminishing return, resulting in more infections, particularly respiratory infections. Up to an hour of aerobics is the amount that seems to stimulate immune cell activity, actually increasing it above normal or average function, and enhances general health.

As usual, the under-one-hour versus over-one-hour is a rule of thumb, something to be aware of rather than follow to the letter. Don't go crazy with it. If your aerobics class is one hour and four minutes, that probably doesn't mean your immune cells are going to go to sleep. Conversely, if you are extremely out of shape and in poor health generally, it's possible that thirty minutes of walking—an amount of exercise that, based on research, should spur your immune system to new heights—could have the effect that a much harder, longer training session would have on a healthier, fitter person. If so, you will want to increase time and intensity slowly.

In general, though, it appears that certain key members of the immune orchestra don't play very well during the recovery period following very intense exercise. The number and potency of immune cells are depleted. One hypothesis is that the elevation of stress hormones that follows heavy exercise may suppress immune function.

Whatever the reason, it makes sense to exercise moderately. This is most easily and simply defined as exercise that leaves you feeling energized and exhilarated rather than exhausted and drained. It's common sense that if you feel sucked dry after a workout, that's going to require a recovery period that sounds very much like the period in which immune function appears to decrease. If you feel vibrant and vital after a workout, you have probably stimulated yourself in a healthy way.

An important note for athletes in high-intensity training: It's important to realize that just because study subjects suffered more infections due to lowered immunity doesn't necessarily mean you have to. What it does mean is that without extra support, your immune system may be weakened by very heavy exercise or training. But there's no proof that you are helpless to counter its effects—it's just that most people don't try to. You can work harder to nourish your body and supplement to compensate for the stressful effects of such training.

Serious training is stress, just like lack of sleep, tough commutes, bad bosses, or screaming children. Herbs can build stamina and endurance as well as sustain immune function during stress. We will discuss stamina tonics later in the book.

Stay Fit and Lean

Good exercise and good diet also indirectly benefit the immune system by helping to maintain a lean, fit body. Such a body may be more likely to have stronger immune function, not only because the habits that lead to its development are immune-supportive, but also because the body itself is hardier. People whose bodies reflect abuses seem to suffer most from an endless string of infections.

Says Lara Pizzorno, M.A., in her article "Power Up Your Immune System," "Obesity has been linked to decreased immune function. The neutrophils of obese people have a decreased ability to kill bacteria, according to studies cited in *Textbook of Natural Medicine* by Joseph Pizzorno, N.D., and Michael Murray, N.D. Blood cholesterol and lipid levels are also usually higher in obese people. Increased levels of cholesterol and certain lipids such as free fatty acids, triglycerides and bile acids inhibit various immune functions including the ability of lymphocytes to proliferate and produce antibodies and the ability of neutrophils to migrate to areas of infection and destroy infectious organisms."[9]

Of course, the lifestyle that contributes to obesity—excess fat and sugar, too little exercise, dieting, and other depleting factors—is probably as immune suppressive as the obesity itself, or more so.

Avoid Drinking, Smoking, and Taking Drugs

Aw jeez, you might be saying about now. No beer, no butts, no joints? Are we taking all your fun away? Well, just remember how much fun it is to be in bed with a red clogged nose, aching head and body, and hacking cough. Remember, every checkmark you put in the "negative influence" column is one more thing you have to overcome or try to balance in your efforts to stay strong and healthy. It's one less advantage, one more disadvantage.

If you enjoy alcohol and it doesn't affect you in any immediate, adverse way that you notice (I don't care for my body's very strong and immediate reaction to it), one drink a day is okay and may be beneficial. The research on alcohol, viewed as a whole, is somewhat paradoxical. One to two drinks a day is often recommended for boosting HDL (good) cholesterol, and as an anticoagulant (blood thinner)—both anti-heart-disease factors. Red wine seems to offer some additional value, because of antioxidant substances in red grapes (these could also be obtained by eating red grapes or drinking red grape juice, though).

However, even two drinks a day has been implicated by some research in breast cancer, so that leaves you at one drink a day. And the American Cancer Society recently issued guidelines saying that people should not drink even moderate amounts of alcohol because of the cancer risk overall, disagreeing with federal dietary guidelines that say one or two drinks a day appear to cause no harm to adults. The ACS said the risk of cancer increases with the amount of alcohol consumed, and may start to rise with as few as two drinks a day.

Certainly more than two drinks a day can increase risk of high blood pressure, stroke, or cancer, damage the liver, raise triglycerides (blood fats), and depress immunity. In general, we wouldn't put "drink more alcohol" high on the list of top dietary health-boosters. If you're doing everything else wonderfully, I certainly wouldn't worry that you're not drinking enough!

Alcohol is a depressant. It depresses the central nervous system. It makes sense that it would also depress immune function, and studies show that indeed it does interfere with white-blood-cell activity. Animal studies show increased risk of infection after alcohol consumption, and alcoholics are known to be more vulnerable than nonalcoholics to infections. I remember years ago when I was feeling "under the weather," a beer could push me over the edge into a full-blown infection. That seemed logical and predictable to me even then. (Alcohol also irritates the gastrointestinal lining, destroys nerve cells, depletes nutrients and interferes with their absorption, and increases bone loss, among other things.)

Drugs of all kinds can lower immunity, whether they are intended to deal with health symptoms or provide a high. Most recreational drugs have so many side effects that it seems almost too obvious to even mention them (i.e., if you're a heroin addict, having a cold may be the least of your worries). But clearly they alter body chemistry in ways that are not exactly conducive to strength and superior health—and the lifestyles associated with recreational drug use are likely to add at least several other risk factors for lowering immunity.

Some prescription and over-the-counter (OTC) drugs can also interfere with the absorption or utilization of nutrients. (This is especially ironic if, for example, you're taking aspirin and cold medicine and losing vitamin C.) More importantly, OTC and prescription medications, by their very design, are often immune-suppressive because they are aimed at quieting symptoms—and symptoms are often nothing more than the immune system's response to an attack. Inflammation, for example, can be an attempt to cleanse the body of a poison, but here come the *anti*-inflammatories. Histamines are produced by the immune system to protect you, but in come the *anti*histamines. Coughs and running noses are attempts to expel the invaders in mucus, but here come the "cough suppressants" and decongestants. These medications might better be called "anti-immune-systems" because they suppress your body's natural defenses.

Much of the mass production of these kinds of drugs is due to consumer demand: In our culture, we simply don't have the patience to wait out our body's natural way of dealing with invaders, and to live with the discomforts that might bring. And most of us haven't been educated about the natural, more gentle, nonsuppressive or immune-supporting remedies that can relieve our symptoms as well as heal our illnesses.

Cigarette smoking is another immune-system enemy. Cigarette smoking can impair the immunity of smokers and bystanders alike. This increases vulnerability to infections, not to mention the well-established links to cancer, heart disease, and lung diseases. Cigarette smoke is known to deplete vitamin C reserves, and children of smokers suffer from more respiratory and ear infections (as well as asthma) than those who live in nonsmoking homes.[10]

Stress and Rest

The word *stress* conjures up many images, and it is indeed a concept that encompasses many possible factors in American life. Almost everyone has his or her own personal definitions of it; almost everyone has complained about it at some point or another. What is stressful to one person may not be to another, but we do know this: If something is stressful to *you*, your immunity pays a price. Stress takes its toll on the immune system, whether it's emotional, mental, social, or spiritual pressure.

Stress is a fact of American life, and our bodies show it. The "fight-or-flight" response was not meant to be a constant waking state, as it is for so many people. It's meant to be a quick reaction to a genuine emergency that increases our strength and response time so that we may act appropriately. It's a problem that so many of us live in a continuing state of low-grade "emergency," pumping out adrenal hormone that is meant to be used literally only in spurts. Remaining suspended in this ever-ready-for-danger state not only wears on your adrenals, but inhibits white-blood-cell activity. In addition to overstimulation of immunosuppressive adrenal hormones, stress also interferes with sleep and relaxation, which are both important to healthy immune function and healing.

Studies show that mental stress sets in motion a series of bodily responses that amount to decreased immunity. Almost everything from colds to cancer may be attributable in part to stress. Many research experiments have tested for common cold susceptibility at different levels of psychological stress and concluded that increased risk of infection corresponds to increased mental stress.

Aside from all the studies, it's common sense that feeling crunched, pressured, and mentally exhausted will leave you more vulnerable to infection. You've probably noticed the phenomenon yourself many times. You were feeling fine until you heard some bad news, had a fight with a close friend, found out your mother-in-law is visiting the same week that big project at work is due and the dog is scheduled for an operation. Suddenly you begin to feel achy, tired, your throat's a little sore . . .

There are two things you can do about the kind of stress that zaps your immune system's potency. One, you can eliminate from your life the consistent, chronic sources of stress. An occasional traffic jam is no big deal, but if you sit on the freeway four hours every day, maybe it's time for a new job. If you fight with your boyfriend six times a day, if you are in an airplane three weeks a month, if your nine community activities and hobbies create constant scheduling conflicts (I'm raising my hand sheepishly on that last one), think about what changes might be in order.

The other thing you can do is to supplement herbally and nutritionally to help you deal with emotional stress. Again, this works better when you are also making supportive lifestyle changes; otherwise you are just employing a crutch, however natural it might be. Still, there are certainly people, events, and situations we cannot simply change, at least not instantly. For those times when extreme stress cannot be avoided, herbs can help calm nerves as well as give extra support to the immune system. (See Chapter 12, "Herbs for Depression, Addictions, Anxiety, and Insomnia," pages 289–312, as well as the immunostimulant herbs covered in the next chapter.)

I have eliminated many stresses that at one time I could actually feel making me sick, but all stress cannot be avoided. During especially busy times, I can feel myself weakening (when you're used to feeling great, you can become extremely sensitive to fine gradations of wellness and can feel "drops" in immunity that others might not notice). When this happens, I can immediately step up herbal supplementation with immune-building tonics until I feel full strength returning.

Breathing exercises and meditation are both excellent ways to relax, bust stress, and maintain immune function. Some studies show that people who meditate regularly are healthier based on several standard health measurements, and they get sick less often. Andrew Weil's *Spontaneous Healing* details some excellent breathing exercises for the beginner. I find it calming and peaceful to read Jack Kornfield's *Buddha's Little Instruction Book*. Possibly the best book on mindfulness meditation I have ever read is Jon Kabat-Zinn's *Wherever You Go, There You Are*. I am convinced that simply *reading* one of its short chapters lowers blood pressure and increases immunity!

Defusing stress involves listening to your body and giving it the rest and sleep it asks for. Studies show that sleep deprivation definitely challenges the immune system, significantly decreasing the number of disease-fighting cells. Not that you needed studies to tell you that—you've noticed it for years, haven't you? Colds, flu, and other infections seem to nail you the week you're finishing a big project at work, working long hours, getting up early, and going to bed late. Two or three late nights or extra-early morning risings, and you can feel your increased vulnerability.

Yet sleep deprivation is as common in our culture as stress; they often go hand in hand. We fill our lives with so many priorities that sleep falls to the bottom of the list. We go to work early in the morning and, thanks to electricity, can stay up until all hours working under unnatural lighting, when our ancestors would have been asleep simply because the lack of light made anything else difficult. We then fly into bed straight from the computer (guilty!), reading, cleaning, or homework and stare at the ceiling, wondering why we cannot wind down and fall asleep. In addition, sleep quality and depth are often poor, and people often don't feel rested even when quantity is high, so quantity definitely isn't the only issue.

"Pushing through" that tired feeling is often what pushes you over the edge. Whenever possible, take the time to answer the call for rest or sleep. When you know what it feels like to be well, you will know when all is not right. Nourish yourself at those times; don't push it.

Part II

Herbs for Health and Healing

6

Health-Building Herbs, Foods, and Nutrients

Natural healing seeks to nourish the body in a way that supports its own disease-fighting mechanisms. Rather than trying to fight infections "without you," herbs incorporate your immune system in the effort.

There is a vast cornucopia of herbs and foods that stimulate, support, and nourish the immune system. Some have been used for thousands of years by other cultures and are now being evaluated by modern research, which confirms the observations of these cultures—that they stimulate the immune system in a nonspecific way so that general resistance to infection and other illness is heightened.

Your immune system can't be too strong. This is distinct from it being oversensitive. The immune system can overreact—but it does so when it is not adequately nourished and is in a disadvantaged position, not when it is strong. When the immune system is prepared to do what it needs to, it doesn't attack a bunch of things it shouldn't, as in the case of allergies.

The herbs, foods, and nutrients overviewed in this chapter are general health builders and unless otherwise indicated can be used to maximum tolerance as needed or desired. More precise dosage information applicable to healing specific conditions is given in other chapters.

TONIC HERBS

There are a few herbs you wouldn't want to take every day, but in the vast majority of cases this is not because of toxicity. For example, as a poisoner of bacteria, goldenseal has little benefit taken indefinitely, so if you know anything about herbs you don't use goldenseal as a tonic. It won't hurt you, because it is so much milder than a pharmaceutical antibiotic and its active compounds are found in many plants that have been around for a long time, so our bodies have evolved with those compounds. You also won't build up a "tolerance" that will make it ineffective later. You will just waste time and money if you don't have a specific job you want the goldenseal to do.

However, there are other herbs you can take every day that will do nothing but benefit you, no matter how much you take or how often and how long you take them. Herbs that are specifically beneficial when taken every day, even over a lifetime, are called **tonic herbs.**

Some tonic herbs are **adaptogens.** Russian scientist Israel Brekhman, M.D., who initiated some of the first research on ginseng in the 1940s, first used the term *adaptogen* and showed the connection between stress and immune function. Dr. Hans Selye gave further definition to the concept and won a Nobel prize for his work in this area. Selye coined the term *adaptations energy,* stating that when this energy is depleted, performance is limited and resistance to disease is reduced.

In order to be classified as an adaptogen, a plant must:

- Raise nonspecific resistance to disease (cell-mediated immunity)
- Be capable of normalizing bodily functions even in disease states
- Be nontoxic and completely harmless; safe for ingestion for long-term, preventive/nutritive consumption

Not all tonics are adaptogens. Adaptogens increase resistance and adaptation to all stresses and build stamina and vitality. Tonics may generally support a specific organ or system—i.e., an herb may be a tonic for the kidneys or bladder, but that doesn't make it an adaptogen.

In terms of herbal energetics and tastes, tonic herbs are usually moistening and usually sweet, salty, and/or sour. Herbs with these tastes are generally anabolic, which means they build or increase tissue mass. (Herbs with bitter, pungent, or astringent tastes are usually drying, light, and catabolic, decreasing mass or detoxifying.) Thus one definition of a tonic—the criterion used in most ethnic healing systems—is an herb that, with long-term use, is "building" in some way.

A different, more scientific definition labels as tonics only those herbs that exert "opposing forces" to influence body processes back to "center," or normal, rather than pushing the body in only one direction. This makes tonics balancing and appropriate for indefinite use. They will never push the body too far in one direction; to the contrary, they will always have the effect of bringing it back "home," into balance.

Drugs push the body in one direction (unidirectional)—back to normal, we hope—when it has gone too far in another direction. The purpose is to increase or decrease a process or situation that is under- or overactive. *There is no reason to use a unidirectional substance unless you are specifically trying to address an underactive or overactive disease process that needs to be reversed.* In a disease state, substances that push only in one direction are perfectly appropriate.

When there is a need for a unidirectional substance to repair such an imbalance, an herb is a better choice for many reasons. Most single, nontonic herbs actually work unidirectionally, but in a much gentler and more nourishing way than drugs, without side effects.

Daniel B. Mowrey, Ph.D., author of *Herbal Tonic Therapies* and *Scientific Validation of Herbal Medicine*, explains, "While the specific purpose of drugs is to restore health, these substances are typically inadequate for the task. In terms of the seesaw model, the weight applied to one end of the board by the drug has a tendency to push the board through the balance point and unbalance it in the other direction. At the same time, it is unbalancing other boards around the playground with unpredictable and sometimes devastating consequences."[1]

Unidirectional substances do not create or keep balance in any system over a long period of time; they are not useful when you are already balanced and want to stay that way. One of the common misuses of herbs is people taking, over an extended period, herbs that are useful for healing specific conditions but will not provide any long-term strengthening or balancing. Again, this is rarely harmful, but it can be wasteful.

The ability of a substance to both push and pull at the same time is very rare indeed, which is why the plants possessing this quality have been long prized by the cultures they come from. Tonics have been a mainstay of Chinese and Ayurvedic medicine for thousands of years.

We like tonic herbs because to us they represent the very essence of what herbs are about, first and foremost: prevention. Tonics are focused primarily on keeping you well (although many have secondary uses as medicines for already sick people). Thus natural medicine is the exclusive domain of tonic substances. Conventional medicine doesn't have substances that perform a tonic (preventive/building/enhancing) function, since it has historically been geared toward disease treatment, not health enhancement.

David Hoffmann, in *The Elements of Herbalism,* writes of tonics: "Western medicine has neglected such ideas as having no basis in fact. This is not so; rather it was a reflection of research procedures that could not recognize such complex and multifactorial processes." In addition, the tonic concept doesn't fit into the orthodox scientific criteria for what makes a drug valuable. Dr. Andrew Weil points out in *Spontaneous Healing* that most doctors only like substances with very narrow and targeted mechanisms of action; to our scientific model, a tonic's lack of specificity bespeaks the lack of an underlying mechanism. And that could mean, as Weil wryly puts it, "the drug could be—perish the thought!—merely a placebo."

In Eastern cultures, the tonics are the most valued medicines in the system. Since in natural healing it is considered superior to stimulate the host's defenses rather than attack external agents of disease, medicines that make people generally stronger are most prized. By contrast, the highly specific, unidirectional "magic bullets" that conventional doctors like so much are considered inferior in Ayurvedic and Chinese medicine.

Ron Teeguarden, in his book *Chinese Tonic Herbs,* notes that medicinal herbs in China "are known as the 'Inferior Drugs' or 'Poisons' which are used only to treat specific problems and cannot be used for a long period of time," while tonics are called "Superior Herbs" and are used to build and maintain health. Even when tonic herbs are used to treat disease states, "according to Oriental philosophy, the change is due to the life-promoting influences of these herbs, and not due to any properties attacking specific disease agents as they are known in the West," says Teeguarden.

It's important to note that only *whole herbs* act as tonics. Purified "active ingredients," even if they are extracted from tonic herbs, are unidirectional. It's the complementary actions of many different components that exerts the opposing push-pull. (See page 466 for a detailed discussion of purified extracts versus whole herbs.)

Tonic herbs are a great way to begin with herbal medicine, to try something new and see what it does for you. Tonics can be taken throughout life. We live in such a toxic and disease-filled world that it cannot hurt to use tonics to strengthen our "shields."

Of course, if you venture into herbal medicine by using tonics, you have to be prepared not to experience a necessarily dramatic result. One of the ironies of taking good care of yourself in this culture is what I call the "no-result" result. We are not accustomed to measuring our success by what *doesn't* happen. We want to see something take place, even if it means being very ill and getting heroically "cured." A shift in thinking is in order here: No news is good news. There are countless all-too-common health catastrophes whose absence in your life will confirm your success.

Your Best Tonics

Just as some herbs have affinity for particular organs, systems, or body processes and are best utilized for healing in those areas, many tonic herbs "specialize" in balancing a specific system or systems.

Because everyone has a limit for daily herb consumption in terms of time, convenience, tolerance, and money, it's not necessary to try to take four or five herbal tonics all the time and work on all body systems or processes at once. It wouldn't hurt you, but it's simply not practical. One or two at a time is sufficient. There are a couple of strategies you can employ when choosing which herbal tonics are best for you and beginning a program of tonic supplementation.

One way to choose your tonics is to think in terms of individual areas of weakness. If you have a family history of heart disease and did not adopt heart-healthy habits until recently, hawthorn berry or the Ayurvedic arjuna might be a good tonic for you. If you tend to have respiratory infections and are a former smoker, a lung-affinity tonic such as schizandra or mullein would be good. If a constant string of varying infections is your complaint, tonics that specifically increase cell-mediated immunity should be included.

If you can't think of a specific area that would help you counter individual disease tendencies, another way to approach tonic use is by rotation. Use one or two for six months, then switch to another one or two, so that every year you are nourishing and balancing two to four major systems.

Here are some tonics (either building or bidirectional) for specific areas or issues. Many of these will be discussed in more detail in the chapters to come, and preparations and dosages will be covered.

> **Immune**: Echinacea, astragalus, isatidis, licorice, pau d'arco, ginseng, ginger, pipali, garlic, guduchi
>
> **Cardio/Circulatory**: Cayenne, arjuna, hawthorn berry, bilberry, tienchi, turmeric, butcher's broom, guggul, garlic, ginger, ginkgo
>
> **Digestive**: Licorice, turmeric, schizandra, ginger, clove
>
> **Female**: Dong quai, chasteberry, black cohosh, red raspberry, shatavari, schizandra, wild yam, triphala
>
> **Male**: Ginseng, damiana, pygeum, muira puama, saw palmetto, ashwaganda, codonopsis, sarsaparilla, triphala
>
> **General Glandular**: Licorice, fo-ti root, lycium fruit, red date, tienchi, poria, cordyceps, saw palmetto, eleuthero
>
> **Nervous System**: Ashwaganda, gotu kola, scullcap leaf, eleuthero, ginseng, valerian, chamomile, hops, passion flower, lemon balm, peppermint
>
> **Urinary**: Buchu leaf, uva ursi, cornsilk, mullein
>
> **Liver**: Boldo leaf, bhumy amalaki, turmeric, baical scullcap
>
> **Respiratory**: Elecampane, mullein, schizandra
>
> **Skin**: Gotu kola, figwort root, Chinese violet leaf, turmeric
>
> **Musculoskeletal**: Turmeric, ginger, alfalfa

Noteworthy Tonics

Astragalus membranaceus

The root of astragalus, a traditional Chinese herb from the pea family, is an extremely versatile and powerful immune enhancer. Astragalus can be used as a long-term tonic as well as to assist healing and recovery in chronic illness or infection. It's a general energy booster (the Chinese call it a master *qi* replenisher, *qi* being a concept of Chinese medicine usually translated in the West as "life force" or "vital energy") and a marvelous guardian of the immune system, useful both to prevent illness and infection and to hasten its departure. It is an adaptogen, increasing our ability to adapt to stress.

Astragalus is especially antiviral (not in the sense that it actually kills viruses directly, which is virtually impossible to do, but because of the ways it boosts the body's own antiviral defenses). And although it is considered a "warm" herb by the Chinese, it does its work without increasing heat (as chilies do) by Ayurvedic standards. Therefore it is appropriate for use by fire types (*pitta*) or in *pitta* conditions. I think of astragalus as being at the helm of my own herbal immune-building and maintenance efforts. It's exceedingly mild, completely nontoxic, and easy to take.

Astragalus is sold in capsules and tinctures, but we prefer to use it the way it is used in Asia, to make a fresh broth or soup that can also have other tasty and healthy ingredients in it. (See the astragalus broth recipe on page 499.) Unlike many medicinal herbs, astragalus is actually fairly tasty and makes an excellent base for soups. If you don't think so, adding bouillon or broth base usually helps.

Dried, sliced astragalus root, which looks like rough yellow tongue depressors, can be purchased at most Asian grocery stores. We recommend checking a major Chinese grocery, perhaps in your city's international district if there is one, because the astragalus there will be much less expensive than at an herb pharmacy. The growing mainstream popularity of astragalus has driven the price up, so you should definitely shop around. My local herb pharmacy, which I trust for most of my herb needs, nevertheless charges eighty dollars per pound for dried astragalus, while the Chinese grocery where I purchase it charges eight dollars a pound! According to Karta Purkh, the differences in quality are negligible despite the exorbitant price spread, because they are of similar grades—both a medium quality. (Chinese herbs are graded: Low grade is cheap junk, medium grade is economical and acceptable quality, and high grade is for connoisseurs and frequently overpriced.)

The immune-building and adaptogenic effects of astragalus have been studied extensively. Modern research has isolated the constituents in astragalus that are believed to be responsible for its effectiveness. Two types of chemical compounds found in astragalus, polysaccharides and saponins, are credited with many of the herb's benefits. But traditional herbalists believe there may be dozens of other active, synergistic, or supportive components.

Astragalus heightens the efficiency of virtually every component of the immune system. Astragalus stimulates phagocytosis (invader-engulfing activity), increasing the total number of cells and the aggressiveness of their activity. Increased macrophage activity has been measured as lasting up to seventy-two hours. It increases the number of stem cells (the "generic" cells that can become any type needed) in the marrow and lymph tissue, stimulates their maturation into active immune cells, increases spleen activity, increases release of antibodies, and boosts the production of hormonal messenger molecules that signal for virus destruction.

Some research demonstrates that astragalus can make "resting" immune cells active, increase cell regeneration, and make healthy cells resistant to certain viruses. Astragalus root has also been demonstrated to increase the life span of human cells in culture, and an extract has been shown to reduce tumor cell growth in mice.

Saponins are antioxidant compounds, and a saponin in astragalus is reported to be especially protective of the liver. This is probably another reason this tonic is prized so highly by the Chinese, since traditional Chinese medicine emphasizes the importance of the liver in healing and recovery, especially during and after infection.

Astragalus is used as an antiviral to decrease the incidence of colds and shorten their course (which research shows it does, typically by half). It also has been tested not only for its general immune enhancement but also for its ability to mitigate the effects of more toxic therapies. Research shows that astragalus can reduce the side effects of steroid therapy and counteract the immunosuppressive effects of toxic cancer therapies such as chemotherapy and radiation.

Says Herb Research Foundation president Rob McCaleb in his paper "Boosting Immunity with Herbs," "Perhaps the best evidence to date for the powerful immunostimulant effects of astragalus come from the University of Texas Medical Center in Houston. There, scientists tested damaged immune system cells from cancer patients, compared against cells from the blood of normal human subjects. Astragalus extracts were able to completely restore the function of cancer patients' immune cells. In some cases, the compromised cells were stimulated to greater activity than those from normal human subjects. The study concluded, '[A] complete immune restoration can be achieved by using a fractionated extract of *Astragalus membranaceus*, a traditional Chinese medicinal herb found to possess immune restorative activity in vitro.' "[2]

Besides its champion immunostimulant qualities, the Chinese say astragalus also builds energy, reduces sweating, increases appetite, cools fever, and is a diuretic and digestive tonic.

In all of the research conducted with astragalus, no toxicity has been reported. It is as safe and mild as it is effective.

Echinacea (*angustifolia, purpurea,* other species)

Like astragalus, echinacea is one of the most researched herbs in the herbal kingdom and thus has been among the first herbs to be integrated into American mainstream medicine in some settings. And like astragalus, echinacea is a versatile herb that can both prevent infection with long-term use, and help your body heal acute infections on a short-term basis.

Echinacea is probably the single most well known herb among U.S. consumers now and is currently one of the five best-selling herbal medicines in the country. (It's also among the most popular herbs in other countries, especially in Europe, where much of the research supporting its efficacy has been conducted.)

Echinacea has the distinction of being near the top of the "favorite" list of nearly every health professional I interviewed. For example, at Dr. Ann McComb's Center for Optimal Health in Bellevue, Washington, echinacea (along with Vitamin C, and goldenseal if bacterial infection is involved) is a standard protocol for all upper-respiratory conditions. Few antibiotics or antihistamines are ever prescribed.

Echinacea's popularity has its good and bad points. It's an effective remedy with a range of documented immunostimulant effects, so if you're going to focus on a single herb, this certainly isn't a bad choice. People trying herbs for the first time are likely to have a good experience with echinacea.

On the other hand, we have observed a downside to echinacea's popularity: For those who really don't know much about herbs, it's all too easy for one herb to become a panacea, the be-all and end-all of herbal medicine. Echinacea seems to have become that herb. "Take some echinacea!" has become a sort of generic battle cry.

Echinacea is not synonymous with herbal medicine. It's a wonderful herb, but it's just that: one herb. And it's a good antimicrobial and decent anti-inflammatory and wound healer, but if you start "prescribing" it, to yourself or others, for relief of muscle pain, headache, laryngitis, or nausea, you're going to be disappointed. We have seen this happen too many times to count.

Unlike many of the popular tonics discussed in this section, which are Chinese or Ayurvedic in origin, echinacea is homegrown. The plant is the purple coneflower, a popular garden flower that's especially common in the Northwest and Midwest. It was used by Native Americans to treat a wide assortment of infections and inflammations, including coughs, colds, sore throats, and wounds. Introduced to Western medicine in the late 1800s, it enjoyed extraordinary popularity as a medicine in North America through the early 1900s, dispensed by pharmacies as a tincture.

By the 1930s, with the discovery of penicillin and other pharmaceutical antibiotics, echinacea had fallen from favor along with other botanical medicines, swept aside in the stampede toward more technologically oriented medicine. By the 1950s the herb had virtually disappeared from consciousness in the United States.

Meanwhile, echinacea use continued to thrive in Europe, particularly in Germany, where echinacea is frequently prescribed by medical doctors (over 180 government-approved botanical formulas in Germany contain echinacea). Research continued in these countries, with Germany leading the way. When interest in natural medicine was revived in the 1970s and 1980s, echinacea was at the head of the pack as botanical medicines were reintroduced to the American public. Now that it's back to best-seller status in the United States, one echinacea species, *Echinacea angustifolia,* is alarmingly close to extinction in the wild and is harder to cultivate than other species.

The healing part of echinacea is the root. It is usually used in tincture form or in capsules, after being powdered or cut, since the dried herb tastes—well, like dirt (my dog will eat it as long as it's mixed in yogurt, but then she eats dirt, too). It can be used for acute infection, chronic infection and inflammation, wound healing, and as a preventive agent. It is an excellent general promoter of healing. Externally, echinacea is used as an antimicrobial and again to promote wound healing.

Despite an extremely pervasive myth to the contrary, echinacea does not lose its effectiveness when taken for a long period of time (this belief was spurred by the misinterpretation of a German study). It can be used as a tonic. The different types of enhanced immune activity shown in echinacea research also suggest valuable long-term effects that may potentially keep cancer as well as infection at bay.

From the scientific point of view, echinacea has earned its popularity. About 400 studies of echinacea have revealed a battery of different immune payoffs. Several active constituents, including polysaccharides and polyphenols, activate or enhance both the quantity and activity of various immune-system components. All the active compounds appear to be antimicrobial and immunostimulant, but the polysaccharides have been the most intensively studied.

Echinacea significantly increases the rate at which phagocytes are created. (Remember, phagocytes eventually yield important cells like macrophages, the large white blood cells that detect foreigners, alert the system, engulf invaders, and help filter and clean up lymph wastes.) Echinacea's polysaccharides also stimulate phagocytosis. This invader-engulfing process is consistently shown in studies to increase by 20 to 40 percent with use of echinacea.[3]

Echinacea also increases white blood cell count—the total number of cells as well as the vigorousness of their activity—and production of interferon and tumor necrosis factor. Echinacea also inhibits the action of hyaluronidase, a bacterial enzyme that punches holes in cells to make way for microbial entry. By binding with the protective hyaluronic acid in our cells, echinacea polysaccharides prevent this important protective acid, and subsequently our cells, from being destroyed by bacteria or viruses. If invaders are denied access to cells, the illness is effectively slowed or stopped from spreading.

Finally, echinacea polysaccharides can increase the activity of natural killer cells, the "freelance" cells that can attack independently of signals from other cells and suppress virus and cancer; and boost levels of neutrophils, the free-roaming white blood cells that attack invaders upon the command of macrophages.

Echinacea polysaccharides are also anti-inflammatory, fungicidal, and accelerate tissue repair and new growth. Echinacea increases fibroblasts, cells which play a role in connective tissue development and thus support new tissue regeneration.

Happily, echinacea has one of the best safety records of any herb, with no cases of toxicity or side effects reported over several hundred years of use. Allergic reactions have been reported, but they are extremely rare and usually mild.

Triphala

Triphala is the most revered general tonic in Ayurveda. Herbalists in Asia may suggest it for literally, every single client. This combination formula is a superb, slow-acting tonic that can be taken from infancy through old age. It is one of the few remedies that can be used to treat all doshas, at all times, and contains all six tastes in balanced proportions.

Translated from Sanskrit as "three fruits," triphala contains the dried powders of amlaki (or amla), bibitaki, and haritaki. Triphala is very high in vitamin C because of the inclusion of amla in the formula (amla is discussed a little later in this chapter). The other two fruits are about the size of a fig, and are sour or bitter and medicinal tasting.

Individually, the herbs in triphala distinguish themselves as follows:

Amla is anti-*pitta*, a nutritive tonic, laxative, aphrodisiac, and hemorrhoid remedy.

Haritaki is a strong astringent, known as "King of Medicines" in Tibet. It is laxative, and is especially good for respiratory conditions (cough, asthma), prolapse of anything, mouth ulcers, heart, liver, skin, and detoxification.

Bibitaki is anti-*kapha*, an astringent tonic; it's good for the respiratory system; treats cough, voice and throat problems; dissolves stones.

Triphala benefits every system and organ of the body, but particularly the skin, liver, and eyes, as well as digestion and the respiratory system. It is a light laxative. It is also good for the cardiovascular system, glandular systems, sinuses, the immune system, and more. You can take 2 capsules a day, every day, on a regular basis throughout your life. In India it is taken as a powder; in America it is capsuled.

Turmeric Root (*Curcuma longa*)

That yellow powder from South Asia that we know as a curry ingredient is powerful medicine, including preventive medicine. Turmeric is active against many types of bacteria, and is antifungal and antiparasitic. It is also a blood cleanser (a concept we will explain later in the book) and a potent antioxidant.[4]

While known to be generally immune supportive, turmeric has been shown to be a potent inhibitor of HIV. A recent study at Harvard Medical School comparing curcumin (turmeric's active ingredient) with chemotherapy drugs demonstrated that it was effective as an inhibitor of HIV replication.[5] Studies also show that, like other antioxidant foods, turmeric reduces the formation of cancers. It inhibits the disease at all stages—initiation, promotion, and progression. In smokers, turmeric given at 1.5 grams per day for 30 days substantially reduced the formation of mutagenic (cancer-causing) chemicals.[6] It is estimated that 500 milligrams (less than 1/2 teaspoon) of turmeric per day in the diet could eliminate

DNA damage characteristic of the development of cancer.[7] Another recent study reported a 68 percent reduction of cancer in animals following treatment with curcumin.[8]

Turmeric has wide applications throughout herbal medicine, including as a tonic or treatment for joints, skin, digestion, and the liver. These are discussed in more detail where we cover those subjects.

Ginseng

Asian ginseng is another tonic herb, very popular and probably the most Westernized—at least, the most familiar—of Chinese herbs. The ethnic (Chinese) name for this herb, *jen shen*, means "man root"—possibly because it is a highly regarded male tonic or because the root's "branches" can resemble the arms and legs of a human figure. The root is not harvested until it is at least two years old; as the root ages, its value increases.

Classified as sweet and warming by the Chinese, ginseng is used as a general energizer and (as the Chinese call it) *qi* replenisher. Like most tonics and adaptogens, though, it has other uses. It has an affinity for lungs and digestive system and an ability to help the body adapt to stress, shock, inflammation, and trauma.

The Chinese value ginseng for the way it affects the flow of energy, the life force, in the body, in ways that are difficult to describe without entering into a discourse on Chinese medicine. Still, ginseng is valued by many other cultures for increasing stamina, endurance, sexual performance, and mental concentration. Research does back those claims.

Ginseng is among the most widely researched herbs, the subject of about 3,000 scientific studies in the past 50 years. Chief constituents of ginseng include polysaccharides and saponins. Ginseng's saponins are called ginsenosides, and dozens of them have been shown to aid the body's adaptation to stress; enhance clarity, alertness, and concentration; regulate blood sugar and blood pressure; decrease anxiety; and reduce inflammation, among other things.

The most well known of the ginsengs is *Panax* ginseng (*panax* means "panacea"). This includes Chinese and Korean red ginseng (the "red" being the result of a special processing it undergoes in Asia). Korean ginseng is considered to be hotter in energy.

Asian ginseng is imported into the United States. There is an American ginseng variety (*Panax quinquefolius*, grown in the upper Midwest and

Appalachia), which unlike the Asian varieties is classified as a cooling herb and is adaptogenic without the sexual tonic effects. Most American ginseng is exported to Asia.

A relatively recent discovery by scientists is *Panax vietnamensis*, a species of ginseng used throughout Vietnam as a tonic. Studies have revealed many of the same chemical constituents found in other species of Panax, plus two components unknown to other ginsengs and one that is found in a member of the gourd family.[9] It has also been found to be strongly antibacterial, specifically against streptococcus.

Eleuthero (*Eleutherococcus senticosus*)

Eleuthero is frequently called Siberian ginseng, but actually is not in the ginseng family. It is, however, ginseng-like in action—a very good stamina-building and immune-enhancing tonic herb. In addition, it is appropriate for both men and women to use on an ongoing basis. Although some women may benefit from Asian ginseng when specifically indicated by individual conditions (as determined by a natural health practitioner), Asian ginseng is considered to be primarily a male tonic in the same way that dong quai (see below) is primarily a female tonic. Eleuthero is milder and less stimulating.

In addition to stimulating the immune system and increasing endurance, eleuthero may also protect the liver and lower blood pressure and triglyceride (blood fat) levels.

Dong quai (*Angelica sinensis*)

Dong quai is a universal Chinese herb that has benefits for both men and women, though it is used widely as a reproductive system tonic for women. In fact, it is considered the quintessential herb for women, kind of the female "master herb" used throughout Eastern cultures. It's recommended in those cultures as a tonic for use throughout a woman's life, although in America it is often used to treat symptoms, particularly those relating to PMS and menopause.

Dong quai is mildly warming and, although bitter, still tastier than many of the medicinal herbs, so it makes an okay tea or broth. It's a member of the umbellifer, or carrot, family. It also can be found in capsules and tinctures.

Dong quai regulates the menstrual cycle and does relieve a wide variety of menstrual and menopausal complaints. It is an antispasmodic and appears to be effective in cases with low estrogen levels. To deal with menopausal symptoms, dong quai is traditionally used for an estrogen-like effect. (See Chapter 8, "Especially for Women: Natural Healing for a Woman's Lifetime," for more on this.) It increases pelvic circulation (and circulation generally) and reduces abdominal pain. Dong quai is also reputed to lower blood pressure, improve digestion, purify the blood, and treat anemia and tinnitus.

Angelica sinensis is not to be confused with the European angelica (*Angelica archangelica*), which has some of the same benefits as the Chinese variety but is more of a stimulant. Chinese angelica is an antispasmodic (one reason it is effective for menstrual cramps, and for stomach cramps as well) but the Western variety is not. Dong quai should not be used during pregnancy.

Licorice root (*Glycyrrhiza glabra, Glycyrrhiza uralensis*)

Licorice root is an extremely useful herb that enjoys a fair amount of Western popularity now, in addition to its prominence in Chinese herbal medicine. It's also another good-tasting herb, which makes it appealing. It makes a good tea (although if it's medicinal strength, it's probably not going to be your favorite beverage because it's outrageously sweet—many times more so than sugar).

Chinese herbalists value licorice as a base for multiple-herb formulas; it's said to help focus the purpose and direction of other herbs as well as mitigate the harsh, bitter, or stimulating properties of other herbs. It's not as warming as many of the other Chinese tonics, so it provides balance. According to Ron Teeguarden in *Chinese Tonic Herbs*, the Chinese variety (*uralensis*) is more calming than the stimulating *Glycyrrhiza glabra*, and thus less likely to cause the rare potential blood pressure increases reportedly caused by large amounts of *glabra*. It's the most commonly used herb in China (poria is second). Children there even chew the root as "candy."

Licorice is a powerful and diverse tonic in its own right. Conditions of adrenal insufficiency are treated well with licorice; it contains compounds that resemble the adrenal cortical hormones. It's an immune activity enhancer and liver detoxifier. It has reproductive-enhancing and -healing properties, is a lung tonic, good for digestion, and is an energizer despite being "cooler" than herbs like ginseng or dong quai. It reduces muscle spasms (especially in the legs and abdomen), cools accumulated heat and inflammation, and has a laxative effect.

Licorice can be used for sore throat, dry throat, or laryngitis (I have found it helpful to swallow licorice powder moistened with honey when my throat is tired from singing). It moistens the lungs and liquefies mucus to relieve dry cough. It makes a soothing cold and flu remedy. Because it is an adrenal builder and lung tonic, it's a perfect asthma remedy.

Studies of licorice have revealed many components believed to be responsible for its wide spectrum of action, especially its immunostimulant properties. These compounds include glycyrrhizin, glycyrrhetinic acid, phenols, triterpenoids, and saponins. Glycyrrhizin can inhibit growth of human viruses and bacteria; glycyrrhetinic acid and glycyrretic acid can do the same and are also anti-inflammatory. The saponins can increase antibody production and interferon production. Animal studies show licorice may prevent breast cancer by triggering liver enzymes that reduce tumor-promoting estrogens.

For women, licorice is progesteronic, which means it supports and regulates progesterone production; thus it is useful for menstrual irregularities related to low activity in the progesterone phase of the cycle.

Licorice root is discussed further in Chapter 11, "Energizing Herbs"; Chapter 22, "Herbs for Digestion"; and Chapter 24, "Urban Myths and Sidewalk Talk."

Other Chinese Tonic Herbs

There are some other tonic herbs from Chinese medicine that are not as common or popular, but are worth knowing about. Many of these, along with astragalus, are becoming respected for their immune-restorative effects with cancer and AIDS patients:

Ligusticum (*Ligusticum lucidum*) is considered to be synergistic with astragalus and to contain some of the same properties. They are often used together. For example, many of the experiments on immune restoration in cancer patients (or cancer cells) have paired the two. Ligusticum alone may inhibit tumor growth. It is also being studied as an AIDS treatment. This bitter and pungent herb is considered in China to be a liver tonic and blood cleanser as well as a circulatory enhancer.

Schizandra (*Schisandra chinensis*, called Wu Wei Tze in China, which means "Five Flavors Herb") is a superb general tonic for men or women.

With all of the five flavors identified in Chinese herbalism, its energetics are extremely balanced. But it's especially helpful as a women's tonic and hormone balancer, almost a "junior dong quai," as well as a superior general lung tonic and cold, sore throat, and flu soother. It's used to treat acute cough and wheezing.

Schizandra is also used for other diverse purposes. It improves digestion, reduces fatigue, increases sexual energy, and relieves insomnia and forgetfulness. It's an adaptogen and is said to calm the spirit.

In the Chinese philosophy organized around *qi*, schizandra's unique function is to stop *qi* from "leaking" out of various organs or energy meridians. Thus it is used to hold back secretions (stops nocturnal emissions, frequent urination, vaginal discharge, night sweats, diarrhea, and so on).

Fo-ti (*Polygonum multiflorum*, called Ho Shou Wu in China, also known as fo-ti root here) is renowned in China for contributing to longevity, energy, and sexual vitality. It's also used for its anti-inflammatory, anti-tumor, detoxification, and sedative abilities. The root is the medicinal part and may be made into a tea or a tincture. We discuss this herb relative to specific health conditions later in the book.

Codonopsis (*Codonopsitis lanceolate*, called Tang Shen in China) has been compared to ginseng in its activity, but is milder and cooler and so may be useful for cases where the body doesn't need a warming agent. It tonifies digestion and treats diarrhea, reduces stress, stimulates appetite, eases muscle tension, increases energy, and stimulates blood production. Like some of the Chinese tonics described earlier, it enhances immunity by stimulating phagocytosis.

Poria (*Poria cocos*, called Fu Ling in China) is the second-most-used herb in China, both as an herb and a food. It's actually a fungus and is often used as a balancing agent as part of other *qi* tonics, to be sure that their warming, energizing effects don't send the body too far in that direction. This would especially be of concern to fire types. Poria cools and acts as a diuretic, treats edema; reduces stagnation of fluids, including excess phlegm; is tranquilizing (treats insomnia and heart palpitations); increases appetite and regulates blood sugar.

Poria grows in North America and was used by Native Americans and early settlers as a survival food. It grows underground and is nutritive.

Atractylus (*Atractylodis ovata*) is yet another sweet, warming herb that is considered a general body tonic but acts especially as an excellent digestive tonic, and can also be used to boost the immune system. It has also shown an ability to augment muscle strength.

Tienchi (*Panax pseudoginseng*), still another "ginseng-like" root, is used in China to improve circulation and calm nerves. It is also considered a blood builder. Research has shown that raw tienchi contains saponins and flavonoids that provide raw materials for synthesis of adrenal and reproductive hormones, and promote nonspecific immunity. It also has a variety of tonic effects on the heart (which we discuss in more detail later). It is a top-notch antibleeding herb, reduces swelling from traumatic injuries, and circulates blood to joints to relieve pain.

The Chinese use these and other tonic herbs in food, as part of their daily diets. Soups are common ways to get the benefits of Chinese herbs while enjoying a tasty meal. Astragalus, due to its warm, sweet, yellow color and flavor—its almost chicken-soup-like and buttery qualities—is a classic soup broth base to try, but dong quai, schizandra, and ligusticum can also be used this way. Ginseng, licorice, and others may be added to soups and stews, or grains can be cooked in their broth. A spoonful of soup helps the medicine go down. Your family may not even notice it's medicine.

Foods/Spices

All of these have general immune-increasing function, even when they are specified as good for particular conditions. For the care and feeding of your immune system, include as many of these foods as you can in your diet, as often as possible.

Garlic, onion, and **ginger** are the basis of all healing food recipes in Ayurveda (except for extreme *pitta* conditions or fire-type people). The three have been dubbed the "trinity roots" by Ayurvedic healing master Yogi Bhajan. All are immune supportive as well as warming. (In fact, these roots affect virtually every body tissue. They're tonics for the hormone-producing endocrine glands, which increase stamina, vigor, alertness, and sexual performance. They also reduce blood pressure and cholesterol and increase circulatory health. They enhance digestion and strengthen the joints.)

Garlic is one of the most widely used natural health products in the world and one of the most researched therapeutic herbs, with hundreds of studies showing one benefit after another. Garlic supplements are a top-selling OTC remedy in Germany, where the government approves its cardiovascular health claims, and it's also a top-selling dietary supplement in the United States.

Garlic is antimicrobial; it poisons bacteria (Louis Pasteur discovered that garlic could kill bacteria in 1895). It's also good for killing systemic yeast. It's been the subject of intensive study for its possible effects against heart disease and cancer. It increases general immune system activity. Studies have shown garlic to be effective in treating AIDS. It lowers blood pressure and cholesterol. It has an affinity for the ear, and garlic oil is excellent to treat ear infections in children. It's a general glandular tonic, increases libido and sexual function, enhances digestion, and is warming. Clearly, for most people, the more garlic the better.

Have a problem with the smell of garlic? You can use deodorized garlic tablets or capsules. Kyolic is the original Japanese product; there are a number of other brands now. Many people have also found that garlic doesn't smell as bad if your body is not toxic; several natural medicine practitioners have observed that people who smoke and eat red meat especially seem to have this odor problem. If you are "clean," it just smells like—garlic. And garlic actually smells tasty to a lot of people.

In natural healing it's generally believed that the smell is based on what your body is doing with the garlic. If the body processes it adequately, burning it up rapidly in the digestive tract, it gets out through the intestines and the smell is negligible. Many people are not doing very well digestively, so it comes out through the skin. If a little bit of garlic creates a strong smell, you may need some work on your digestion.

Onions include green onions as well as red, yellow, and white. Chives and shallots are separate "alliums," not onions. They all act pretty much the same, though the greens are a little sweeter and less "hot" in energy than the white and yellow. Onions have a particular affinity for the lung. They are milder than garlic, but offer many of the same benefits. They have not been studied as intensively as garlic, but they have traditionally and clinically been observed to produce many of the same results that garlic does, particularly as a warming, antibacterial, and antiviral and immunostimulant remedy.

Ginger is another valuable kitchen herb that is very trendy in scientific circles now; it's being scientifically verified as anti-inflammatory, a use for which Asian medicine has revered it for thousands of years. It's a classic rejuvenator for joints and increases circulation particularly to joints. It's good for digestion too, and beats just about anything for the relief of nausea (a couple of capsules does the trick for most people). It's also a good staple in any antiyeast program. It's warming, immunostimulant, anti-inflammatory and good for colds, congestion, and coughs.

Most people find the taste of ginger pleasant, though more pungent and stronger than most of us are used to. It can be used as tea (you don't need to peel it—just slice it up and simmer a few pieces the size of a quarter in hot water for about twenty minutes), juiced into fruit or vegetable juices, steamed or sautéed, diced or grated into stew, rice, soups, and broths. The fresh powder can be capsuled for maximum convenience. Powder can be used to make tea as well (I add ginger powder to chamomile tea as an after-dinner beverage that's warming, pleasantly calming, and a digestive tonic).

When buying powder, beware of old ginger that has been spoiled by exposure to air, heat, and light. It won't hurt you, but it probably won't help much either. It's best to get ginger powder from an herb pharmacy or health-food store specializing in herbal medicine, one that turns enough volume so you know the herbs are fresh. Ginger should be a little oily; some of its active components are oils, which give the herb its pungent taste. Oily ginger will "clump" when pinched between the fingers. Powdered ginger should not look or feel like gray dust.

Research has recently focused on isolating the compounds responsible for ginger's medicinal effects; those identified include gingerols and shogaols. However, it's unlikely that pills made out of these compounds will be pursued for synthesis and marketing, because ginger powder from the spice aisle of the grocery store for thirty-five cents an ounce is so effective.

The trinity roots are synergistic—as a threesome they provide more powerful immune support than each does on its own. For this reason you might want to add a little of all three to an herbal tea or broth.

The trinity roots are not good for children, because garlic and onion are sexual stimulants and ginger is extremely pungent. They are fine to use from puberty on.

Chilies include cayenne, red peppers, jalapeño, habanero, and other hot varieties. They have actions similar to those of the trinity roots. In addition, they are exceptionally antiviral—the best broad-spectrum, widely available, well-tolerated antiviral around. Jalapeños appear to be particularly antiviral for some reason.

In all chilies, the active ingredient is the hot stuff—the much-studied capsaicin. Their ability to warm us is probably key to their antiviral activity. Viruses have evolved to infect us at a certain temperature. Thus there is a significant increase in immune function for every degree of body temperature increase. (Your body has its own mechanism to produce this warmth that is so inhospitable to viruses. It is called a fever.)

You can treat a cold very effectively with nothing but chilies if you can get enough down. In our culture, we eat a relatively bland diet, using the fewest spices and medicinal herbs of just about any culture around the world. Therefore, most of us haven't built up a tolerance that allows us to accommodate medicinal amounts when necessary. Chilies are a regular staple in most other cultures' cuisine; for example, the four-star rating system for "hot" food in American Thai restaurants is actually the bottom of a ten-star system in Thailand.

If you get your body used to eating hot foods day to day, you will be able to use enough to fight virus effectively when the time comes (if it comes). Most of us eat so little of these kinds of warming foods that we don't need to worry about a "too-warming" effect. For most people, chilies will provide a warming and immune-supportive effect; it's rare to find someone "abusing" warming substances.

Stomach upset can occur if you take way too many chilies too fast. If they burn when they're being excreted, your body is not producing enough of the digestive substances (mainly enzymes) it needs to break down those compounds before they come through. Unless you are very *pitta*, you should be able to eat unlimited quantities and not experience much discomfort, if any at all, once your body's used to it.

Cayenne pepper is high in capsaicin. Cayenne pepper also contains cartenoids, flavonoids, and vitamin C, and is antiseptic. You can take it in capsule form, which means you won't have to taste it and thus are more likely to be able to get enough in your body to treat the viral infection.

Root vegetables include beets, carrots, and radishes. They can be juiced or eaten raw or cooked; generally, the less cooking, the better. Root vegetables have an affinity for the liver and are especially detoxifying. (They are discussed more fully in Chapter 14, "Herbal Renewal: Cleanse, Detox, Rebuild," pages 325–340.)

The liver is under stress when you are fighting an infection, especially a viral infection. In Western medicine, this is often ignored; almost no one thinks of the liver when you have a cold or flu. You're concerned with your headache, your stuffy nose, your sore throat, or your body aches, and conventional remedies for these infections are made to mask those symptoms. There are no conventional remedies to support your body in the cleanup and rebuilding after the "fight."

Eastern healing systems have always recognized the need to support the liver in the aftermath of an infection and include some sort of liver tonic in treatment of infection. Interestingly, nature seems to have the same idea in mind; many immune-supportive herbs are, conveniently, also effective for liver support, protection, and building. For example, Chinese medicine has licorice root and baical scullcap root, and Ayurveda uses turmeric, bayberry root, bhumy amalaki, guduchi, and kutki.

Tubers—potatoes of all kinds, including yams and sweet potatoes—are a great energy source. They provide nutrient-rich complex carbohydrates and help avoid problems with grain metabolism. (Americans overconsume wheat and often develop allergies to it; although we should theoretically be able to digest whole grains well, we typically eat so many processed grains that the body is overstimulated and overreacts. Tubers provide a great complex carb alternative for the allergic.)

Cruciferous veggies are a huge family that includes cabbage, broccoli, kale, and Brussels sprouts. They are currently being regaled by much of the scientific community for their antioxidant sulfur-containing compounds—sulforaphanes—which appear to boost production of anticancer enzymes and detoxify foreign substances, including carcinogens. Sulfur has been prized since antiquity as preventive medicine—something that mainstream cancer organizations and antioxidant research now support.

In addition to sulforaphanes, other sulfur-containing phytochemicals include allyl sulfides (found in the allium family, including garlic and onions), thiols (garlic and crucifers), and isothiocyanites (watercress and crucifers).

For the immune system, these vegetables are also mildly antibacterial generally, and contain assorted immune-supportive and antioxidant vitamins and minerals.

Cabbage is also great for ulcers—a tall glass of juice each day reduces pain. An enzyme sometimes called vitamin U may be responsible for its ability to repair mucous membranes and/or help fight the bacterium now believed to be a factor in at least some ulcers. (See page 431 for more on ulcers.)

Yellow and orange vegetables such as carrots and yellow squash contain *carotenes,* the vegetable cousins of vitamin A. The body turns carotenes into vitamin A, but the carotenes themselves provide a different antioxidant effect than vitamin A. Beta-carotene, which is probably the most commonly talked-about carotenoid, is just one kind. There are many kinds of carotenoids, such as lycopene, lutein, and zeaxanthin, which are also considered to be antioxidants. A high food intake of beta-carotene appears to stimulate T-helper-cell activity to arrest cancer-cell development, especially in lung and colon cancer, and people with a high intake of food sources of beta-carotene have lower cancer rates, although research on synthetic beta-carotene supplements for cancer prevention has produced mixed results.

Ajwain seed is a member of the huge family known as umbellifer (carrot/parsley family). The carrot is the root; celery is a stalk. Leaves and seeds are also used. This seed is crescent-shaped (like dill or fennel, also from this family). The taste is like that of caraway, but stronger. The seeds are a staple in India—Indian restaurants usually serve a mound of rice with ajwain seed. The seeds are immune building and antiviral. In the recipe section of this book, you'll find a recipe for "immune pancakes" made with ajwain seed, onion, garlic, and chilies.

Mushrooms from Japan—specifically, shiitake as a food, and reishi and maitake (which are currently available in the United States only as extracts)—offer a host of immune-system benefits.

Shiitake mushrooms have been shown through research to have impressive immunostimulant properties. Their polysaccharide, lentinan, appears to be the immune booster (like many polysaccharide compounds, although lentinans have an unusual shape that may be significant to their effectiveness).

While research is usually conducted using an extract of the root, it certainly can't hurt to include the whole vegetable regularly in your diet. Shiitake mushrooms are dark, meaty, and flavorful. I use them in soups and stir-fries (they used to be imported from Asia but are now grown in the United States) as a "multitasking" way to boost my immunity and enhance a good meal at the same time. Shiitake can also be taken as powder or in tablets or capsules.

Shiitake mobilizes the immune forces in ways that help us fight viruses, bacteria, cancer, and even parasites. Research shows that lentinan stimulates T-cell production and aggressiveness, and anti-tumor activity (by increasing interferon production). It's also anti-aging and may lower blood cholesterol levels.

Maitake appears to be effective against AIDS and cancer, and reishi against arthritis. All of these mushrooms appear to be liver protective (especially useful in a program to heal hepatitis B) and also to offer cardiovascular benefits.

Juice

Juice is a good way to consume many of the healing foods listed in this section, especially if you might find it difficult to "fit" that much food into your diet (or your body) every day. You don't need to go to extremes: We *don't* recommend you live on juice, except for a very short period once in a very great while, if you or your natural health practitioner feel that such a "juice fast" helps you.

In general, you need the fiber that comes from whole food, not to mention the experience of eating. Whole foods are important. But after you have consumed as much whole food as you are going to get down, juice allows you to concentrate the nutrients available in these foods in an easy-to-consume form.

Fatty Acids

In *BodyFueling*® I offered a basic overview of how, when, and why fat is—and is not—made, stored, conserved, or used as fuel. This is important for understanding how to eat to stay lean. I also tried to present a big-picture view so that you would understand that all fats are not inherently evil—it's their misuse and abuse that leads to disease. I have tried to curb the tide of fat phobia that has many people thinking a low-fat diet is the single magic bullet to heal all ills; that low-fat means no-fat; that cutting fat, by itself, leads to instant leanness; and that fat-free products are always better. (None of this is true.) Now it's time to learn a few new things about fats.

All fats are not created equal. Saturated fats, primarily animal fats consumed in excess, have been implicated in the cause and progression of countless diseases. They should be minimized in the diet.

Among unsaturated fats—plant or vegetable fats—there are a number of further distinctions. Some plant fats are better for us than others. Some can actually be as harmful as animal fats, or more so, though in different ways and for different reasons. Others have proven not only to be harmless, but are actually helpful in preventing or treating disease. *The source and form of a fat determines its ability to heal or hurt us.*

What this means is that a diet moderately low in fat (not compulsively, retentively approaching fat free) is healthiest, and that the fats we do eat should be chosen carefully, to provide optimum healing power and to avoid harm. By no means is it ever helpful to be overfat or obese, or to get half of all your calories (fuel from food) from fat. This is not a suggestion to gulp massive amounts of fat. It is a suggestion, based on research to date, that neither a 5 percent fat diet nor a 55 percent fat diet is healthiest—and that there's more to it than number of fat grams.

The new distinction here is that a diet whose calories are comprised of 20 percent harmful fats is *less* healthy than one comprised of 30 percent "helpful fats." The total percentage of fat calories does count for leanness (which is also important to health), but the type of fat can make the difference between health and disease, too.

In addition to providing fuel (either burned immediately for energy or stored, depending on circumstances) for the body to run, fats are also involved in the synthesis of hormone-like messenger substances that include prostaglandins and leukotrienes. The manufacture of these messenger molecules requires fatty acids. Fatty acids are the major building blocks of fats, similar to the way amino acids are the building blocks of proteins.

At one time there was believed to be only a single prostaglandin. In the 1930s, a Swedish scientist discovered a substance in the prostate gland not identified before, and named it "prostaglandin." Now about forty prostaglandins have been discovered to play a role in every body cell, dictating a whole range of system responses. There may be hundreds more as yet undiscovered. These substances regulate virtually all body processes, both harmful and necessary ones.

Leukotrienes have a purpose, too—they signal white blood cells to accumulate in an infected area. But protracted oversecretion of them spells inflammation, immune suppression, and oversensitivity.

Herein lies some of the power of "good" and "bad" fats: Certain types of fatty acids create prostaglandins and leukotrienes that do good things for us (or at least are benign), and other types of fatty acids go to build prostaglandins and leukotrienes that signal for inflammation, cell damage, or other destructive processes. The ratio of helpful prostaglandins to destructive ones at a given time has great bearing on your overall health.

Essential Fatty Acids

Essential fatty acids (EFAs)—linoleic acid (LA) and alpha-linolenic acid (ALA)—are used to synthesize cell membranes and make prostaglandins, the hormone-like messenger substances that regulate body functions. They are also involved in many other important body functions.

We need to consume LA and ALA, in food or supplements, because our bodies cannot manufacture them. When you consume LA, the body converts it to gamma linolenic acid (GLA), the form it takes before conversion to prostaglandins. GLA is found in no food other than human milk. Without GLA, we can't make prostaglandins.

Various factors such as too much alcohol, saturated fat, cholesterol, sugar, or processed oils may block the LA-to-GLA pathways. So can diabetes, cancer, infections, and deficiencies of zinc, magnesium, niacin, B_6, or vitamin C. In such cases, supplements containing already formed GLA—such as borage oil, evening primrose oil, and black currant oil—may be used. (Borage oil contains three times as much GLA as evening primrose oil. Evening primrose oil has been studied extensively, however.) GLA oils have been shown to give relief from PMS, arthritis, and eczema, as well as to lower blood pressure and cholesterol levels.

Flaxseed oil contains some LA and is also nature's richest source of ALA. Hemp oil contains both LA and ALA, and is considered to have the most balanced proportion of the two.

LA is an omega-6 fatty acid and ALA is an omega-3 fatty acid. Our bodies need both of these types of fatty acids—but from healthy sources and in the right proportions. Let's look at what that means.

Omega-6 Fatty Acids

Fatty acids in meat and polyunsaturated vegetable oils such as corn, safflower, and sunflower oil are omega-6 acids. Omega-6 fatty acids include arachidonic acid, an inflammatory substance that has been blamed for a wide range of sickness-producing reactions, including the joint damage found in several forms of arthritis and allergic or asthmatic reactions. These fatty acids end up as damaging prostaglandins and leukotrienes that give cells instructions that lead to damage and disease. The more of these overactive messengers you have running around giving orders, the more breakdown and illness you are likely to have.

Our bodies need some omega-6 fatty acids, such as from LA. But polyunsaturated oils are easily damaged, and damaged oils make damaged cells. Although polyunsaturated oils were once heralded as a healthful choice, it is now recommended that you avoid corn, safflower, and sunflower oil, especially for cooking, frying, and baking and in food products that are fried or baked. (*High-oleic* safflower or sunflower oil, which is specially processed and now showing up in some healthy, alternative snack products, is acceptable.)

"Trans" Fats

Hydrogenated and partially hydrogenated cooking oils and margarines (which are not only sold by themselves but can be found among the ingredients of a vast array of packaged foods) are purified with strong chemical processing that not only taints the product but removes nutrients. Even more important, they are exposed to extremely high temperatures that twist the fatty-acid molecules. This processing changes their shape from a *cis* configuration to what's called a *trans* form.

The rise in cancers and other illnesses has been attributed in part to Americans' increased use of these highly processed, "deformed" fats. This is logical, since the fat we eat is what our cells become. Since fats are used as materials to build cell membranes, it makes sense that misshapen, twisted fatty-acid molecules will create messed-up cells. "Good" fats with the correct structure fit into the membranes properly. But "bad" fats with their irregular shape fit into cell membranes like a broken key. The unnatural fatty acid disrupts the cell's functioning, locks out the natural-form fatty acids that are actually needed there,[10] and leaves a defective problem cell. Further, trans fats block the conversion of LA to one of the helpful prostaglandins.[11]

This is also the probable reason for the "mystery" of why even those countries consuming a diet relatively high in saturated fats don't have the same high rates of cardiovascular disease and cancer that we do. Even Americans at the turn of the century did not experience our current levels of these illnesses. The answer appears to lie in the way our food processing practices have changed over the last 100 years. Omega-3 fat intake has plummeted—as these fatty acids are lost or damaged through processing—while omega-6 fat intake has stayed the same or increased. It seems that people who eat a fair amount of saturated fat, but who consume enough "good fats" and don't use damaged fat (trans fat and altered polyunsaturated oils), can keep their good prostaglandins outrunning the bad ones.

This doesn't mean saturated fats are optimally healthy and it doesn't mean you should put the unlimited green light on saturated fats. (It's still healthiest to be lean and to keep total fat intake moderately low—and saturated fats trigger less-than-ideal reactions of their own.) But it does lend some proportion to the picture.

All of this has led to what the public perceives as a major flip-flop on the part of health authorities: While once margarine and other hydrogenated fats were touted as being healthier substitutes for saturated-fat spreads such as butter, trans fats are now being revealed for the dangers that they are. Butter in large amounts is not great, but butter is better for you than margarine, despite the fact that butter has saturated fat—because butter is natural. Not surprisingly, our body simply does better with nature-made food than processed, altered substances.

The "Good" Fats:
Omega-3 Fatty Acids and Monounsaturated Oils

Omega-3 fatty acids (rich sources being fish and flaxseed oil) and monounsaturated (oleic acid) oils such as olive, canola, and almond oil are the "good" fats. They should make up what fat is in your diet, if you're interested in prevention and excellent health.

Research is piling up with accolades for these fats—not only because they don't actively harm (unless we eat huge amounts and get overfat), but because they actually have healing properties that can block or reverse the damage done by their troublemaking cousins. They go into the synthesis of "do-gooder" prostaglandins that give orders for repair and regeneration instead of destruction. Adequate amounts can prevent arachidonic acid from conversion to unfriendly prostaglandins and leukotrienes.

One reason these fats may be used for the body's good while those described above wreak havoc on normal processes is that our bodies evolved ways to handle the "good" fats. When we consume something that the human body has been exposed to for millions of years, our bodies know what to do. When we consume something that our ancestors didn't, we're on our own—because they never needed to develop, and thus didn't pass on, any apparatus for dealing with the newcomer substance. In the big picture of history, foods with these beneficial plant fats have been consumed since the times of our earliest ancestors, while the processed oils used excessively in our culture today are relatively new.

For the healthiest diet, make fat from fish, flaxseed, and olives the lion's share of your total fat intake. Fish fats are best obtained from eating fish itself, rather than fish oil capsules, because you can't control the source of the fish when you take capsules, and unfortunately there is a significant risk of hazardous toxic contaminants in much of the fish available today. Saltwater fish is less likely to be contaminated by pollutants than freshwater fish (and saltwater fish, from the coldest waters, also tend to be the richest in omega-3 fats). Salmon, sardines, herring, and mackerel are good sources. Younger (generally smaller) fish have had fewer years of exposure to toxins, suggests Jean Carper in *Food: Your Miracle Medicine*, and eating a variety of fish lets you rotate sources just in case one is contaminated.

Fish fats appear to raise levels of HDL (good) cholesterol, lower triglyceride levels, and thin the blood to reduce clotting—all factors that lower risk of heart disease. They also may prevent and even help treat a wide variety of autoimmune, inflammatory skin and other disorders.

If you don't want to consume fish (because you don't like it, are vegetarian, or worry about contaminants), flaxseed oil is consistently proving to be a worthy omega-3 alternative with many of the same benefits. It's generally a cheaper source, too. It can be purchased in capsules or the seeds themselves can be ground into cereal or salads. If you buy the oil, it must be refrigerated.

Olive oil is also a winning fat. Again, we don't need 150 grams of it in our diets every day (we can survive on a minimum of 3 grams of fat daily and thrive on somewhere between 35 and 70 grams, depending on the individual). Get your 35 to 70 grams a day from olive oil, and you're doing more than simply avoiding damage—you're lowering LDL (bad cholesterol), boosting HDL cholesterol, and interfering with the deadly oxidation of LDL cholesterol. Oils from almonds, macadamias, pistachio, rapeseed (canola oil), and avocados are others rich in monounsaturated fatty acids.

Choose unrefined, cold-pressed oils (to avoid those processed with heat or chemicals) and preferably from organically grown nuts or seeds.

Don't strive for getting less than 10 percent of calories from fat. This can lower levels of HDL cholesterol and cause menstrual irregularities and other health problems. Extremely low total cholesterol (below 140) may eliminate any risk of heart disease (no person with a cholesterol level known to be 150 or below has ever had a heart attack), but it causes other problems. Cholesterol does have a purpose, such as cushioning cell membranes. Without that cushion, cell walls may be weakened and can burst, causing cerebral hemorrhaging. (However, cholesterol levels that low are extremely uncommon in the United States).

Besides, such extremes are not necessary for leanness and health. Think moderation! *BodyFueling*® was so much more than a "low-fat diet" because elimination of fat is not the key to everything. Lowering excessive fat consumption is one small part of a larger strategy of understanding and working with your body on many levels. I personally am not fanatical about fat. I get an average of 20 percent of my calories from fat (about 40 to 45 grams a day), probably on some days dipping a little lower and on many days somewhat higher. Most of my added fat is from olive oil and a little sesame oil; most of the source fat is from plant products.

This is obviously a complex subject and, though we've only been able to overview it here, an important one. We encourage you to educate yourself even more thoroughly on this subject. The books *Fats That Heal, Fats That Kill* by Udo Erasmus and *Optimal Wellness* by Ralph T. Golan, M.D., are two we recommend for more in-depth explanations of these issues.

7

Colds and Flu:
Dodging the Immune
Breakdown Epidemic

WHEN THE IMMUNE SYSTEM
FALLS DOWN ON THE JOB

Let's say you've been doing all the right stuff, as discussed in the preceding pages, but life and stress simply get the better of you and you can feel the beginnings of an infection. Or let's say you've only just learned about these ways to boost your immune power and haven't had a chance to implement them for very long. It can take some time to "clean up your act," and initially you may find yourself still stuck in the cycle of infection. Now your throat is scratchy, your head aches, you're starting to feel glassy-eyed and feverish. What can you do to stop the infection in its tracks—or at very least, to keep it from overtaking your life while it runs its course? A wide range of herbs from around the world can be used to combat viral and bacterial infections as well as soothe their symptoms.

THE THREE FACES OF BREAKDOWN

First, realize that there are three types of immune failures we experience. The first is *infection*, and for many of us, this is the evidence of immune breakdown we'll face most commonly day to day. Cold and flu are some of the most common—and, for many people, disruptive and annoying—infections we experience on a recurring basis.

The second is *allergy*. The immune system, responsible for determining what is us and what's foreign, sometimes overreacts and attacks foreign substances that are not genuine threats—cat hair or pollen, for example. That usually happens when the immune system is overexposed to something at a time when it is not nourished, balanced, and taken care of properly.

For example, my former allergy to chocolate probably developed during that time in my life when it was just about all I ate. There I was, ignoring or abusing my body in every way possible—lack of nutrients, rest, sleep, relaxation—and in addition, I was bombarding my body with a substance it doesn't need. When your body is concerned that it's not going to be able to police invaders effectively enough, it gets defensive and launches a full-scale attack on something like pollen grain or a strawberry. (Also see Chapter 16, "Herbs for Allergies.")

The third type of immune dysfunction is *autoimmune disorder*. This type of disorder is like an allergy—the body mounts a full-blown campaign against something that's not really a threat—but instead of the "foreigner" being an outside catalyst, like dander or chocolate, it's part of *you* that gets attacked. For some reason—probably a combination of factors, most of which are still mysterious to medical science—your immune system sees that tissue as foreign.

There are many suspected autoimmune diseases. Rheumatoid arthritis, lupus, and Hashimoto's disease (a condition in which the body produces specific antibodies against its own thyroid tissue) are examples. Multiple sclerosis is also considered to be an autoimmune disorder by many experts, although there are other theories (such as viral infection). Any part of your body can be attacked by the immune system in an autoimmune disorder.

All three manifestations of immune-system weakness need treatment individualized both for the person and for the particular body system or part involved. However, fundamentally, the underlying issue is the same with all of them: Your immune system needs support.

WINNING YOUR NEXT CLOSE ENCOUNTER

Ideally, you'd have an immune system so strong that as soon as a new virus comes in, the body cranks out new antibodies by the millions and deactivates the virus. You then have immunity, and don't have to go through fever, muscle ache, headache, and so on. *This is possible.* It may take some time to get there, but cold and flu are *not* inevitable facts of life. It is possible simply to not get sick.

For example, at the time I was working on this book, I had an almost inhuman schedule: a tight editorial deadline requiring many months of long nights, working part time on several statewide health-care projects, rehearsing and performing in a play, singing in a chorus, actively volunteering for two community organizations, and taking yoga classes. That was in addition to my share of everyday household and social responsibilities. During this period I was highly exposed to illness—in play and choral rehearsals (half the group had respiratory flu, the other half a stomach virus), on buses, in libraries, stores, and so on. I was getting less sleep than usual and feeling constantly pressured for time. Yet I did not get sick. This was not "luck." I absolutely attribute it to the way I eat and the herbs I take.

As you begin to work with botanical medicines, you may find at first that you still get sick, but herbs can help you get through it faster and more comfortably. Then you get sick less often, and it's less severe. Then you feel yourself just barely start to get sick and you're able to knock it before it goes anywhere. Finally, you just plain won't get sick—or at least only rarely.

Karta Purkh describes his experience with this process. First, he got to where he could shorten the cold or flu from weeks to days. Then it got so he could knock it in twenty-four hours. Then he developed those fine antennae for "something being amiss" and was able to stem the tide of symptoms in advance. Finally, nothing ever got "amiss" to begin with—and it's been that way for close to two decades.

When you get to this point, good diet, exercise, relaxation practices, and general (tonic) supplementation should be sufficient to maintain excellent health. Ideally, you don't need to use specifically therapeutic things to treat disease states all the time. However, if you don't do something special—conscientious self-care that's better than average—you're likely to get sick just like everyone else.

Listen to Your Body

It's important to be in touch with your body. If you don't know what it feels like to truly feel good, it's hard to know when you're starting to feel bad. It appears to us that many Americans live in a low-grade state of discomfort all the time, so there's no differentiation. If you're generally worn out all the time, it's hard to tell if an extra-exhausting day is the flu—or just another day. By the time you figure it out, symptoms may be full blown. Making some of the basic health-building changes described in the previous section will help with this.

If you're accustomed to really paying attention to how you feel, you'll notice subtle changes that could give you a head start in staving off infection. Learn to spot "pre-symptom symptoms" that are more subtle than the glaringly obvious cough, runny nose, or headache. For example, when an infection is incipient, sometimes I get a puffy, achy feeling in my eyes, like the fluid in them or behind them is infected. Or I get a twinge of pain in a lymph node in my neck, like it's gunked up with extra garbage. Or I can't ride uphill on my bike as fast as normal.

Ninety-nine percent of the time, that's as far as it goes. When I notice a "symptom" like this (or am highly exposed and stressed), I don't ignore it. I take echinacea, drink a pint of astragalus broth daily, and take isatidis (a Chinese immune-boosting herb that is synergistic with astragalus) and vitamins. I lay off exercise for a day or two, except perhaps for short walks (depending on how concerned I am), avoid all sweets, and make sure to get extra sleep. As a result, the invader gets only far enough to cause the whisper of trouble that alerts me.

Once or twice, the messages from my body have been more serious: Once I woke up in the middle of the night with a sore throat, and once with a stuffy nose and phlegm in my chest. In both instances, I got out of bed, took an assortment of botanicals and lots of vitamin C, made my broth and drank it, then went back to bed. In both cases, I woke up symptom-free. To me these are like small miracles. It may sound inconsequential, but think for a minute about how your last cold or flu disrupted your life—and how helpless you may have felt.

Many other times, I'm sure, the microbes are doing their level best to make headway, but they simply can't get far enough past my defenses to create even a telltale twinge. Once during a routine checkup, my dentist exclaimed when he looked in my mouth, and asked if I had a sore throat. I didn't. He said my tonsils were red and inflamed. I never did develop symptoms.

As you start to care for your body holistically, you will know enough to get suspicious and reinforce your immune cops before a riot breaks out. Eventually, the most that the rabble-rousers will be able to provoke is a peaceful demonstration—before you effortlessly show them the door.

TYPES OF INFECTIONS

There are differences among the invaders that attempt to penetrate our defenses and cause us to experience uncomfortable symptoms. Knowing what type of interloper is scavenging about is important, because it can determine the specific herbal remedy that's best to use. Some herbs "specialize" in dealing with specific infectious saboteurs: bacteria, virus, yeast, or fungus.

This chapter will deal primarily with colds, flu, and bacterial infections, because they have become so everyday and far-reaching, and too many people are needlessly resigned to their intrusion in our lives. Other infections, such as yeast and fungal diseases, will be dealt with in later chapters.

Bacteria

Bacterial infections are caused by microbes we call bacteria, little one-celled organisms that have a body of their own and a life of their own. They are large compared to our cells. They can be poisoned to death, just like any other living thing. Drugs like penicillin kill the bacteria without killing the host. The advantage of using herbs to treat bacterial infections is that there's much less likelihood of side effects, and they can enhance our health in many other different ways, which drugs simply do not do.

Some herbs offer a safe, nontoxic way to kill bacteria directly by poisoning them. Others work by stimulating the immune system so that the appropriate immune cells kill the bacteria and engulf them faster and better than they would otherwise. Herbs of both types can be used in combination to enhance the action, getting the work done at both ends.

What About Antibiotics?

Drugs that kill bacteria were exciting drugs to have at the time they were introduced, when bacterial infections were a primary cause of serious illness and death. But to heal many illnesses today, especially the increasingly common chronic immune-system-related diseases—and even more importantly, to stay healthy—we need different approaches. We especially need to know how to make ourselves functionally stronger, to resist or overcome a wide range of potential illnesses. To focus only on external, chemical weapons overshadows our potential as individuals to help ourselves heal and keep ourselves well.

Certainly, in the case of some bacterial infections, antibiotics may remain the best choice. However, antibiotics have many risks and disadvantages and are best used sparingly—and besides, in many cases, herbs are simply more effective as well as less damaging.

Virus

A virus is not a living thing in the way that a bacterium is; there is scientific disagreement over whether a virus is a living thing at all. In the conventional sense, it really is not. As such, it's pretty much unlike anything else we know on earth.

A virus has no cell or metabolism of its own. It's a little hunk of genetic material (nucleic acid) with a fatty coat. Since a virus is not a viable life form by itself, it can't function independently for very long (though it can survive outside your cells on something inorganic for a short period). To maintain itself and proliferate, however, it needs you! It can only function inside a host cell, where it takes over the cell's internal metabolism.

A virus is so small, unlike a bacterium, that it can penetrate any tissue in the body. Once it gets into your body tissue, it sheds its fatty coat, penetrates into the middle of the cell, and attaches to the nucleus of the cell. It then turns your cell into a virus factory. Essentially, it takes the cell hostage and tells it to crank out a million copies of the virus. And your cell has no choice but to do so.

The poor hostage cell is done for. It fills up with virus, bursts open, spills out all the virus copies it has manufactured, infects its neighbor cells—and there you have your problem. Your body recognizes the problem, of course, and performs various functions to flush it out. How soon and how fast your body is able to overtake the busy production of these little portable gene factories depends on—you guessed it—the efficiency of your immune system.

The scary thing about viruses is that they can kill us—and we can't externally poison them. They aren't "alive" in the first place—they have no metabolism—so there's nothing to poison. Our only recourse is to gobble them up: Our immune cells must attach to and engulf them. And viruses can proliferate very rapidly, so it takes many millions of immune cells on vigilant patrol to apprehend all the troublemakers. Then, once the little antagonists have been deactivated, the body's cleanup crew—the toxic elimination system—has to dispose of them.

That's why herbs called antivirals are really just superb immune boosters. As far as we know, the herbs aren't going in and killing the virus itself. They are supplementing, enlarging, and exhorting your immune system to do the job with maximum efficiency. They make you "bigger"; they don't make the virus "smaller."

That's why there are few drugs that work antivirally, and why we don't have a medical cure for the common cold. Drugs don't nourish you or your immune system. They don't make you a healthier or stronger match for the virus. Drugs either do the killing themselves, directly, or they salve symptoms.

Many health experts predict a viral epidemic the likes of which we have never seen before—if it hasn't already arrived. The prevalence of many different viruses, old and new, has increased dramatically in recent years, from the likes of AIDS to chronic fatigue syndrome. Each new cold and flu season seems to bring an ever more serious period of viral illness. Even in a normal year, 25 million to 50 million Americans catch the flu, and roughly 25,000 die from it.

Again, your own immune function is your most valuable weapon against this viral onslaught. That's why we cannot emphasize enough the importance of treating your immune system right, and doing all you can to protect and nourish it. Fortunately, as we've seen, good health practices *can* support and rejuvenate the immune system, even in the most serious situation. And herbs can contribute enormously to your immune "armor."

Herbal healing has a tremendous repertoire of effective therapies for infectious disease, including cold and flu, the aggravating and persistent maladies most people struggle with every year. In fact, viral illness may well provide the most dramatic examples of the effectiveness of herbal medicine in our time. In the absence of effective conventional drug treatment for viral infection, such as cold and flu, herbal medicine is internationally known to be of great benefit.

So Which Is It?

It can sometimes be hard to tell by symptoms or tests if your infection is the result of an invading virus or bacteria. Even medical testing can be inexact and is open to clinical interpretation. But there are ways *you* can learn to recognize what type of infection you have, allowing you to choose the most effective herbal healing method.

Bacterial infections are often characterized by some sort of a colored discharge—yellow or green pus, for example, rather than clear fluid. Bacterial infections also usually occur close to a body opening—hence bladder, kidney, throat, ear, eye, and gum infections are typically bacterial.

Viruses are usually what we think of as "sick all over" kinds of sicknesses, rather than being localized. Here is a comparison of the telltale characteristics of the two infection types:

BACTERIA	VIRUS
Local	Widespread/systemic
Stays where it started:	Spreads all over:
Near surface of body/opening	muscles, digestive system,
(bladder, ear, sinus)	lung, nose
Short, high fever spike	Long, low-grade sustained fever
Thick, sticky, colored mucus	Thin, clear mucus

While any herb that generally stimulates your immune system—or cell-mediated immunity—is going to be beneficial before or during any type of infection, some herbs are better choices than others for cutting down specific infections. Let's look at the viral hindrances we know as cold and flu.

COLD AND FLU: VIVA LA VIRUS!

An adult American can expect to get, on average, 2½ colds a year. Small children average eight to 10 colds a year.[1] There are over 250 varieties of colds known to researchers, and the flu virus mutates constantly. You can be reinfected with every single one. The body develops an immunity to a particular cold virus once you get it, but there are 249 more out there that can still infect you, and new versions are always evolving. We can't hope the "supply" will run out.

Cold and influenza ("flu") share many of the same symptoms, especially at onset, and may be hard to tell apart. A little way into the infection, though, there are telltale differences. While both infect the respiratory tract, the flu is generally considered to be a more serious infection. Both can cause runny nose, sneezing, sore throat, cough, and fatigue, although the fatigue is usually more severe with the flu. Both can cause a headache, but the flu also causes body aches. The cough produced by the flu usually worsens and lasts longer, and may be more productive. The flu usually causes a fever, even in adults, while a cold rarely causes fever in adults. The fever will usually spike suddenly and can go quite high. Flu, unlike colds, can involve stomach symptoms such as nausea or vomiting.

A cold usually lasts four to ten days; the flu can linger for two weeks. Both can result in a secondary bacterial infection; this seems to be more likely in the sinuses or ears with a cold, and more likely in the bronchi/lungs with flu. People with weakened immune systems frequently develop bronchitis or pneumonia following the flu.

The onset itself is also different; a cold may take one to three days to present itself fully, while the flu hits hard and fast, usually within a period of twenty-four hours and often more quickly than that.

Both of these viruses are obviously very disruptive to health and life, and are best avoided or reduced in severity whenever possible. Botanicals can help ease the discomfort of symptoms (without being immune suppressive) and build immunity and strength.

Let's look first at emergency tactics to stop the infection in its tracks. Then we can look at ways to make the situation more bearable if it does get past your front line of defense. (And then you can go back and look at the preventive immune-boosting suggestions in the previous section and chapter.)

KARTA PURKH'S "SQUELCH-IT" EARLY ANTI-FLU ROUTINE

You can knock the flu! If you act fast, when you feel the first stirrings of symptoms—muscle ache, fever, headache—and hit it hard with this kind of program, you can be done in twenty-four hours, stop the otherwise inevitable progress into full-blown disease, and skip the ten days of bed rest.

Karta Purkh devised this shotgun, four-step anti-flu routine—which is

not strictly herbal—to include something for everyone. It is not individualized, and you may not need all four steps. But it is a general program that
people have found beneficial for early counteraction.

1. *Herbal antiviral combo.* This would be any combination of herbs
specifically designed to support immune-system activity. Some examples
are isatidis and astragalus (my favorite); a capsule with boldo leaf,
jalapeño, cayenne, cubeb berry, rose hips and garlic; or a capsule with
jalapeño, echinacea, and cubeb berry. (Specific herbal antivirals are listed
later in this chapter.) Some hot or spicy ingredient should be included, if
you can tolerate it. Take as many capsules as possible—10 to 15 a day,
maybe even 20. Just get down as many as you can, as fast as you can. The
effect is cumulative, so the faster you take them, the better you'll feel. One
or 2 every hour with water may be the best method. For many people, this
step alone does the job.

2. *Zinc lozenges.* These allow zinc to be absorbed directly into the
mouth rather than going through the digestive tract (zinc is poorly
absorbed through the gut so it essentially gets wasted, and it also produces
queasiness). Lozenges also bathe and saturate the whole respiratory area
with this antiviral mineral. Studies show that zinc shortens colds and
reduces symptoms, theoretically by preventing viral replication, stimulating
immune activity, and/or stabilizing cell membranes. Use up to 10 per day.

3. *Vitamin C.* Karta Purkh does not find much use generally for vitamin C as an antiviral, because although it is a good, safe, general substance
to use, there is frequently an herb that does a better job at everything vitamin C does, for less money. Still, for a shotgun approach that's directed
at everyone, it's not a bad remedy to include. It needs to be used in very
large doses to be effective. In these situations, you take vitamin C to what's
called bowel tolerance. (I learned what that means one time after taking
10 grams a day for a couple of days.) When it starts to give you the runs,
cut the dose back.

Most people have a bowel tolerance of 5 to 10 grams a day, but it goes
up proportionally with the severity of a viral infection. People with very
serious infections like AIDS can have bowel tolerance of 50 to 60 grams.
Dr. Andrew Weil notes that he takes 4 to 5 grams of vitamin C a day, and
had a patient with no bowel problems at up to 54 grams a day.[2] Basically,
the bigger the infection your body is fighting, the more vitamin C is depleted and the more you can tolerate—because it's definitely being used.

Even though research shows that vitamin C may inhibit zinc absorption, they are both recommended here because they are both useful for colds, they can be taken separately, and one is taken orally while the other is used to saturate the site of infection.

4. Cinchona bark. This antiviral herb is especially potent against colds and flu. It's also useful after you have full-blown symptoms (discussed coming up), especially in synergy with willow bark for pain. Take it in capsules, up to 10 per day, as it is too bitter for use as a tea.

ROBYN'S FAVORITE ANTI-INFECTION "RAID"

I, too, have a personal favorite anti-infection routine. It has worked for me every time but once—when I had a two-day cold that marred my current seven-year "record." It's more extensive than Karta Purkh's knock-it-back strategy, to account for either virus or bacteria (even though most of the infections we experience as being cold- and flulike are, in fact, viral).

Try it, or your own personalized variation, next time you feel "under the weather." (But remember, don't expect this to work in a general environment of abuse. Depleted systems need this sort of nourishment all the time.)

1. Antiviral soup. This has a base of the immunostimulant adaptogen *astragalus*, discussed at length in Chapter 6. Simmered in this broth is one *garlic* bulb, peeled and sliced; one large chopped *onion*; and about 1/4 cup sliced *ginger* or several tablespoons of ground ginger. Then add as much *black pepper* and *cayenne* as you can stand. Watch out—this is pungent stuff! (As a fire type, I only use this on a "special-occasion" basis.)

2. Antioxidant vegetables. To the soup I also add vegetables rich in vitamins A and C and those known to have powerful healing phytochemical compounds or immunostimulant properties. For example, I might include *broccoli, carrots, cabbage, beets*, and *shiitake mushrooms*. I generally try to include vegetables with carotenoids, root vegetables, and some from the cruciferous group. This soup then becomes my food for the day.

3. Herbal immune-boosters and blood cleansers. My favorites are *echinacea, astragalus*, and *isatidis* (the latter two are synergistic). *Licorice root, ginger root*, and *boldo leaf* would round out my routine in this case.

4. *Grapefruit seed extract*. This is a powerful, unique antimicrobial. It is lethal for bacteria, but also works for yeast, fungus, and anything else that's killable. Some herbalists and naturopaths have also found clinically that it's an effective antiviral, although the mechanism is still a mystery—whether it is immune stimulating or actually offsets viral replication no one knows. The unique thing about GSE is that somehow it manages to snuff out only the "bad guys" and leaves the friendly flora unharmed.

Nutribiotic is a common brand of the liquid extract. Any health-food store should have it. I squeeze it into capsules (I find it irritating to mucous membranes and think the recommendation on the bottle to mix it in water is misguided—I can barely swallow for an hour after I do that). GSE is also available powdered in capsules.

5. *Vitamin C*. In a "raid" such as this I will take 6 to 8 grams—1 gram every 2 to 3 hours.

Just imagine some poor microbes trying to function under this kind of load! I figure with a routine as varied and aggressive as this, those little critters don't have a hope of surviving.

Note: An addition to either of these routines that may be worth trying, though neither of us has yet personally tried or observed its use, is a syrup made of *elderberry* (*Sambucus nigra*). Elderberry was a cold and flu remedy for centuries in Europe, but more recently has become popular here since it was scientifically proven as antiflu by the doctoral work of an Algerian-born Israeli named Madeleine Mumcuoglu. In the early 1980s, as her dissertation for her Ph.D. in virology, Mumcuoglu investigated the antiviral potential of the herb (at the suggestion of her adviser, Jean Linderman, the scientist who discovered the body's own antiviral chemical interferon).

Mumcuoglu found two chemicals in elderberry that prevent the flu virus from invading throat cells (its only way to reproduce), thus preventing infection. When Mumcuoglu returned to Israel, she developed an elderberry syrup containing the two compounds, naming it Sambucol. A flu outbreak in 1992 gave Mumcuoglu a chance to test the remedy. Half the residents were given 4 tablespoons of Sambucol a day at the first sign of a fever. The other half took Tylenol and cold formulas. After 3 days, 90 percent of the Sambucol users felt well again. The other group took twice as long to heal.[3] Sambucol quickly became popular in Israel and is now marketed in other countries. Many U.S. health-food stores carry it. Follow package directions.

All this may seem like a lot, but compare this effort to the lost time and productivity that comes if you actually succumb to your infectious adversary. Most of this stuff isn't even bad tasting, and if you make the soup your meals, you've eliminated one other task for the day.

Whether you use Karta Purkh's routine or my "raid," please remember too that it helps immensely to do other common-sense things like rest and lay off any immune-suppressive habits. These tactics are not designed to sustain you in the face of a sixteen-hour workday, four-hour commute, a pack of cigarettes, an evening on the StairMaster, dinner at Burger Bob's, and a fight with your roommate. The results will be much better in a total healing environment.

IF YOU ALREADY HAVE A COLD OR FLU

If you do fall prey to the latest "thing that's going around," be assured that your natural-remedy medicine chest has a powerful set of tools to put you back on your feet in short order—and make you feel better until you are. Many of the same herbs and foods already discussed as generally immune boosting or infection blocking are also useful for helping your body rise to the occasion during those times when the immune-boosting just wasn't enough.

First, a Note about Symptoms

The cold and flu symptoms that everybody is so familiar with are reactions that our body produces. This may sound too obvious even to mention, but do you ever think about that when you're scrambling to make them go away? Mucus discharge, headache, fever, inflammation—these are not symptoms that the invader itself creates or "does to you"; they are reactions that the body creates to cripple the invader, to drive it from your body.

Microbes can do damage. It is not good to have our cells converting to virus factories. Bacteria dine on our tissues, cells, and nutrients. It's a good thing that the body responds to the trespassers. But we don't like how that feels, so we try to make the symptoms go away.

Ideally your body should respond quickly, efficiently, and aggressively without having to resort to those symptoms, without you even knowing that the invasion happened. As we have said, this is definitely possible. However, if the trespassers do manage to establish themselves, the body goes to the next stage. Unfortunately, you will feel the tactics it uses in this phase. But we don't want to focus on getting rid of or suppressing these symptoms. We want to emphasize getting rid of the invader, and helping your body to do that.

You can make a choice about how much you want to treat symptoms, something that can be done very adequately using herbs. Sometimes you may have a more pressing need than letting your body do its work at the expense of comfort. You may have a class to teach or a trip to take. You can't have a headache or a runny nose or be vomiting. Treating symptoms for those reasons, in and of itself, isn't so terrible.

What doesn't work long term is the illusion that the symptoms are the problem. They are not. They are a sign that your body is responding to an infection. The problem is that there was an opening that the invaders could drive a truck through. If you don't address that, you will keep getting infected, and you will always be treating symptoms.

If possible, once you're infected it really is better to let the body do what it's going to do, because it's the body's natural way of getting rid of those things. Case in point: An elevated body temperature is created because viruses have co-evolved to live with us in a very narrow range of temperature, at body temperature. Viruses that affect humans generally only affect humans, although there are some viruses that can be transmitted from animals to humans—rabies is an old one; the ebola virus was more recently discovered. Viruses don't function very well at 100° or 101°, and they die. The body has evolved to increase our temperature as a defense mechanism for that very reason.

Take a bunch of aspirin to bring your fever down, and you lose that benefit and ability. You thwart what your body is trying to do. And so it goes with many other cold and flu "treatments." When you have a runny nose, you *want* that mucus there, flushing out nasal membranes so viruses don't penetrate farther, and to get rid of dead invaders and cells. Suppress it and dry it all up by taking a decongestant, and you give the virus just that much more chance to continue to penetrate into your nasal membranes. You make the course of the disease potentially longer and more serious when you medicate away your immune response.

When considering the value of a particular treatment, consider that the superior treatments are those that help eliminate the cause of the problem. Ask yourself how effective a remedy is that doesn't actually heal or make you healthier.

When Your Body Gets Sick, Look at Your Life

With natural healing, I have learned to think about health and my body very differently. If I get a patch of fungus on my leg, I don't think, "What can I put on this to get rid of it?" I may want to apply something natural and gentle topically, to help heal it, but I certainly don't stop there. What I think is, "What is going on with my body and in my life that left this opening in my defenses for something foreign to make its home on me? What can I do to give my immune system a boost? What changes have I experienced lately? How can I adjust my life right now to reduce stress and promote rest and healing?" I don't want to shove it down; I want to find out what its message is.

Cutting Your Cold or Flu: Victorious Antivirals

Once you have a cold or flu, your goal should be to shorten its duration and intensity as much as possible, and to make yourself feel and function better (but not at the expense of immune functions, as with OTC drugs).

Here are the best herbs for the job(s). All of these can be mixed and matched to your convenience, though you certainly don't need them all. Try one or two at a time and see what works for you best and what you like.

With all of these, the general rule is to work your way up gradually. It might take two or three times of working with an herb to get a feel for how it functions in your particular body, and how quickly. Take with food, divide the doses (don't take a full day's worth all at once), and work up to the amount that produces the result you want with no negatives (such as queasiness).

Chilies

Chilies, as we have mentioned, are potent antivirals. Eating more of them in the diet is fine for general preventive purposes, but to get enough down to knock back an invasion quickly, capsules are usually necessary. Increase gradually as you become comfortable with the effects.

Cayenne pepper is probably the best, most available, and most effective antiviral. Take as many capsules as you can tolerate. Unfortunately, unless you're used to taking it, your digestive tract probably won't tolerate enough cayenne pepper to treat the virus. That's why it may be useful to start integrating more and more chilies into your diet *before* you get sick. Then, if you need it, you'll have more of a tolerance for high doses.

Cultures all around the world have long observed that substances that warm up the body help fight infectious disease. Not surprisingly, many (though not all) foods and herbs known as antivirals are hot and pungent—for example, onion, garlic, ginger, chilies, and cubeb berry.

There are two groups of people who should probably look elsewhere for herbal antiviral activity: children and *pitta* (fire-type) constitutional body types. Non-warming antivirals are better in such cases. These include cinchona bark, guduchi, isatidis, and astragalus, which is technically warming, but very mildly. If you are a *pitta* and use chilies, be prepared for the effect of their heat on your already-hot systems. You can counteract this somewhat by taking it in small doses with plenty of food—starches and fats are best—and water. Still, you may experience a burning sensation in your stomach (peppermint tea may provide some relief in this case) and "acid stools."

To quell an occasional cold or flu before it can take hold, you may be willing to put up with these side effects. I've done it a few times, and I can attest to the fact that fire types will experience these discomforts. (I didn't get the cold, though!) You won't sustain long-term damage doing this, but hot, pungent foods and herbs would not be a great thing for fire types to consume on a long-term basis.

My husband, with his *vata* (air-type) constitution, is able to tolerate cayenne in much higher doses—in fact, he takes a tablespoon or two of cayenne every day of his life as an immune tonic and for the circulatory boost. This is probably one reason he hasn't had an infection of any kind for more than six years. And if he needs to up the dose in order to knock back a potential infection in its early stages, he's "conditioned" for the heat, just as if he lived in a culture that consumed these kinds of foods regularly. (Another bonus: He can also order five-star-plus dishes at Thai restaurants.)

Trinity Roots

Onion and garlic, as discussed in detail in the previous chapter, are hugely successful immune stimulants and can be consumed in very high quantities—as much as you can stand—in the immediate effort to kick an infection in the early stages, as well as throughout the illness to speed healing. Again, garlic in the form of capsules (up to 20 daily) may be necessary to get these very high medicinal dosages quickly. Garlic is probably more potent than onion, and is available in deodorized form. Both garlic and onion can, of course, be used as food to maximum tolerance, and onion can be juiced as well.

Ginger root, the classic immune-system and respiratory-system tonic, is synergistic with onion and garlic, so all three in a soup works well. Ginger will also provide relief for virtually all of your cold and flu symptoms, from fever to sinus congestion to sore throat to stomachache and nausea.

Cubeb Berry

Cubeb berry is a large peppercorn. It's dried and can be taken in capsules—5 to 10 a day, or more during the course of an illness. You can also make a tea out of it and use it as a culinary spice; it's pungent but rather tasty, like a piney, aromatic black pepper. The *Piper* genus has hundreds of peppercorn-type herbs, which are used medicinally all over the world.

Other peppercorns that work well antivirally include pipali (*Piper longum*, or "long pepper"), an Ayurvedic herb also related to black pepper (*Piper nigrum*). Pipali is better for long-term viral protection than black pepper, though, and is a superb blood purifier. Both are warming herbs, but pipali is more of a tonic than black pepper because it is moistening and building. Black pepper is drying and contracting; this makes it better for acute issues such as nasal congestion.

Cubeb has many benefits as a cold and flu treatment. It's generally antiviral (immune supportive), has a particular affinity for respiratory tissues (both sinus and lung; it's an exceptional long-term lung-tissue builder), and is an adrenal builder. This is very important because the adrenal glands secrete hormones that control the immune system. Adrenals are also our fight-or-flight regulating glands; they mastermind how the body will respond to stress (which a viral infection is). It's an excellent idea to nourish these glands generally, and especially during and after a viral infection. Take up to 10 capsules per day for acute conditions or 1/2 ounce as tea for long-term building purposes.

Black Walnut Hull and Gum Benzoin

This nonspicy, nonwarming antiviral combination works synergistically. When the two herbs are taken together, the effect is greater than either taken individually.

Black walnut hull is a Native American herb. The hull of the walnut is the fruit; the nut is the seed inside the fruit. The dried hull/skin is powdered and used in capsules. It's also a good liver tonic—again, a plus, because the liver is stressed when you have a viral infection. It should only be taken in capsule form because it's irritating to the tongue and skin and tastes bad.

Gum benzoin is the pitch, or resin, that exudes from the bark of a plant grown in Indonesia. You can't make tea out of gums and resins, so it too is capsuled.

Five to 10 capsules a day of the combo is usually an effective dose for cold and flu.

This pairing is a great example of the concept of global herbology discussed in Chapter 1: "Herbs: The Original Medicine." Modern communication and transportation methods give us the opportunity to put together combinations like this North American and Indonesian one, and to confirm through clinical use by herbalists around the globe that they work more effectively when combined.

Cinchona Bark and Willow Bark

This is another synergistic pair of herbs that is outstanding for cold and especially perfect for flu. Not only do they enhance each other's effectiveness, but each has a special job it can do: Cinchona bark works antivirally, bumping up your disease-fighting power, and willow bark is a pain reliever, good for headaches as well as muscular aches and pains.

Cinchona bark is what quinine originally came from. Quinine is pretty close to what it is in the plant; it wasn't tinkered with too much to make the remedy (which is now off the market due to lack of evidence for its claims as a leg-cramp treatment, according to the FDA). Cinchona bark was also at one time used as a treatment for malaria.

In addition to its antiviral activity, cinchona bark is a muscle relaxant—good for muscular pain and spasm. It's also relaxing and sedating, which can help you get more rest when you're sick. Four capsules an hour of willow/cinchona combination capsules can do wonders for acute muscle pain. (Cinchona bark is very bitter, too terrible for tea—capsules are the way to go.)

White willow bark is the kind of willow bark usually used. Willow bark is not antiviral. But it enhances the effects of the cinchona bark, and has all the benefits of aspirin without the problems. It reduces pain, inflammation, and fever without any digestive distress.

Karta Purkh had one student in a class who was taking pharmaceutical anti-inflammatories, with unpleasant side effects, to control muscle pain from an injury. He now drinks 1 cup of willow bark a day and that takes care of it. He is also treating the underlying healing issues, but while he's doing that, his pain relief comes from a natural source instead of a drug.

Willow bark tastes okay, and since it is mild, tea is the best way to take enough of it to be effective. It has a springy, spongy texture, so you really can't get enough in a capsule to be convenient. Besides, you'd have to take a lot of capsules—it wouldn't be like taking a couple of aspirin. Brew it as strong as you can take it. A very strong concentrate of willow bark will last a week or so in the fridge (as will most teas).

For optimal synergism, take 2 parts willow bark to 1 part cinchona bark. The amount you need for desired effect may vary. These are safe things to experiment with, so just work up to tolerance or until you get the desired effect.

Note: Reye's syndrome is a neurological condition that develops in children taking aspirin when they have a viral infection. There is no evidence that willow bark can have the same effect. However, to be on the cautious side, avoid using willow bark, as well as aspirin, for children during viral illness.

Astragalus and Isatidis

These two Chinese antivirals are synergistic, and capsuled combination formulas can be found in natural food stores. They work well for cold and flu, and astragalus is especially valuable for stubborn, long-term viral illnesses that are hanging on. Isatidis (sometimes called "woad") is particularly good for mumps or hepatitis (it reduces swelling and liver inflammation) but is excellent for any virus. The nice thing about these is that neither is spicy, hot, superstrong, or aggressive, so they're good for children or anyone who can't tolerate heat or intensity (i.e., *pitta*).

While warm and sweet astragalus makes a good tea or broth, bitter and cold isatidis tastes bad and is best used in capsules. (I combine the two by drinking or eating astragalus soup and taking isatidis capsules that I make myself out of powdered isatidis from a Chinese doctor.)

Astragalus can be consumed daily at 1 to 2 ounces as tea, or 10 to 20 capsules for acute conditions. Long term as a tonic, try 1/2 to 1 ounce as tea, or 5 capsules. Isatidis can be taken 5 to 15 capsules per day in acute situations.

Other Antivirals of Note

Echinacea root has become extremely popular for staving off colds and flu, both at the onset and to shorten the duration once the infection is in full swing. Echinacea does stimulate nonspecific immunity and is therefore by definition helpful against virus, and many people achieve good results with echinacea for this purpose. But while echinacea is an extremely well-studied and safe immunostimulant, in our experience it is not necessarily the most potent. Many other herbalists agree that for antiviral purposes—particularly to knock back a cold or flu—some other herbs and foods (including those mentioned on the previous pages) are actually more powerful than the trendy and often overpriced echinacea. That means that you could well achieve better results with something else—without having to take as much or spend as much. Echinacea is an outstanding antibacterial, however. (See p. 183.)

Ajwain seed is a potent antiviral seed that, like chilies, can be taken to maximum tolerance during cold and flu season. A good way to get enough down is to use the ajwain/jalapeño pancake recipe on p. 498.

Pau d'arco bark is good for chronic or repeated viral illness (1 ounce as tea daily).

Red raspberry leaf tea is a mild antiviral, a good long-term tonic (1 to 3 ounces as tea daily).

Licorice root is another long-term immune builder, through the adrenals (5 capsules or 1/2 ounce as tea daily).

Amur cork tree bark is a mild Chinese antiviral for acute conditions (5 to 10 capsules daily).

Eleuthero root is another good long-term builder for chronic or repeated illness (3 to 5 capsules daily).

Guduchi is an Ayurvedic immune tonic (long-term rebuild and short-term acute), good for fever and supports and rebuilds liver function (5 to 15 capsules for acute treatment, 1 to 3 long-term).

Reishi, shiitake, and *maitake* mushroom extracts or powders are all proven antivirals and are used as immunostimulants around the world for everything from colds to cancer. Follow package directions.

Yogi tea is a blend of spices used heavily in Ayurvedic healing, including cinnamon, cloves, and black pepper. You can purchase it preblended in natural foods stores, or make it yourself (recipe on p. 496). Ayurvedic lore has it that during a flu epidemic in India, an army officer who also happened to be a yoga practitioner knew about yogi tea and arranged for the canteens of the soldiers around him to contain only yogi tea instead of water. The epidemic swept through the army and leveled everybody else, and this officer's group was the only one left standing.

Helping Your Liver Clean Up after the "Bust"

As mentioned earlier, the liver has a great deal of work to do during and after a viral infection. There are herbs that nourish and boost liver functioning (covered in detail on pages 330–335).

Interestingly, many liver herbs also treat fever: astragalus, Ayurvedic kutki, Chinese bupleurum root, Chinese rhubarb root, Chinese licorice root, isatidis root, baical scullcap. From the Eastern healing point of view, this makes perfect sense. First, both fever and liver inflammation reflect *pitta* (fire) excess and are typical *pitta* problems. The standout herbs for healing either of these conditions are typically cooling or cold herbs. By cooling *pitta*, they restore balance. Many liver herbs are also bitter (reducing) as well as cold.

Many liver herbs also turn out to be immune-support and antiviral herbs. This is also logical because the liver is such a crucial station in the immune system, and is particularly occupied with disposal work in the wake of viral illness. By supporting the liver's cleansing and detoxifying work, you support the efficiency and smooth operation of the whole system.

A few examples:

Boldo leaf (Peumus boldus), from South America, is one of the best liver tonics in the world, and also has an affinity for kidneys and bladder. It was very popular around the turn of the century as a kidney tonic, right before natural healing was forced out of the picture. It makes a drinkable tea, and combined with goldenseal (to kill the bacteria) is excellent for kidney and bladder infections.

Bayberry has the advantage of being a mild liver builder in addition to a warming and drying cold remedy.

Again, for a complete list of liver tonic herbs, see pages 330–335.

Bacteria Takes a Beating

Goldenseal (*Hydrastis canadensis*)

Goldenseal is one of the most misunderstood herbs among "sometime herb consumers," and as a result is the nucleus of a great deal of myth and misuse. Goldenseal is not a great immune booster. It is not a long-term tonic. It is a poisoner of microbes and an anti-inflammatory (especially for mucous membranes). There is no purpose in taking goldenseal unless you have a bacterial or parasitic infection, gastrointestinal problem, or membrane inflammation.

That said, if you do have an acute bacterial or parasitic infection, goldenseal is probably the ultimate choice of any herb in the world. It can help wipe out bacterial infections of all kinds: sinus, bladder, kidney, skin, gum infections, strep throat, eye and ear infections, and just about any other bacterial invasion.

Goldenseal may also be good for colds (it's very commonly combined with echinacea in commercial herbal cold formulas) because it's astringent and a membrane healer which may help dry up excess mucus and soothe inflamed tissues. According to Herb Research Foundation president Rob McCaleb, one of its compounds has been found to have an antihistamine effect, which may further support its use in colds and flu.[4] However, we think there are other more effective (and less expensive) ways to deal with colds, as described earlier.

A North American herb, originally used by Native Americans, goldenseal grows in Appalachia and the forests of the upper Midwest, Wisconsin, and Canada. It's the root that's medicinal. Goldenseal is exported; it's a favorite remedy in other countries' herbal medicine chests.

Goldenseal is quite bitter and thus is rarely taken as tea. In addition to capsules, it is often found as a tincture in alcohol. However, some herbalists feel that the active ingredient of goldenseal is inhibited by alcohol, and its large molecules may not be soluble in alcohol. (The same is true of echinacea's polysaccharides.) With both of these herbs going for upwards of $120 to $150 a pound in some herb pharmacies now, you want to make sure every molecule you pay for gets into you. Therefore, we think capsules are the way to go.

With excellent-quality goldenseal, for a typical acute infection, you might try 10 a day short term (a week or so). For a very drastic problem such as extreme sinusitis, 15 to 30 capsules a day is appropriate.

One of the problems that comes of being so effective is that goldenseal has become well known and trendy. This does happen to some very effective herbs. Thus the demand rises, the supply plummets, and the price skyrockets. Goldenseal today costs more than ten times what it did a decade ago, and may not be worth it at this price. You could use other, milder herbs and treat the infection just as effectively for less money.

Goldenseal is also extremely overharvested and nearing extinction, and much goldenseal is illegally poached from the wild. For these reasons, many herbalists feel it should never be used anymore unless it is *the* perfect remedy and nothing else will do. Sometimes this is the case—such as for a very dramatic, active, acute infection where you need rapid action at a high dose. An example would be antibiotic-resistant staph infections.

Karta Purkh recalls one woman who had a staphylococcus infection in one of her toes. She said she had been given three different courses of antibiotics, and none had worked. Her doctors told her the infection was antibiotic resistant and there was nothing they could do. She was told to "watch it." (Watch what?) A year later, the infection had spread to another toe. It occurred to her that she was going to lose her foot a few years down the road if this kept progressing.

After attending a class taught by Karta Purkh, the woman decided to try goldenseal and took 25 capsules daily. She reported that the infection was completely gone in both toes after one week. Necrotic tissue popped out of the infected areas, leaving a pink depression which was treated successfully with topical arnica, pine extract, and vitamin E.

Another problem besides price when an herb gets trendy is quality. A huge demand inevitably motivates some people to sell junk to make money. Goldenseal is therefore often adulterated. This is easy to do with goldenseal in its powder form, because you never get to see the whole root. It's yellow, so adulteraters can throw in other yellow herbs. Growers may also grind up and powder the whole plant (even though only the root is medicinal).

Neither is color always a good indicator of purity or strength. While this herb is usually deep yellow, with a lime green color meaning the tops of the plant were ground in, one year Karta Purkh found a source that was excellent, potent quality but just happened to have a greenish color. Sometimes a brownish color can be good too.

In the average health-food store, commercial-quality goldenseal is mostly low quality. In most cases it's good enough that it will work, but because it is lower potency it takes more to do the job—which is more expensive.

Goldenseal's alkaloid compound berberine is credited for its powerful antimicrobial and anti-inflammatory effects. Berberine may work by preventing microbes from attaching to cells, rather than directly killing the microbes itself. Berberine is found in other less expensive and more abundant herbs, such as the North American herb barberry (the name berberine comes from the plant's botanical name, *Berberis vulgaris*) and Oregon grape root (*Berberis aquifolium*). These are both good alternatives to goldenseal. The herb goldthread is also becoming a more popular alternative. In fact, herb expert Rob McCaleb says some of these have been used as adulterants in commercial goldenseal and suggests that the adulterant may actually be as effective as or more effective than the authentic herb.[5]

Still, goldenseal is definitely a "buyer beware" product right now. If you consult or know a professional herbalist (always a good idea) who has the scoop on sources and crops from year to year, you can make better choices. Unfortunately, the average layperson without inside information will have a hard time determining what's good, which is why we encourage you to shop around for sources, get to know experts you can trust, and keep educating yourself. (Quality and source issues are discussed more fully in Chapter 23, "Living It: Herbs in Practice.")

Goldenseal has virtually no side effects. Again, you don't want to take it long term, but that's mainly because it has no special long-term benefit. Some suggest that theoretically, as a natural antibiotic, long-term use could conceivably result in depletion of friendly bacteria in the intestines and/or reproductive tract. But this herb is not only incredibly mild in comparison to antibiotic drugs, it also contains active ingredients (berberine and hydrastine, which may also be anti-inflammatory) that are found in many other plants, so our "good" bacteria likely evolved to accommodate these compounds. In practical experience, Karta Purkh has never seen this depletion of friendly bacteria happen, and no one he knows knows anyone else who has seen it happen, either.

Twenty capsules a day or more of goldenseal for acute situations is perfectly safe—but you may only need 10, so work up gradually to find out. This makes early detection critical. Hit it right away when a bacterial infection is coming on. Then you will know exactly how it works for you personally and can go right up to the dose you need in the future.

Echinacea

This Native American herb from midwestern prairies has already been discussed at length relative to prevention (as a tonic and nonspecific immunostimulant) as well as for treating infection. Echinacea is both antibacterial and antiviral, since it stimulates production of white blood cells.

Like goldenseal, echinacea has become so popular—possibly the trendiest herb in the herbal kingdom and certainly one of the hottest-selling—that everyone is using it for everything, and it doesn't work very well for everything. And it's expensive, so you can spend a lot of money and not get great results. But it's very appropriate for antibacterial use. Clinically, many herbalists find echinacea to be even better as an antibacterial than as an antiviral.

For an acute bacterial infection, 5 to 15 capsules a day works well for most people. (See pages 137–139 for more on echinacea.)

Grapefruit Seed Extract

This notable remedy is described earlier in my "Anti-Infection Raid" routine (page 169). Again, it's not a tonic, but it's a great short-term "hired gun" that can be used to deactivate any and all invaders. It's a tremendous antibacterial, though it's also good for wiping out yeast, fungus, or parasites. And it spares the immune squad, taking out only the interlopers.

GSE has many other uses. It's combined with boric acid to make a natural external flea remedy for pets and homes. It's also fantastic for dissolving kidney stones. One man who worked with Karta Purkh had passed several stones, and X rays showed forty more intact in his kidneys. When he felt the beginnings of symptoms, he began taking GSE daily. A few days later he passed a mushy glob. Then he never passed a stone again. Subsequent X rays showed that the rest of the stones had disappeared.

Even though grapefruit seed (or other citrus seed) extracts are not normally recommended as long-term immune boosters, and the exact mechanism by which this remedy disables virus is not known, grapefruit seed extract is nontoxic and very powerful (fairly small doses are effective) so it's well worth using with infections of uncertain cause.

Use 2,000 milligrams per day of GSE to treat acute infection. This would amount to about 8 capsules of powder or 1 to 2 teaspoons stirred into water or juice. (Dilute adequately to avoid mouth and throat irritation. Take capsules with plenty of water and "chase" with food. Do not take on an empty stomach.)

Chaparral

This common herb grows in the desert Southwest, covering millions of acres of desert. It originally came to the notice of the scientific community as a potential cancer treatment. There have been claims that it is a cure for that disease, and Native Americans used it for that purpose. In fact, the largest herbal company in the United States, Nature's Way, is a family company that started when one of the family members reportedly used chaparral tea to bring on a cancer remission that lasted twenty-five years after she was sent home to die in the mid-1960s.

Chaparral is known by herbalists to be effective against a wide variety of infectious agents: bacteria, viruses, and yeast. It's a good immune-system-supporting herb in general, a very potent antimicrobial, and a blood cleanser. (*Blood cleanser* or *blood purifier* are general terms referring to substances that assist the body with removing waste material from the circulatory system and getting it processed and excreted by the liver, kidneys, and large intestine. Another term used to describe such herbs is *alterative*.)

Chaparral tastes *very* bad. It has an unmistakable smell. A few hearty souls may use it as tea, but capsules are much better for most people. If you want to take it on a long-term basis as a general tonic, a couple of capsules a day is fine. If you're doing temporary cleansing and immune-boosting in an acute situation, you could take 5 to 10 capsules for a short-term time. To bring up T-4 counts with AIDS, aggressive treatment of 20 or more capsules a day is necessary. This must be done gradually, to bowel tolerance, as this dose can cause queasiness and loose stools.

(Caution: Chaparral has been a focus of controversy over its safety. See pages 489–490 for an analysis of this issue.)

Garlic

Garlic is one of the most well known, widely studied, reliable, and effective antibacterials. We have discussed it at length already. For acute infection, take deodorized capsules at 10 to 20 per day (unless you can down at least one or two bulbs, fresh, each day—as I have been known to do, garlic maniac that I am!). German health authorities have established the effective medicinal daily dose of allicin, an identified active antibacterial compound in garlic, as being that which is contained in about 4 grams of fresh garlic.[6]

Garlic can also be used effectively in combination with echinacea and/or goldenseal.

Other Antibacterials

Isatidis root, mentioned above under antivirals, is less well known for its antibacterial properties but functions well against both kinds of "bugs." Like goldenseal, it is bitter and cold, a common characteristic of many antibacterials. In acute situations it can be taken in the same doses as goldenseal capsules, described earlier on page 180.

Baical scullcap root is discussed elsewhere as a liver herb and for its anti-inflammatory properties, useful in allergy or arthritis treatment. It is also a good antibacterial. It is taken in capsules, up to 10 per day for acute bacterial infection.

Chinese violet leaf is another bitter, cold antibacterial that is particularly good for reducing heat and swellings, red swollen eyes, and sore throat. It is considered in Chinese medicine to have an affinity for sores and abrasions.

Bayberry root is an excellent choice when you have a cold or flu. This Ayurvedic herb is antibacterial, not antiviral, so it won't help you attack cold or flu "bugs" directly, but it may help prevent secondary bacterial infections (such as sinus). More importantly, it is pungent, astringent, and warming, thus controlling *kapha* energy (cold, wet, mucusy). An excellent warming and drying cold relief solution from Ayurveda is bayberry combined with cinnamon and ginger.

SYMPTOM SOOTHERS

The following will help relieve specific, acute symptoms, regardless of the type of infection.

Sinus Remedies

These are excellent upper respiratory remedies; many are appropriate for use as tonics as well as acute symptom relief.

Eyebright leaf is antimucus, astringent, anti-inflammatory, and excellent for sinusitis; it's especially good combined with goldenseal for sinus-membrane rejuvenation. Eyebright tea can be taken up to 1 ounce per day for tonic purposes and up to 2 ounces for acute conditions.

Yerba santa leaf is a Southwest desert herb that's somewhat greasy, and extra good when you have sticky, goopy, thick congestion. Up to 2 ounces per day as tea for acute conditions.

Honeysuckle flower has an affinity for lungs as well as sinuses, so it's a good choice when you have stuffy nose and cough. It's also a mild relaxant, a fever-cooler, and reduces swelling and inflammation. Up to 1 ounce as tea daily as a tonic; for acute conditions, up to 2 ounces.

Rose hip has an affinity for sinus tissue as a builder and tissue healer; it's also a source of vitamin C and bioflavonoids. In addition to tea (1 ounce as tonic, 2 ounces acute) it can be taken as capsules (2 to 5 daily) or in a paste that is commercially available (1/4 teaspoon).

Elder flower has an affinity for the head area, so it's good for sore throat or sinus congestion; it's also cooling and reduces fever. As a tonic, take up to 1 ounce as tea daily; for acute conditions, up to 2 ounces.

Chinese chrysanthemum flower is a cooling anti-inflammatory that makes a tasty beverage tea and has special affinity for upper respiratory tissue; it also lowers fever and relieves headache. As a tonic, take up to 1 ounce as tea daily; for acute conditions, up to 2 ounces.

Chinese magnolia flower releases respiratory mucus, reduces nasal congestion, and is warming. Up to 1 ounce as tea per day as tonic; up to 2 ounces for acute conditions.

Boneset leaf is a Native American herb that gets its name from the disease it was used to remedy, an epidemic flu so strong that the muscle contractions it caused broke people's bones ("breakbone fever"). This tea would relax the contractions. It's a cooling upper-respiratory remedy, eases aches and pains, lowers fever, and is antiviral, so it's ideal for cold and flu. While it was trendy in the past and is still widely available, it hasn't yet been "rediscovered" and is quite economical. Boneset can be taken at a dose of 1 to 2 ounces as tea daily for acute conditions.

Ma huang (ephedra) is a classic Chinese herb that works both as a nasal decongestant and bronchial dilator for asthma. Psuedoephedrine, the active ingredient in OTC decongestants like Sudafed, was synthesized from this herb's alkaloid compounds. It can be taken as a tea or used in capsule form. Begin carefully, as it can be very energizing, and increase the dose gradually to your personal comfort. Try 1 to 3 tablespoons a day of crushed herb made into tea.

Nettle leaf is another excellent remedy for respiratory symptoms, and works especially well as a natural antihistamine and for hives. A nourishing blood cleanser (alterative), it also helps clear clogged lymph nodes. When dried, the sting is neutralized, and it can be made into a very drinkable tea (which smells like grass clippings).

There are two ways that nettle can be used as a respiratory remedy. The method of drying determines the use. The usual method of shade-drying nettles neutralizes the antihistamine properties, but it is still effective for other types of respiratory issues (including lung). To get the antihistamine effect, nettles must be freeze-dried or otherwise specially processed. There are no side effects when using nettles in this way—no drowsiness, for example. It may take five 300-milligram capsules all at once to suppress symptoms. For other purposes, nettle can be taken as tea (up to 2 ounces daily for acute conditions or 1 ounce as a tonic), or steamed like a vegetable.

Watercress is a sinus-tissue healer; it also provides bioflavonoids and sulfur for immune building and blood cleansing. Take 2 to 4 capsules daily.

Lemon grass is yet another herb with affinity for sinus tissue; again, 2 to 4 capsules daily.

Tulsi, an Ayurvedic herb, is a species of basil; it means "holy basil" in Sanskrit. In addition to drying up mucus in sinuses and lungs, it is antiviral, promotes sweating, and treats fever, making it another ideal cold and flu remedy. (Other kinds of basil also have the same general effect.)

For sinus congestion, the following can be used as inhalants (sniff a small amount into nostrils): *onion powder, garlic powder, ginger, gotu kola powder, salt water,* or *glycerine.* (Most of these will cause you to sneeze.)

A paste made of ginger and water, or ginger and *eucalyptus* oil, can be topically applied to the skin over the sinus pain location. Eucalyptus oil or peppermint oil alone can also be used (they can be used full strength, but if you find them too strong, you can dilute using another oil or lotion).

Pulmonary (Lung) Herbs

The average dose for each of these lung tonics and remedies is 2 to 3 ounces of the herb daily for acute symptoms, or 1 ounce daily for building and tonifying, unless otherwise indicated.

Coltsfoot flower—This herb was used by Roman soldiers in ancient Europe. It's an excellent lung tonic, supporting the tissue of lungs and bronchi, and thus is useful for colds, flu, asthma, bronchitis, and pneumonia. It's a cooling expectorant, liquefies mucus, suppresses cough, and is also a long-term respiratory builder. It tastes reasonably good.

Elecampane root—European herbalists would probably call this their number-one lung tonic. It's warming for a cold, wet cough. It doesn't suppress the cough, but increases expectoration.

Ma huang—As mentioned above, this is also a sinus decongestant; dilates smooth muscles of the bronchi.

Ginger—Tea is the best form for coughs, and is faster, safer, and less expensive than the chemical expectorants found in OTC cough remedies. According to herb expert Rob McCaleb, the Chinese draw a distinction between the action of dried and fresh ginger for different conditions; either is okay for stomach conditions, but dried and powdered ginger is essential for coughs. The taste of ginger also stimulates secretions that help bronchial congestion, so capsules are not the best choice for coughs.[7]

Honeysuckle flower—A Chinese herb, mildly relaxing and cooling. Good for a cough accompanied by fever and anxious jitteriness. Use as tea as described above or take 5 capsules.

Yerba santa leaf—Spanish for "blessed herb," this Native American remedy is also good for sinus as mentioned above.

Mullein leaf—This lung tonic is also very good for the bladder (lungs and bladder share similar structure—both are big bags of moisture with mucous membrane lining).

Eyebright leaf—Very nourishing to lung tissue. It's astringent and dries up mucus, is anti-inflammatory to tissues, and can be combined with goldenseal for excellent membrane rejuvenation.

Nettle leaf (dried)—as mentioned earlier, an excellent lung tonic and nourishing blood cleanser. Up to 2 ounces for acute conditions, brewed as tea or eaten steamed.

Blue vervain leaf (also called *verbena*) has properties similar to nettles and is a relaxing antispasmodic and diaphoretic (induces sweating). It can be taken in the same forms and doses as nettles.

Irish moss is an expectorant and membrane soother (bronchi as well as digestive, so it's good for flu with cough and stomach upset). Take 1/2 to 1 ounce as tea.

Fenugreek seed is an expectorant and mucilaginous membrane soother.

Lemon balm (also called *Melissa*) is a mildly relaxing respiratory soother.

Turmeric—Traditionally used in Ayurveda as a respiratory herb, turmeric can reduce coughs, especially when mixed with *coriander* and *cumin*. (As an astringent and anti-inflammatory herb, turmeric is also effective as a gargle for sore throat and is especially good for severe sore throat with fever. Its anti-inflammatory and antibacterial properties make turmeric ideal for treating bronchitis.)

Hyssop leaf is cooling, loosens mucus, and is a demulcent (membrane soother), and is good for bronchitis.

Tummy Soothers

When flu or other viral illness involves stomach symptoms, you may not be able to eat much, if at all, or keep down your remedies.

Many people have their own special routine when experiencing stomach distress. My favorite is a popular and long-revered remedy: *ginger tea.* Fresh ginger root is great, but in a pinch I will use plain powdered ginger in boiling water, or in a hot cup of chamomile tea. I find this incredibly soothing. Ginger will help with gas, stomach pain, nausea, and vomiting.

An Ayurvedic remedy for intestinal distress as well as symptoms of nervousness is a spicy vegetable dish called *subzee*. It contains fragrant spices that are calming, soothing, warming, and good for digestion, as well as delicious: cinnamon, nutmeg, cardamom, and cloves as well as garlic and onion. The recipe is on page 501. The spices can also be used singly or in any combination to make a tea.

Slippery elm bark, powdered and mixed with water to make a gruel, is a good throat and respiratory as well as stomach soother.

Peppermint leaf is a good, cooling stomach soother. It relieves pain and can help with nausea. It's also antispasmodic.

Meadowsweet leaf soothes and protects stomach membranes, and relieves nausea and pain.

Other Symptom Soothers

Chinese notopterygii root, a bitter warm herb, couldn't have been better designed for calming flu symptoms: It reduces pain, fever, chills, headache, body aches, and pains. Up to 10 capsules a day can be taken for acute conditions.

WHEN INFECTIONS REQUIRE MEDICAL CARE

Natural healing has become so sophisticated that it can effectively treat almost any infectious disease. However, if you are going to use botanicals to deal with very serious infections, you do need to know what you're doing or have the assistance of a natural health professional. If you have something you want to treat on your own, be careful that you go into it conservatively and do whatever you might otherwise normally do if it's not responding. *You do not want to let infections go without being treated effectively.* Don't experiment at the expense of your own health or life. If anything feels or seems dangerous, seek medical attention.

Kidney infection, for example, is not something to play around with, and if you suspect you have one, unless you have experience successfully self-treating it, it can become serious very fast and damage your kidneys. It's not that such an infection can't be treated herbally—it can be and has been. But you need to know exactly how to do it, and you need to be certain that your infection and your general health are at such a point where treatment can be carried out quickly enough to be safe. And you need to have enough experience—or, preferably, your natural health practitioner does—in order to dose the right substances properly to produce safe, fast results.

But if it's not urgent—if it's a cold or fungus or stye in your eye, something you've had a million times before and you know it will go away eventually but will just be miserable until it does—try some of the herbs indicated for the condition and see if they work. Often you will find that the response is greater than it was to drugs and other methods that had ceased to work for you anyway.

8

Especially for Women: Natural Healing for a Woman's Lifetime

n terms of self-care, there are botanicals and nutrients that are especially suited to a woman's body and the achievement of glowing health. There are safe, natural, and effective alternatives for dealing with PMS, yeast infections, menopause, and ovarian and uterine conditions as well for dramatically increasing the odds for a comfortable and trouble-free pregnancy.

BASICS FOR WOMEN

Foods

In addition to a balanced whole-foods diet as we have described earlier, there are special foods that are particularly nourishing or tonifying for women.

Eggplant is known as "God's ovaries" in Ayurveda, and Karta Purkh learned about eggplant for women from his Ayurvedic teacher, Yogi Bhajan. It's a warming circulation enhancer, excellent for physiologically "cold" women. In Karta Purkh's experience this is the single greatest food for women's healing (and it worked tremendously well for me personally). Eggplant has not been studied for this purpose as far as we know, so the mechanism is unclear, but eggplant may contain phytosterols (steroidlike plant compounds which may mimic or act as precursors to sex hormones) like those being discovered in many other foods now.

Ginger, onion, and *garlic* are all hormone-enhancing, circulation-enhancing tonic foods, covered earlier on pages 146–148.

Flaxseed, olive, sesame, and *almond oils* are good oils that go into formation of helpful hormones and hormonal messenger molecules. Flaxseed is an exceptionally rich source of lignans, phytochemical hormone precursors.

Celery has two different uses for women. The vegetable (best juiced) is relaxant, anti-inflammatory, and anti-irritant, so it may be useful for anxiety and PMS. The celery seeds contain phytosterols and are estrogenic, as are many other seeds in this family, including *fennel.*

Parsley and its juice are especially good for the kidney and help reduce water retention (edema).

Watercress is another good kidney food as well as immune booster and cancer fighter.

Sage is a hormone-balancing spice that contains phytosterols. It should not be used for breast-feeding women because it dries up breast milk, but can be useful for reducing lactation when a woman initially stops breast-feeding.

Herbs/Teas

Here are general female tonics from various cultures. Their actions are similar; they either contain phytosterols that act as "hormone food" or they increase utilization of existing estrogen. All are generally balancing in action. Although some may favor estrogen or progesterone, these are all tonics in that they will push processes toward "center" or "normal"—slow fast cycles or speed slow cycles, decrease or increase bleeding as necessary, and so on.

A typical maintenance dose for any of these would be 1 to 5 capsules a day or 1/4 ounce as tea (where applicable). Larger doses are required for acute conditions, such as 10 to 15 capsules per day, or 1 to 2 ounces as tea.

Red raspberry leaf—Women around the world value red raspberry leaf as a general hormone balancer. It is very mild and is best used as a tea.

Dong quai—Chinese medicine's premier women's tonic is discussed on pages 142–143. (See "Tonic Herbs.") Over a lifetime, a woman could take 1 or 2 capsules a day as a tonic. It is believed to favor the estrogen cycle. It is *not* to be used during pregnancy.

Wild yam—This herb comes from Mexico, although it also has grown in the southeast United States and Appalachia. It is part of the yam family, and some of its constituents were used to synthesize birth-control pills and steroid drugs. It is believed to be progesteronic (supportive of the body's progesterone cycle) but is a useful tonic for a variety of women's conditions. (Note: despite myths to the contrary, wild yam has no progesterone in it, though it does contain steroid precursors. "Wild yam creams" often actually produce results through so-called "natural progesterone," which is actually a chemically altered substance made to match human progesterone. Check the label carefully!)

Black cohosh root—This excellent Native American tonic is widely used to prepare the uterus for pregnancy. It is reputed to soften the cervix and strengthen the uterus for better contractions. It is *not* to be used during pregnancy, except near labor to make delivery easier, under the advice of a practitioner. This is actually a good glandular tonic for both men and women (see page 286).

Chasteberry—This is the main female tonic in European herbal medicine, used for a wide variety of conditions as well as general tonifying. It's excellent for PMS (we'll get to details on this shortly).

Partridgeberry leaf—This herb is sometimes called squaw vine, but it shouldn't be; this is a racial slur against Native Americans. Unfortunately, that's the name under which you may find it. It makes a reasonably good-tasting tea. It relaxes the uterus and reduces abdominal irritation.

Schizandra berry—We discussed this herb in the "Noteworthy Tonics" section, in Chapter 6 (pages 144–145) since it is good for both men and women, but it's very balancing for female hormones used long term, a sort of "junior dong quai." It makes a tangy, refreshing tea (from dried berries) or can be purchased in capsules.

Shatavari root—This Ayurvedic herb from the asparagus family means "hundred lovers" in Sanskrit. The premier herb for women in Ayurveda, shatavari is similar to dong quai in its action and effects, but is not a "connoisseur herb" like dong quai, so it's not as expensive. (It's extremely inexpensive in India.) It's only just started to appear in herb stores here, but is likely to become more and more available. Shatavari is also a blood tonic and builder, increases milk production, and is demulcent (soothes mucous membrane). It's especially good for *pitta* (fire) types.

Chinese three edge root and **Chinese ox knee root**—Both are general female hormone regulators and treat amenorrhea (absence of menses) and dysmenorrhea (painful menstruation).

False unicorn root—A general glandular tonic with hormone precursors. This herb is so outrageously expensive that it's impractical. Any of the others above will work just as well and be more economical.

MENSTRUAL ISSUES

Undesirable menstrual symptoms indicate underlying health problems, and successful treatment must restore overall health in addition to eliminating these discomforts. Usually, women want and need immediate relief, even as they work on the underlying long-term imbalances. Fortunately, there are herbs you can use to obtain short-term relief almost instantly, as well as to initiate or accelerate healing.

The long-term treatment for *all* of the issues below is lifestyle-based—the diet, exercise, and supplementation we have already discussed, including use of the long-term women's tonics outlined above. From an energy perspective, women have "extra organs" clustered in the pelvic region and it is desirable to increase circulation through that area. In both Ayurvedic and Chinese medicine, most women's health problems go along with "cold, stagnant blood" in the pelvis. The tonics can help in that area.

Cycles

In Ayurveda, the proper length of a woman's cycle is considered to be 29½ days, the length of the moon cycle. Anything beyond slightly more or less is considered undesirable, an indicator of imbalance. Herbs and nutrients can be used to shorten or lengthen a cycle.

For a short cycle, herbs with cooling energetics are used to slow things down. Red raspberry leaf tea is relaxant, cooling, and reduces "squeezing." Calcium and/or magnesium would also have the same effect.

For a long cycle, warming herbs that promote contraction are used. (Be sure you are not pregnant before using these herbs.) **Blue cohosh root** is the queen of these. Blue cohosh is unrelated to black cohosh; cohosh means "root" in the languages of the Native American tribes that used these herbs. They are two different plants in which the root is utilized.

Blue cohosh, unlike black cohosh, is not a long-term tonic. But it is a source of hormone precursors and will virtually always initiate menstruation. Capsules are best; blue cohosh's solubility in alcohol for the purpose of tinctures is not great, and as a tea this herb would irritate the throat. Seven to 8 capsules a day appears to be the dose at which most women will begin a period (within days).

Pennyroyal leaf is in the mint family and makes a good-tasting tea. It's milder than blue cohosh, but can be taken in capsules also—you might need to take a few more than blue cohosh. Note: We are not talking about pennyroyal essential oil, which women have reportedly used to induce abortions. We do *not* recommend this practice.

Alfalfa leaf is rich in phytosterols and believed to be estrogenic. It's very mild, so the challenge is to get enough in. A "solid extract" concentrate from the leaf is available in jars—take 1/4 teaspoon daily.

Excessive Bleeding

Herbs can be used in situations where bleeding is continuing for too long, such as at the start of menopause when hormones get wacky and cause bleeding for several weeks, or with a period that won't quit.

Shepherd's purse leaf tea has a long history as a universal remedy for this problem. It is extremely effective—it will work in hours or even minutes. Use 1/4 ounce or 1/2 ounce brewed as the tea. It tastes horrible, but slug it down and the reward will be quick.

Red raspberry leaf is astringent and promotes drying, but it's much milder than shepherd's purse, so the dose needs to be much higher to get anything done. Three ounces of herb-brewed tea per day would be the minimum for this purpose in most cases.

Cranesbill root, another astringent herb, could be taken in a dose of 10 to 15 capsules per day until symptoms respond, and *turmeric* is a classic astringent herb that is excellent to stop bleeding or any other kind of "leaking." Turmeric can be taken in capsules or as a paste with various uses (see recipe on page 497).

Cramps or Painful Periods (Dysmenorrhea)

Menstrual cramps, or dysmenorrhea, plague many women. The pain for some women is so severe that it interferes with normal daily functioning. Like PMS, it is extremely treatable with gentle, natural herbs.

Menstrual cramps can be relaxed like any other muscle cramp. Some of the best remedies are:

Calcium and/or *magnesium*—A glass of warm milk can do the trick if you don't have supplements handy. 1,500 milligrams of either of these (or both in a 2:1 ratio of calcium:magnesium) works well.

Cinnamon may be the best home remedy for cramps there is. Karta Purkh has talked to women who said they suffered with severe cramps for twenty years or more and the first month they used cinnamon it knocked the problem flat, and they never suffered again. Cinnamon is a circulation enhancer generally, but it increases circulation preferentially to the uterus and to the joints. (It's also an excellent antidiarrheal and antibleeding remedy, though for some reason it doesn't appear to curb menstrual bleeding.)

Cinnamon can be used in liberal amounts in tea and in food, though this alone will probably not be therapeutic for this condition. To be effective for menstrual cramps, it's important to get enough in fast enough—12 to 15 capsules a day is usually necessary and it works best if you start intake before the period actually arrives. If you know when it's coming, you can start the dose a day or two before to get the body saturated with it. You may need to take the dose up through the first and possibly the second day of the period.

It's much better if you can get medicinal-quality cinnamon at an herb pharmacy than the stuff in the spice aisle at the grocery store, but that will do in a pinch. Fill "00" size capsules purchased at an herb or health-food store.

It may take a couple of cycles to figure out the best time to begin "cinnamon therapy." If your period is totally unpredictable, you may need to start well in advance—and that's fine; cinnamon won't hurt you. Start with lower doses and work up until you know how many capsules will have the effect.

Cramp bark, a Native American herb used as tea (it's too spongy for capsules), has a reputation for effectiveness with this condition, as is obvious from the name. It's a remedy that is fast and strong enough to use on the day that the cramps are actually happening. One ounce per day brewed as tea should be effective, but more can be used as needed. *Black haw bark* is a close relative of cramp bark that may be substituted.

Red raspberry leaf is an excellent mild uterine relaxant.

Dong quai, even if not being used long term as a tonic, can relieve cramps on a short-term basis.

Black cohosh and *wild yam* are best to resolve this issue long term.

Willow bark and/or *cinchona bark* basically relieve the pain.

PMS

For millions of American women, the words *premenstrual syndrome* describes a monthly torture that makes them dread each new turn of the calendar. Premenstrual syndrome, or PMS, can refer to any of a diverse range of possible symptoms. Essentially, though, it is a condition of hormone imbalance that produces discomfort during the time immediately preceding the woman's menstrual period. Depending on the individual woman and her condition (including such factors as overall health, age, diet, and family history), PMS can last for one day or for up to two weeks before menstruation.

Sometime after midcycle ovulation, from fourteen days to a week or less before the period, PMS symptoms gradually make themselves known. Obviously, every woman experiences her own unique set of symptoms, but the periodicity makes it a syndrome (a nonspecific collection of commonly experienced symptoms). Physical symptoms of PMS can include abdominal pressure, nausea, headache, bloating, water retention (edema), fever, and fatigue.

Most women, however, find the emotional symptoms to be the most distressing and disruptive: crying, depression, anger, irritability, mood swings, and a feeling of wanting to "jump out of the skin." If these symptoms gradually increase until menstruation, and are relieved when the period arrives, it's PMS.

It is certainly normal for a woman to feel characteristically different at different times during the monthly cycle. However, from the perspective of natural healing, at no time during the month does a woman need to feel the slightest lack of health and vitality—let alone the outright suffering that many women experience. PMS and menstrual cramps can be two of the most disruptive conditions a woman experiences in her life, and it is heartbreaking that anyone ever has to suffer so terribly and so needlessly, because they are some of the easiest conditions to treat herbally.

There is such an abundance of natural remedies available to deal with the causes and symptoms of PMS that it is also a shame to find pharmaceuticals being routinely prescribed in many cases of PMS. The antidepressant drug Prozac is often prescribed for PMS-related irritability and anxiety. Xanax, a tranquilizer, is also used to treat the emotional symptoms of PMS as well as some physical symptoms like headaches and insomnia.

Pharmaceutical drugs with side effects and the risk of dependency are usually completely unnecessary. Frequently, these drugs are prescribed without even trying simpler, safer remedies or even dietary changes.

Karta Purkh has seen literally hundreds of women triumph over previously debilitating monthly PMS, simply through changes in lifestyle and sometimes with support from herbs as well. Some of these women have had PMS for twenty or thirty years, and the very first month they try herbal remedies, they find their symptoms can be completely controlled—safely and easily.

Feeling Better Premenstrually

This is our standard disclaimer, but even before you consider using herbs to treat these symptoms, take a hard look at your lifestyle and how it may be influencing your condition. In the case of PMS, countless women have found relief simply by eating a high-complex-carbohydrate, low-fat diet; eliminating sugar and caffeine; and exercising regularly. Because these factors, along with a variety of nutrients, repeatedly prove effective, PMS is increasingly considered to be simply one of many manifestations of the body-unfriendly "American way"—an inevitable outcome of being inactive, stressed, or undernourished.

This handful of lifestyle basics goes a long way toward lessening PMS symptoms; if you have not already made such changes, you'll be fighting an uphill battle even with herbs. These were the first steps I took toward improving this condition close to ten years ago, and even then they made the difference between unbearable and tolerable.

Once you have set the stage for healing through healthy diet and exercise, try these remedies to eradicate the last vestiges of PMS from your life.

The Chinese herb *ephedra (ma huang)* is excellent for water retention and also provides an energy boost. (Please see pages 483–487 for more detailed discussion of this herb and related issues and cautions.) Also good for reducing water retention are *potassium* (most come as 99-milligram tablets; about 500 milligrams is an average dose), *mullein leaf* tea, *parsley* (juiced), and *cornsilk* (the stringy material you pull off the ear of corn when you shuck it, which is dried and made into a tea that's an excellent kidney and bladder tonic).

Premenstrual fatigue can be treated with *kola nut* (or any of the other herbal energizers discussed later in Chapter 11, "Energizing Herbs").

Premenstrual depression can be treated short term using the same herbal depression protocols described later, on pages 291–294. A 100-milligram **B-complex**, plus extra B_6 and B_{12}, can be especially beneficial, as can **vitamin E** and **manganese**. GLA-containing fatty acid supplements such as **evening primrose, borage oil**, or **black currant oil** are also useful with depression, and studies have found them to be effective with PMS specifically.

Chasteberry (*Vitex agnus castus*), an herb relatively new to American herbology but widely used in Europe, is showing powerful effects in treating PMS. It may be the most effective single PMS remedy for nearly every type of symptom.

Originally used by a group of nuns in Europe who used it successfully to treat women's problems (hence the name), the berry of the chaste tree has become very popular for treating women's hormonal and reproductive discomforts from menstruation to menopause—and with good reason. As a tonic, it will influence body processes back to "center," or normal balance, regardless of which direction the imbalance has taken. As a result, chasteberry exhibits a wide range of activity that both relieves symptoms and regulates glandular function long term.

Chasteberry is primarily progesteronic. It helps your body increase its own progesterone production through pituitary support, rather than taking synthetic progesterone orally as is conventionally prescribed for moderate to severe cases of PMS. It increases progesterone production by stimulating the pituitary to release one hormone (luteinizing hormone) and inhibit another (follicle-stimulating hormone). Since a low progesterone-to-estrogen ratio is responsible for many PMS symptoms, especially the emotional and mood-related ones, an increase in progesterone relative to estrogen relieves many of these symptoms.

Chasteberry also inhibits prolactin, and elevated prolactin is usually associated with amenorrhea as well as PMS.[1] Finally, chasteberry appears to be sedative and antispasmodic, something many PMS and menstrual discomfort sufferers can use a little of. Studies have shown that chasteberry can stimulate lactation as well. There are many studies confirming that chasteberry produces PMS relief, menopausal relief, and increase in lactation with no hazard to nursing infants, according to Herb Research Foundation president Rob McCaleb.[2]

While chasteberry can relieve many of the immediate symptoms of

PMS, particularly depression, anxiety, moodiness, and sleeplessness, it can take six months to a year to see long-term permanent changes (where you experience improvement even after you stop taking the herb).

Chasteberry alone can be taken in a dose of 2 to 8 capsules per day. The tea is not bad (dose would be 1/2 ounce per day). We recommend these two forms, though it's also available in tinctures and extracts (we recommend full herbal extracts—see pages 466–469 for a discussion of extracts).

A great combination for a wide range of PMS symptoms use three herbs: *fo-ti root (polygonum), wild yam,* and *blue cohosh.* The capsules should be made in the following combination: three parts fo-ti, two parts wild yam, and one part blue cohosh. Take the capsules as soon as you begin to feel premenstrual problems, possibly midway through the cycle or a little after. Divide the doses throughout the day. Try 1 or 2 capsules in the morning and 1 or 2 in the evening. If symptoms continue, add another. Gradually increase the dose, as necessary, over that 10-day to 2-week period of PMS as the symptoms escalate. A typical dose would start with a couple of capsules, working up to a high of 8 to 12 on the worst day (usually the day before the period starts).

The nice thing about this particular remedy is that it has both short-term and long-term action. Initially it treats the symptoms, such as moodiness and bloating (that's mostly the blue cohosh). The wild yam and fo-ti are longer-term builders, and this routine will stabilize the hormone levels month after month, so that you find you need less and less to achieve relief. Within a year or so, you may find that you are maintaining hormonal balance sufficiently on your own to experience few or no symptoms even when you stop taking the herb.

Ginger can be added to the formula also to increase blood circulation. Like cinnamon, ginger is preferential to the uterus and joints.

Celery juice is an excellent relaxant and can be used in quantities of 1 pint to 1 quart per day during PMS time for irritability and anger. *Valerian root* can be used for this purpose too (see section on relaxant herbs, pages 304–309, for still more suggestions).

The minerals *calcium* and *magnesium* can be especially helpful in cases with pain and anxiety. Many studies suggest that marginal magnesium deficiency is a possible cause of PMS. A processed diet, with high intake of sugar and other refined carbohydrates, is often partly to blame, since magnesium is stripped from grains in the refining process. This may be one of many reasons why women who eat processed, simple-carbo diets have worse PMS, and feel better when they replace sugars with wholesome complex carbohydrates from grains, legumes, vegetables, and fruits.

Chocolate cravings may be due partly to chocolate's high magnesium content, but chocolate candy is not the best choice to solve that problem because of its fat and sugar. If you must have chocolate, try unsweetened cocoa powder mixed into yogurt or a blender drink. If you feel up to trying an alternative that gets you away from chocolate completely, chilies contain magnesium (they're Ayurveda's top chocolate-craving remedy), and chilies also increase endorphins, which can be helpful with moodiness.

Amenorrhea

Amenorrhea is the absence of menses. It can occur for many reasons: stress, extremely low body fat, poor nutrition, or the use of hormones or drugs that throw the body's natural hormonal rhythms out of whack.

The menses are a cycle that is dictated by the rise and fall of certain hormone levels. If these hormones are not produced in the appropriate amounts or ratios to one another and at the right times, the building up or sloughing off of the uterine lining does not occur. From the onset of menstruation through ovulation, estrogen is on the rise. At ovulation, when the egg drops down from the ovary and is available for fertilization, estrogen should drop and progesterone should rise.

Anything that interrupts, interferes with, or changes this precision-tuned hormonal relay can cause missed periods (as well as other PMS symptoms). However, some of the things traditionally thought to cause amenorrhea would not necessarily do so if the body were well nourished.

For example, it's assumed that high-performance athletes with extremely low body fat (less than 15 percent) should expect to cease having menstrual periods. This is not necessarily the case. Often, it's the burden of the strenuous activity that created the physique—not the physique itself—that shocks the body out of its routine. A well-fed, well-supplemented athletic woman can have extremely high muscle mass and low body fat and still have normal periods if she eats and supplements specifically to compensate for the stresses of training, and to "refill" what's depleted.

There are a number of herbs and foods that naturally bring these hormones back into adjustment and stimulate menses to occur. Some of them are tonics that are useful for a wide range of menstrual and premenstrual discomforts, and tend to maintain existing balance as well as restore it when it's "off." In other words, if you're menstruating they make it work better, and if you're not they make it work better.

Other herbs are specifically indicated for absence of menses. Many of the herbs that relieve PMS symptoms also show up on this list, because an herb's ability to enhance the progesterone period of the menstrual cycle will often stimulate the onset of menses as well as eliminate premenstrual tension.

Eggplant is considered in Ayurveda the most potent of all foods for feeding and supporting a woman's glandular systems and hormonal processes. For amenorrhea, it needs to be eaten regularly—half of an eggplant daily—to produce results.

Chasteberry pops up again as a standout herb for restoring regularity to the menstrual cycle. Because chasteberry is progesteronic, it's especially good for amenorrhea that is due to low levels of progesterone (since progesterone is the hormone that rises in the second half of the cycle to signal the shoughing of the uterine lining). Take 5 to 10 capsules per day.

Wild yam is also progesteronic and can help this condition. Take 5 to 10 capsules per day.

Blue cohosh, again, is superb for initiating menstruation, though in the case of long-term amenorrhea it cannot be expected to work as quickly as it will when simply trying to shorten a long cycle. Six or 7 capsules, divided throughout the day with food, will usually produce results expediently.

Motherwort leaf, mugwort leaf, and *cramp bark* can all stimulate menses, even though they may be better known for their ability to relieve cramps in an already menstruating woman. They are especially good used in combination. **Chinese rhubarb root** is yet another good amenorrhea remedy.

Any of the other general glandular tonics listed earlier would eventually work too, though perhaps not as quickly.

As I mentioned earlier, when I first took a class with Karta Purkh I had not menstruated for over two years and had been offered all sorts of synthetic and invasive conventional treatments (ranging from hormone replacement to exploratory surgery), which I instinctively declined. The periods had ended after I stopped taking birth-control pills at the age of twenty-two. Obviously, pulling the plug on the artificial hormone regulation that had crutched my system for several years was a shock. Worse, I pulled that plug in a maximum-stress environment: the end of a six-year relationship, a ninety-hour-a-week job, undereating, and overexercising. I lived on caffeine and doughnuts, and I broke my foot while running about a month later. I wasn't having a great time, and my body knew it.

By the time I met Karta Purkh, my life was much healthier and so was my body, but the amenorrhea remained as a legacy of my former abuse. Based on what I learned, I worked on several levels: tonics to nourish the female reproductive system directly, shorter-term kick-starters, and heat (my basal body temperature was hovering around 95°!). I ate half an eggplant every day, grilled under the oven broiler with tomato sauce and lots of garlic. (No, I don't like eggplant.) I ate at least a bulb of garlic daily. I took schizandra, chasteberry, and blue cohosh (though I admit I was not consistent with the blue cohosh because it made me queasy; had I been, I might have gotten results even faster). I also sat in a hot tub daily for half an hour.

Two months later, I had my first period in 2½ years. I had periods every sixty to seventy days for the first four to five months. During the next four to five months, my cycle settled between forty and fifty days apart. At that point, I stopped taking the herbs but continued eating eggplant several times a week. By the following year, I was menstruating every twenty-nine to thirty-five days. I stopped taking all of the herbs and foods, and my cycle eventually stabilized at about thirty-two days (with a fraction of the PMS I'd had before the amenorrhea, incidentally). I now have a perfect twenty-nine-day cycle: I ovulate exactly fifteen days from the first day of my cycle and menstruate exactly fourteen days after that. I never did need synthetic hormones, drugs, or exploratory surgery.

> Caution: Women who are pregnant or intending to conceive in the near future—six months or less—should not take herbs that induce menses. In high quantities they may be abortive. In addition, we do not recommend using herbs to attempt to induce abortion.

Endometriosis

Endometriosis is characterized by the growth of uterine (endometrial) tissue outside the uterine cavity. It is common in excessive estrogen environments, and excessive cramping and bleeding are typical. The tissue can grow into the abdominal cavity, causing digestive symptoms or even affecting the bladder or lungs. More commonly it grows onto fallopian tubes and ovaries. It appears to be sustained by female hormones but not necessarily activated by them. IUDs aggravate it. The conventional treatment is drugs and sometimes surgery.

Natural medicine is successful at treating this condition, so you should have hope. Generally, herbal treatment for endometriosis includes herbs to promote hormone balance and astringent herbs to dry up tissue, draw back tissue building, and reduce bleeding. However, this condition is too complex to self-treat. You should seek the guidance of a natural health practitioner who has had experience in treating this condition holistically.

PREGNANCY

Herbal health enhancement for pregnancy ideally begins before conception, and should be undertaken by both male and female to ensure the optimum environment for the growing child. A healthy hormonal balance and reproductive system are crucial to a healthy pregnancy, and can be reached and maintained with the help of herbs.

Pregnancy can be one of the happiest, most exciting, and healthiest times in a woman's life. However, the many physical changes that are inherent in pregnancy can be stressful to a body that is already drained or poorly cared for, driving imbalances further awry and creating larger health deficits. The child may also suffer as a result of developing in an environment of scarcity.

As we have already discussed, the stresses of American life, including unhealthy food, overwork, lack of sleep, overstimulation, under- or overexercising, toxins, and so on can interrupt and unbalance our systems, including the reproductive system. Ideally, a couple preparing to conceive would take at least a year to get the diet in order (go back to pages 107–117 for the basics) and use general glandular tonics to ensure that the body is functioning in balance.

Attitudes about pregnancy can also color a woman's experience of this time. The way we deal with pregnancy here is considered very crude by other cultures. We treat it like a sickness requiring medical treatment. A great deal of fear is fostered by the Western approach to pregnancy and delivery. Such a natural, joyous experience—borne by women the world over for millennia without "birthing suites"—in the last century became a condition requiring routine hospitalization, and midwifery became "alternative." Why do we go to the hospital to have babies: Are we ill?

I have had no children, but I have witnessed pregnancies and births among a number of friends, and my observations have been very consistent. The mothers who ate carelessly and were in a general, low-grade state of un-health were troubled by numerous discomforts during pregnancy and had difficult births; those who ate a healthy diet and were in good condition had minimal to no discomfort or complications.

When Karta Purkh's wife was pregnant with their daughter, now four, the attending midwives constantly marveled, "We've never seen a pregnancy like this. We've heard about them, but we've never seen one." She simply experienced *no negative symptoms whatsoever. Ever*. This need not be a "lucky fluke." You too can minimize or even eliminate many of the supposedly inevitable discomforts of pregnancy.

Morning Sickness

The nausea that some women experience in early pregnancy is much less prevalent in other cultures. Morning sickness is an accumulated-waste issue. Mom's body is dealing not only with her own toxins but with the wastes of the fetus, and that new added load pushes the already stressed liver over the edge. It can't process it all, and the circulating waste causes symptoms. So does hormonal imbalance (the liver processes hormones too). Being generally and genuinely healthy is the best prevention for morning sickness.

To treat morning sickness symptomatically, ginger is a standout remedy. Ginger has been extensively studied for nausea, including morning sickness specifically, and beats just about any drug that goes up against it. Many women have used it safely and effectively for this purpose, both here and in other cultures traditionally.

Some health professionals and herb books caution against ginger use during pregnancy, probably because the monograph on ginger from Commission E, the health agency of the German government, recommends women not use ginger during pregnancy. However, other natural health professionals recommend it without reservation.

It is pointed out in an article in *HerbalGram* (No. 38, Fall 1996) that no scientific or medical references explaining the caution accompany the Commission E monograph; that as a food and spice ginger has been used in substantial amounts from childhood on by millions throughout human history with no toxicity; that millions of pregnant women in other cultures consume large quantities of ginger without any adverse effects; and that other than the Commission E monograph, no other health authority or medical body recommends avoiding ginger during pregnancy.[3] No studies in the literature nor clinical observations report adverse effects.[4] Further, Commission E monographs give the same caution about most other herbs as well, and the ginger monograph itself states "no adverse effects."[5]

At any rate, low doses can be very effective; many women get results from a couple of capsules or from sipping some tea throughout the day. Most practitioners who do recommend it suggest using only whole-plant preparations (either fresh or dried).

Keep in mind too that FDA-approved pharmaceuticals for treatment of nausea are all strong drugs with serious side effects that definitely cannot be used during pregnancy without harming the fetus. So in the case of severe morning sickness that is impairing normal function of the mother (hyperemesis gravidarum), ginger may be the best option.

We recommend not using any herbs during pregnancy except on the advice and monitoring of your own health practitioner. Consult your health professional first.

Vitamin B$_6$ has also been shown to be effective even at the basic 50 milligrams per day. Some natural health practitioners use higher doses; consult your own health professional.

Other Conditions

Other conditions related to pregnancy can also be treated very effectively through natural means. However, because each individual's pregnancy is unique and it can be an unpredictable time for a woman's health, we recommend you see a natural health practitioner to work out a plan for your pregnancy. We recommend that everyone avoid self-treating with herbs during pregnancy; use herbs during pregnancy only on the specific advice of, and under the guidance of, your own natural health practitioner.

Fertility Issues

Again, basic health is the first and most important step in dealing with infertility. Use of diet and general glandular tonics should first be undertaken if a couple is having trouble conceiving, especially if no work has been done in that area and they are consuming the standard American diet.

Specific issues related to infertility can be treated well using herbal medicine, but it is useful to know what the exact problem is. Suggestions for increasing the male's sperm motility (which studies show can be impaired by vitamin C or zinc deficiency, for example) will be different from suggestions for regulating the woman's cycle or preparing the uterus. This requires a diagnosis. If a medical examination can give you more information about the specific nature of the infertility, you can then decide how invasive or heroic you want to get, and if you wish, take your diagnosis to a natural health practitioner for views on natural alternatives.

MENOPAUSE

By the year 2020, about 60 million American women will be at or through menopause. It is a subject receiving a great deal of attention right now and one that is of great concern to many women as well as health professionals.

There are entire books out just dealing with the subject of menopause and how to handle it naturally. Several are listed in the "Recommended Reading" section for further reference. Here we will overview the chief issues that concern most women before and during menopause, and how herbal medicine and related natural healing methods can play a helpful role.

A New Outlook on Menopause

First and foremost, it might help to start with a viewpoint that may be considered radical by some: *Menopause is not a disease*. It is a time in a woman's life that can be as rewarding and fulfilling as any other. It is also a time of physiological changes, some of which can be uncomfortable. These discomforts are highly treatable with herbal medicine.

Well-known women's health physician and author Christiane Northrup, M.D., writes, "I believe menopause is a time when a woman's power, wisdom, and creativity pushes to the surface, calling for her attention. . . . We are being sold a bill of goods. Huge amounts of money are being made by hormone companies that frighten women into thinking that menopause requires a doctor's treatment. And many of those treatments . . . are based on dubious research. *Doctors have never studied a group of nonsymptomatic, healthy menopausal women.*"[6] (Emphasis added.)

Karta Purkh agrees, noting that in the cultures he has studied, menopause is a time of transition into "wisdomhood," when a woman becomes an even more respected member of society, a wise woman revered by her juniors. Thus we will heretofore call the physiological markers of menopause "characteristics" of this stage in life, rather than "symptoms," as if it were a sickness.

According to Dr. Michael Murray, N.D., women in traditional cultures do experience the same hormonal changes that American women do, yet they do not experience many menopausal discomforts, either physical or mental. Once again, the mind/body connection works its wonders. Diet probably also plays a role. Cultures that eat a primarily vegetarian diet experience fewer menopausal symptoms. The experience of women eating a plant-based diet in the United States corroborates this. Later in this section we will look at specific foods that cut the risks as well as the sometimes annoying physical hallmarks of menopause.

Another issue associated with the cultural view of menopause has to do with issues of youth and femininity. As Dr. Andrew Weil writes in his *Self Healing* newsletter, "there is an unstated selling point that is quite clear in pharmaceutical company advertisements: that it is a chemical fountain of youth offering persistent beauty, attractiveness, and satisfying sexuality in the face of advancing age. These claims are dismissable, because it is just as easy to find attractive, sexually fulfilled postmenopausal women who are not on ERT as who are on it."[7]

The bottom line, says Karta Purkh, is that without question a woman is going to feel different at this time in her life. At no time does she ever need to feel uncomfortable. If discomforts surface, they can be treated very quickly with mild herbs. Even better, if a woman prepares for menopause by eating well, taking general good care of herself, and using long-term glandular tonics well before menopause, the passing into this phase will be much smoother.

To Replace or Not to Replace?

That is *the* question facing millions of women before and at menopause. Hormone replacement therapy (HRT) involves ingestion of synthetic estrogen and progesterone. These are the two reproductive hormones whose levels drop sharply in women, usually beginning between the ages of about forty-five and fifty-five.

Replacing these hormones artificially to maintain premenopausal levels can reduce the discomforts that some women experience as the body adjusts to this change. Because estrogen also provides some protection against heart disease and osteoporosis—two conditions for which many American women may be at high risk, especially after menopause—HRT is often heralded as The Answer for menopausal women. Many women reportedly feel pressured by their doctors to take the hormones.

However, HRT is not the magic pill for bones, heart health, and hot flashes that it's been cracked up to be. With its protections (which many natural health practitioners feel are overhyped, since the conditions they protect against are preventable as well as treatable through natural means) come risks. Doctors who prescribe the therapy may be gung-ho about the benefits, but women should be absolutely clear about the risks—especially since diet, exercise, and natural therapies have been shown to offer many of the same benefits without the risks.

Increasingly, women are unwilling to assume these risks. According to *Health* magazine, only a third of menopausal women in the United States actually try hormone replacement and half of them eventually drop it.[8] Still, there are 10 million women every year opting to take the hormones, and that's big business. Wyeth-Ayerst's postmenopausal synthetic estrogen, Premarin, is the nation's best-selling prescription drug.[9]

Many women feel confused about the risks, and have a frustrating time deciding whether to choose HRT, because the reporting and interpretations of research present a typically conflicting and contradictory picture. We recommend that you research carefully and thoroughly when making this decision, ensuring that your information is coming from an impartial source.

It may be helpful to remember that women have been dealing with menopause in some way or another probably since women appeared on earth. Until the pharmaceutical boom in the middle of this century, women basically ignored it, didn't make a big deal out of it, or used botanical medicine for discomforts. There *was* life before HRT.

What You Can Do Regardless of Your Choice

There is no doubt that the decision to take or forgo HRT is a complex one. Either choice comes with both risks and benefits, and an evaluation should be made with full understanding of all those risks and benefits—preferably with the assistance of a well-informed, open-minded, and trusted health practitioner who will not pressure you either way.

Women who already have symptoms of either osteoporosis or cardiovascular disease at menopause should consider HRT. There are no botanicals that will rapidly reverse the negative effects of these conditions if you are already suffering from them, and you probably do need all the protection you can get. (That is why we want to encourage those who still have time to make changes premenopause and avoid these problems.)

If you do opt for HRT, make every effort to get the natural progesterone instead of the synthetic Provera, as this will reduce side effects and offer better protection against estrogen's risks. It is also very important to get regular gynecologic checkups and screenings for the various side effects and potentially serious illnesses that can result from the therapy. There are also lifestyle changes and herbal interventions that can help offset the increased risks you may experience as a result of taking the hormones. These are detailed below.

If you elect not to go with HRT, you can deal naturally with the characteristics of menopause that may cause discomfort, and there are a number of lifestyle changes that can be made to compensate for the loss of protections that estrogen once offered. For example, synthetic estrogen is hardly your only option for protection against heart disease! There are many ways to lower cholesterol and triglycerides with diet, lifestyle, and herbs. These are also discussed below.

Whether or not you opt for HRT, it is wise to seek the advice of a health practitioner who is interested and skilled in working with the full range of solutions for menopausal issues. Many women's health centers are beginning to offer integrated therapies, bringing together the services of medical gynecologists, naturopaths, herbalists, massage therapists, acupuncturists, nutritionists, homeopaths, and psychotherapists to offer a truly holistic approach to menopause.

Health Program for Women Taking HRT

If you do decide that your health condition warrants taking hormone replacement therapy, take heart. There are ways to address its side effects and possible risks—naturally.

First of all, make as many changes as you can that will improve the condition for which you are taking HRT. For example, if heart disease risk was the chief factor in your decision, make changes that will lower your risk of heart disease. The viability of this is now well established; if the actual disease can be reversed through lifestyle interventions, surely heart disease *risk* can be reversed!

Of course, stop smoking if you smoke. Adopt a low-fat, high-complex-carbohydrate, high-fiber diet. Begin exercising if you don't already. (*Body-Fueling*® has great basic information and guidance on making positive diet and exercise changes—and making them fun.) Also, the fat that remains in your diet should be from monounsaturates and omega-3 oils, which can actually lower LDL ("bad") cholesterol.

Combine these practices with herbs and nutrients that will help you lower serum cholesterol and reduce the oxidation of LDL cholesterol (which is partly responsible for the buildup on, and hardening of, artery walls). There are lots of natural ways to do this.

- Eating *garlic* lowers cholesterol levels, reduces oxidation of LDL cholesterol and reduces blood clotting.
- *Antioxidant vitamins* (A, C, E, and beta-carotene) will help reduce oxidation of LDL cholesterol.
- The Ayurvedic herb *guggul* (also called guggul gum or guggula), can be bought in capsules or as a powder to make capsules; it is extremely effective at lowering serum cholesterol.
- The B vitamin *folic acid* (400 milligrams daily) reduces levels of homocysteine, an amino acid that can injure blood vessels when it appears in very high levels in the blood, causing hardening of the arteries.
- To increase circulation, take *ginkgo*.
- To strengthen and steady the heartbeat, take a cardiotonic like *hawthorn berry* or *arjuna*.
- To lower blood pressure, try *hawthorn berry* or *arjuna* and *cayenne*, *garlic*, and *nutmeg*.

Secondly, integrate all of the anticancer practices and foods and nutrients into your life that you can, to offset any increased risk of breast or uterine cancer from the hormones. Anticancer strategies include:

- a moderately low-fat diet, eliminating saturated fats and favoring monounsaturated fats
- less or no smoking, alcohol, and drugs
- consumption of large amounts and wide variety of fruits and vegetables for the benefit of cancer-preventive phytochemicals
- supplementation with antioxidant vitamins and minerals, including carotenoids; vitamins A, C, and E; the mineral selenium
- use of long-term immune-enhancing herbal tonics such as astragalus and others described on pages 134–146
- use of female glandular tonics described at the start of this chapter

All of the above recommendations are healthy recommendations whether you are taking hormones or not.

If you can improve the high-risk condition that made HRT the right choice at first, you may later be able to discontinue taking the hormones without risk. (This can be done through *incremental dosage reduction* over a period of time, under the guidance of a health professional.)

Health Program for Menopausal Women Not Taking HRT

Lowering Your Risk of Heart Disease

Whether you take hormones or not, the bottom line is the same for heart health. See the recommendations above. If you are not taking the hormones, it will be even more important for you to pay attention to these guidelines. If you are healthy and fit and already living consistent with heart-healthy guidelines, you're fine, but adopting a few of those suggestions that may be new to you wouldn't hurt.

Preventing Osteoporosis Naturally

If you don't take HRT, you should eat as little animal protein as possible (a high-protein diet hastens demineralization of bones and "leaches" calcium from the body, and meat's sulfur-containing amino acids are especially damaging; in one study, eliminating meat cut urinary calcium losses in half). Sodium and caffeine also increase calcium excretion.

Smoking and alcohol are associated with bone loss; alcohol may actually destroy bone cells. Avoid processed foods and cola soft drinks; their phosphates can also cause calcium loss and excretion.

Get plenty of regular weight-bearing exercise (using large muscle groups—walking, running, skating, tennis, weightlifting, etc.)— the maximum you can comfortably and happily do.

Herbs for bone maintenance and mineralization include *nettle, alfalfa, slippery elm, oatstraw,* and *horsetail* (these latter two are sources of digestible silicon, a trace element crucial to building of bone and other tissue). *Algae* are a rich, broad-spectrum source of minerals as well.

Studies show that milk is *not* great for osteoporosis. In fact, the countries with highest osteoporosis rates are those that have the highest milk consumption. Absorption and retention, not intake, are the issues.

Loss of bone mass is typically caused by excessive calcium loss, not inadequate calcium intake, according to the Physicians Committee for Responsible Medicine (which has filed a complaint with the Federal Trade Commission against the popular "celebrity milk mustache" advertising campaign). And excessive calcium loss is linked to consumption of animal protein—such as milk.

Besides, a glass of carrot, parsley, spinach, or other green juice has twice the calcium of milk, without the fat or the protein. In fact, three glasses of carrot, parsley, or spinach juice exceeds the U.S. RDA for calcium (which is, at any rate, more than double the World Health Organization recommendation). Drink these juices and/or eat plenty of carrots, dark green vegetables, and seaweeds (sea vegetables). Soy products, sesame seeds, and molasses are all good sources as well.

You can take a calcium supplement, up to 1,500 milligrams daily, if you do feel your diet is not providing adequate calcium. Calcium hydroxyapatite is expensive, but the best. Calcium citrate is probably the best compromise—moderately priced and decently absorbed. (The carbonate form is antacid and, ironically, inhibits mineral absorption.) To support calcium absorption and metabolism, make sure you get adequate *zinc* (supplement up to 50 milligrams per day) and *mangesium* (take half the calcium dose). Also take 25,000 IU of *vitamin* A and 400 IU of *vitamin* D.

Boron has been shown to have a positive effect on calcium *and* active estrogen levels in postmenopausal women. One study showed that supplementation with 3 milligrams of boron daily reduced urinary calcium excretion by 44 percent, and increased estrogen levels. Another study on athletic college women showed that boron supplementation lowered serum phosphorus levels, and high phosphorus is another factor associated with osteoporosis.[10] Fruits, vegetables, and beans are the best natural sources of boron, which may help explain why vegetarian women have less osteoporosis (besides the lower protein content of a vegetarian diet).

Eat as many soy foods daily as you can manage. As we will discuss below, soy foods contain estrogenlike compounds that may offer protection against bone loss in the same way your own estrogen does.

Maximizing Continued Hormonal Activity

There are natural ways to keep as much estrogen available in the body as possible, and for as long as possible, and/or to increase estrogenlike activity.

Don't get too over-lean (meaning this is not the time in your life to try to look like Linda Hamilton in *Terminator II: Judgment Day*). Estrogen is stored in fat cells. (Note: this does not mean get fat!)

The liver processes estrogen, so take a mild liver tonic for general support. Liver tonics include burdock, yellow dock, dandelion, and others listed on pages 330–337.

Black cohosh (unrelated to blue cohosh) has been studied extensively and is probably the most well documented natural alternative to hormone replacement therapy (for example, in one article Dr. Michael Murray, N.D., cites five different studies in which black cohosh performed better than drugs or placebos[11]). It's the best-selling women's herbal product in Germany.[12]

Black cohosh lowers luteinizing hormone (LH), and increased LH production is believed to cause many menopausal discomforts. (When estrogen levels drop, the pituitary secretes more LH.) Black cohosh is effective for hot flashes, vaginal atrophy, night sweats, depression, anxiety, and lowered libido, among others.

Other herbs with estrogenic effects include *dong quai, burdock root, blue cohosh, Chinese ox knee root, Chinese three-edge root, sage, alfalfa concentrate*, and *motherwort*. All of these are especially good for hot flashes; blue cohosh is probably the best of those.

The normalizing tonic *chasteberry*, with its emphasis on boosting the body's own progesterone production, in particular has been reported to mitigate a wide range of unwanted physical and emotional effects of menopause, just as it does with PMS.

Any of the herbs on the general tonics list at the beginning of this chapter can prolong hormonal activity somewhat and reduce the side effects of lowered levels. Among those, according to Karta Purkh, the best herbs for long-term use to increase estrogen activity are *dong quai* and *shatavari*. He recommends 3 capsules a day long-term in preparation for menopause, or 10 to 15 a day if already at menopause. Dr. Murray writes that he feels the four most successful herbs for increasing estrogen activity are *donq quai, licorice root, chasteberry,* and *black cohosh.*[13]

Essential fatty acids are important for maintaining production of helpful prostaglandins, balanced brain chemistry, and healthy cell membranes. Good sources for EFAs are *flaxseed, borage, evening primrose,* and/or *black currant* oils. Flaxseed oil also contains lignans, antioxidant phytochemical compounds that are believed to be hormone precursors (discussed on page 115). Lignans may bind to estrogen receptors in breast tissue and interfere with estrogen's cancer-promoting activity there. Studies show that women who excrete more lignans in their urine (presumably from increased consumption of lignans), have much lower breast-cancer rates.[14]

Ayurveda also emphasizes *sesame* and *almond* oils for women at this time—they are light, sweet, warming, easy-to-digest oils.

Many foods contain phytoestrogens (plant estrogens). Of these, soy is emerging as such a powerful winner that we will discuss it in its own separate section next. However, other foods that may contain plant hormones, since they are valued specifically for women by other cultures, are listed at the start of this chapter.

Note: Most foods or herbs with phytoestrogens are normalizing in either direction. If levels in the body are low, the phytosterols can be precursor substances out of which the body can make its own hormones. If levels are already high in the body, the plant hormone can bind the receptor cells, so that receptors are not responsive to the high levels in the body. Thus "estrogenic" plant substances do not necessarily contain estrogen or increase estrogen production, but can assist in a number of different ways.

The Soy Solution

Soy is a food that has garnered a great deal of attention for its apparent abilities to mitigate all manner of health concerns, from breast cancer to heart disease to uncomfortable characteristics of menopause. Soy has many valuable properties: Several compounds in soy have been shown by numerous studies to lower cholesterol, slow bone loss, and block breast-cancer activity.

Most of the studies showing soy's cholesterol-lowering effects (soy protein beats out a low-fat diet alone) have been on men, but recent research has focused on benefits to women, and not only for heart health. The fact that soy contains phytoestrogens makes it especially significant to women, and even more so at menopause. Plant estrogens can fill in naturally to some degree for the body's decrease in estrogen production. This may help prevent some kinds of cancer, improve the odds against heart disease and/or osteoporosis without the increased risks linked to those hormones, and reduce or eliminate some of the characteristic discomforts of menopause.

Isoflavones are the phytochemicals in soy that have received the most attention. These plant estrogens are found in other foods, but soy is one of the richest sources. Genistein is soy's special "brand" of isoflavone, and has powerful antioxidant properties. It appears to block certain tumor-supporting enzymes as well as starve the blood supply to tumors by blocking angiogenesis—the formation of blood vessels—that would feed tumors.

The National Cancer Institute is already studying the potential of purified genistein as an anticancer drug. In the meantime, you don't have to wait for genistein pills to reap the benefits. If population studies in other countries are of any value, simply eating more soy foods can slash your cancer risk.

Mark Messina, the former program director in the Diet and Cancer Branch of the National Cancer Institute, believes that one serving of soy a day, such as a glass of soy milk or a half-cup of firm tofu, can significantly lessen cancer risk, and that twice that "dose" (about 25 grams of soy protein) could significantly lower cholesterol.[15] According to Michael Murray, N.D., one cup of soybeans containing about 300 milligrams of isoflavone would be the equivalent of about one Premarin tablet.[16] Some researchers believe that soy protein will eventually become a widely accepted alternative to estrogen replacement therapy.

While ideal "dosages" of soy would probably vary from person to person based on individual health and risk levels and physical makeup, the idea is not to get some perfect amount of soy or "medicate" yourself with it in a precise manner. Rather, the point is to integrate it into your diet as much as possible so you can relax and know you're doing yet one more thing to eat your way to health naturally.

Certainly, the countries in which high soy intake is linked with low breast-cancer rates (as well as lower cholesterol) are not measuring out soy as an antidote. It's simply a part of people's lives, a dietary staple. For example, the traditional Japanese diet, extremely high in soy (they typically eat it every day), may be why Japanese women simply don't suffer through menopause the way American women seem to. Blood levels of phytoestrogens are 10 to 40 times higher in Japanese women than in their Western counterparts, and Japanese women don't complain about hot flashes.[17]

Again, as with much of natural medicine, getting out of the American one-pill dosage mind-set takes some doing. To get enough soy to make a difference, you will probably want to try it in many different forms. I use seasoned soy in many grain dishes; we have it cubed in scrambled egg whites for breakfast, in burritos, rice stir-fries, and on pasta. We also use soy cheese, and soy milk on cereal. Tempeh and baked goods with soy flour or soy protein are other ways to get soy into your daily diet.

Some researchers have actually been reported as saying that soy's value is not certain enough to warrant advising women to eat more of it. But why not try to find ways to incorporate tofu or soy milk or flour into your meals? With this much data, it would seem unconscionable not to make that recommendation. It's not as if soy were a toxic drug that should only be used as a last resort.

Miscellaneous Menopausal Discomfort Solutions

Hot flashes: Almost three-fourths of American women experience hot flashes to some degree during menopause. For many women this is the chief physical complaint during menopause. Fortunately, it is extremely treatable naturally. First, get plenty of exercise. Avoid hot, spicy foods. Also limit alcohol, sugar, and animal protein. (Interestingly, these are all good bone-protective measures as well. Funny how that works.) Use the herbs mentioned earlier (blue cohosh chief among them) and also try mixed citrus flavonoid supplements.

Depression or mood swings: *St. John's wort* is an herb that has been useful for depression generally. *Motherwort* is another good one. Try *red chilies* and the amino acids *tyrosine* and *phenylalanine* as supplements too. See pages 291–294 for more on herbal and nutritional depression treatment.

Here's a fun one: Regular sex is thought to help slow the decline of sex hormones that heralds the onset of menopause. Rina Nissim's *Natural Healing in Gynecology* claims that the little-known but best way to counteract shrinking and drying of vagina is to continue to have orgasms.

For vaginal dryness, *wild yam* cream and *vitamin E* suppositories have been effective with many women. Karta Purkh has observed that most women have the best success with a 1,000 IU capsule of vitamin E used as a vaginal suppository every night or every other night. Vitamin E is better absorbed than some other products made specifically for this issue, which can be messy. The Red Hot Mamas, a nationally-known menopause support group, suggest introducing "sexual oils" into your sexual repertoire before menopause so that when the time comes, it will not seem like "menopause treatment."

The increase in estrogenic activity from soy has been shown to increase the number of superficial cells lining the vagina. This relieves the common complaint of dryness and atrophy.

"Restless legs syndrome" can be treated with any of the following taken before bedtime: *calcium, magnesium, potassium,* and *vitamin E.*

For intermittent bleeding during or after menopause, try *shepherd's purse* tea, *red raspberry leaf* tea, *cranesbill root,* or *turmeric.*

It is helpful to deal with the psychospiritual aspects of menopause. Talking with other women not only about the physical changes but the broader perspectives on aging and womanhood can be enormously helpful. Menopause support groups are not uncommon.

Cautions

It is not understood how purely botanical preparations relieve menopausal symptoms, although it is clear that they have this capability. For women at high risk of breast cancer or who have or have had breast cancer, some scientists are concerned that the estrogens in plants may be as aggravating or dangerous as the estrogens we produce ourselves or the synthetics we might take.

However, others argue that the estrogens in plants are so much weaker and more dilute than the synthetics, or even those found in our bodies premenopause, that they cannot do damage. Even though isoflavones behave like human estrogen and provide many of the benefits, they do not seem, preliminarily at least, to carry the same risks. One reason they are theorized to raise rather than lower a woman's risk of cancers is that they may plug estrogen receptors on cells or tissue, yet not have the potency to stimulate the cells the way "real" estrogen might. The effect has been compared many times to that of a key that fits but doesn't open the cell. It jams the lock so the "real" keys can't get in.

So if the weaker estrogens bind to estrogen receptor sites on cells and "lock out" the stronger estrogens, that seems to be a good thing. If the botanicals stimulate our own estrogen production, however, that may be a different story. Since the mechanism of symptom relief is not known for many of the botanicals, women with breast cancer (or at high risk of the disease) may want to avoid natural estrogenic therapies as well as synthetic ones.

Overall, however, the risks seem clearly much higher for synthetic hormone replacement than for taking mild, health-enhancing herbals and favoring particular foods for relief of discomfort. After all, if soy and other foods containing phytoestrogens were actually to increase cancer rates rather than decrease them, that would be reflected in studies of other populations. Japanese women would have more breast cancer, not less.

The important thing for you to know is that the potential discomforts of menopause are easily treated by natural means, using herbs in combination with diet, exercise, mind-body techniques, and other supplements. Incorporating as many of the above foods, herbs, and teas as possible into your diet and routine will help. The more you do, the more results you will notice.

CYSTS AND FIBROIDS

First and foremost, any lumps, thickening, or other changes in breast tissue should be evaluated by your physician, as should any excessive bleeding from the uterus.

If the diagnosis is a benign cyst or fibrocystic breast disease, or a uterine fibroid, you may want to seek the advice of a natural healing practitioner (if the diagnosing physician is not one) because these conditions can be treated naturally in many cases.

They can also be prevented. Good basic nutrition is, yet again, critical to prevention of these conditions, and is likewise part of the treatment. Caffeine, sugar, fat, and alcohol should be avoided (Gee, where have we heard that before?), and antioxidant vitamins and minerals at therapeutic doses may be helpful.

Like everything else, abnormal growths of any kind often occur in an environment that is toxic, immunosuppressive, and stressful, both inside and out. Poor diet, lacking in nutrients and excessive in negative influences, contributes greatly to a toxic internal environment. Myriad chemical and pollutant exposures create a poisonous external environment. All of this can stress and burden the liver, whose job it is to process and eliminate all kinds of wastes. Hormonal imbalances can result, since the liver is too preoccupied or tired to manage circulating hormones. If it does not dispose of hormones properly, fibrocystic diseases can result. These conditions are influenced by estrogen, just as some breast cancers are.

There is an interesting theory, proposed by Dr. Catherine Kousmine in Rina Nissim's *Natural Healing in Gynecology*, that cysts of these kinds represent the body's attempt to deal with toxic overload and liver overwhelm by creating a "second liver," a little storehouse of tissue where toxins that cannot be dealt with presently can be stored. She observes that such cysts are often present with other liver-toxicity symptoms such as constipation, acne, headaches, and bloating. Because of this, she strongly suggests that you don't just lop off the growth without changing the factors that led to its development, because it may actually be performing a maintenance function.

In Ayurveda, conditions of excess growth or tissue accumulation are considered to be characteristic of *kapha*, so any treatment program would include anti-*kapha* herbs, foods, and lifestyle habits. Astringent herbs such as *gotu kola, turmeric, black walnut bark*, and *haritaki* would be used, and *dong quai* or *shatavari* would be recommended for hormone balancing. *Castor* oil packs would be used externally to reduce tissue mass. (Poke root infused oil is an effective Native American external remedy that can be substituted. Do not use poke root internally.) Root vegetables such as *beets, radishes*, and *carrots* would be used as juice to flush the liver.

Many natural health practitioners believe that dietary, exercise, and herbal therapy should always be a first resort, and that lumpectomies and hysterectomies are often performed unnecessarily in these cases. It is worth trying other remedies first because they are going to be cheaper and less traumatic for everyone concerned. Again, however, such conditions should be diagnosed and monitored by your doctor.

Ellen: Healing from the Inside Out

Ellen Dart, a thirty-nine-year-old student of Karta Purkh's, is an inspiring example of what's possible when you approach disease both naturally and from a systemic point of view.

Ellen found a breast lump in 1986. She saw two different doctors, both of whom wanted to remove the lump, give her chemotherapy and radiation if it was cancerous, and do nothing if it was benign. As the daughter of an MD who strongly believed in natural medicine, she was dissatisfied with these options. "I grew up believing, as my father said, that all doctors should be interrogated and that people give away too much of their power to doctors," Ellen explains.

Ellen felt that by dealing only with the lump, "we were dealing with a branch. I wanted to pull out the problem by the roots. I just felt very strongly that something was behind it, and I wanted to deal with that." Ellen was frustrated that none of her doctors shared this intuitive sense.

Ellen located a doctor of Chinese medicine in Boulder, Colorado, where she lives, and saw him on and off for three years. During that time, while the lump did not grow, neither did it disappear. She used acupuncture and Chinese herbal teas, but still felt that something else was going on. For example, she had terrible facial acne, "almost like boils," she remembers. Finally, she stopped seeing the Chinese doctor and conceded to having the lump surgically removed. It was found to be a fibroid, and nothing else was recommended.

A year later, the lump came back. "I really wasn't surprised. All we did was cut off the branch. I wasn't doing anything about why it grew there." In addition, Ellen became increasingly fatigued. "I have two daughters, and I didn't work—I couldn't have. I was constantly exhausted. Doctors were unable to give me any answers."

Determined to get to the source of the problems, Ellen sought treatment from a naturopath, who diagnosed chronic systemic candida (yeast overgrowth). She ate a special diet and took supplements to kill the yeast. "It definitely helped," Ellen says. "I felt a flash of health and energy I had not felt since I was sixteen." But still, she says, "I knew the candida was not the whole story. I still had the breast lump, I still had acne. I also had allergies and caught every cold and flu that came my way." When she began to develop more breast lumps, Ellen says, "I knew I had gone as far as I could with the naturopath. I knew there was more, that somehow the entire picture had not all been put together. I wasn't giving up."

Soon after that, Ellen saw a flyer promoting a class that Karta Purkh was coming into town to give. "It was an absolutely intuitive thing. The instant I saw his picture, I knew this was the person who could help me." Through what she learned, Ellen was quickly able to determine the likely source of her problems. Ellen's liver was so congested and burdened with toxins that it was not breaking down, processing, and eliminating wastes and other substances properly—including the estrogen that was "sent through" monthly during her menstrual cycle. The buildup of estrogen was causing the skin problems and breast cysts, as well as the fatigue and susceptibility to infection.

Ellen began taking herbs for hormonal balance, immune building, and liver detoxification. She took astragalus as an immune system restorative; shatavari and chasteberry for hormone regulation; burdock, bhumy amylaki, and dandelion root for liver detox; ma huang for short-term energy, fo-ti root for long-term energy building, and dried stinging nettles for allergies. She ate foods such as eggplant for female hormone regulation, and root vegetables and green vegetables for liver cleansing.

Within nine months of beginning this herbal and nutritional work, Ellen says, "the breast lumps and acne were gone." That was three years ago, and Ellen says proudly, "I haven't been sick since. I don't get colds and flu, I don't have allergies, and I have all this robust energy. My skin, quite frankly, is gorgeous—totally clear and smooth. I still take some herbs, and I expect in the next year and a half that will fade down to a maintenance level."

One of the things about Ellen's story that interested me, and which could relate to, was the fact that after the first lump was removed ("Whi I now regret," Ellen admits, "since there was nothing productive or h ing about that procedure"), she never had any of the subsequent lumps removed or biopsied. "I just felt, you know, I am going to heal, and I am going to heal whether it is cancer or not. Either way, I knew I was going to take the same path and do the same things. So what did I need with the stigma of a cancer diagnosis? That's such a heavy burden to bear. It carries a toxic weight that I know would have affected my healing, my immune system. I didn't need the fear and the pressure. I just went ahead and did what I knew I needed to do to heal my *whole body*. And I did heal."

Ellen says she constantly struggles to communicate to people the underlying, holistic philosophy that led to her healing. "I feel fortunate because I had the wisdom and the intuition to take the time to go through this and knew it would be worth the investment and occasional unpleasantness. I have noticed people really do want to take one or two capsules and have the problem be over with. And if it doesn't go away after one or two capsules, they think it must not be working. I sat down every night in the beginning with a bowl of herb capsules and mugs of tea.

"And to me, while nine months is not a long time for healing compared to all those years I suffered, some people think that's an incredibly long time for medicine to work. That really is the problem with the thinking that our medical system has encouraged. Big-picture thinking is what it takes to turn around your entire physiology, if you really want to heal from the inside out."

BREAST CANCER

We would like to raise briefly the extremely complex issue of breast cancer, because it is difficult to discuss women's health without at least touching on this topic. Obviously, there are many complicating factors surrounding this volatile issue. Rather than delve into them here—something that would require a whole book on its own—we simply encourage you to consider all of the preventive lifestyle options available to us day to day. There is weighty evidence for their effectiveness.

Like most cancers, breast cancer is a complex illness that in every case probably has a variety of environmental and genetic factors at its nexus. Still, even given the same sets of circumstances, some women develop breast cancer while others' immune systems arrest the disease before it can develop.

We already know that there are some basic choice-related risk factors for cancer in general. Dietary fat has been linked to a large handful of cancers, including breast cancer, even though you'll hear researchers continue to hem and haw about whether the data is "conclusive." Dr. Robert M. Kradjian, M.D., author of *Save Yourself from Breast Cancer*, criticizes the medical establishment for downplaying the strong dietary connection and for encouraging the myth that all breast cancer is genetic. (Kradjian's own exhaustive literature review shows that 80 percent of breast cancer patients have no relatives with the disease.)

Champions of real prevention (*"early detection" is not the same as prevention!*) have cited these facts repeatedly: The lower a nation's fat intake, the lower the breast-cancer rates. When a country's fat intake increases, breast cancer rates soar in kind. Migration studies show that women who move here from other countries increase their risk as they adopt our diet, and their daughters have the same rate of breast cancer as other Americans. A high-fat diet boosts blood levels of estrogen, and estrogen is believed to fuel at least some breast cancers as well as other types of cancer. What more do you need to know?

Large population studies also show a protective effect from plant foods. A National Cancer Institute review of worldwide studies found over 125 studies linking fruits and vegetables to cancer protection, with the lowest intakes corresponding to the highest cancer rates. (For other general healthy diet recommendations, see pages 107–117.)

We also know that the immune system can be supported and strengthened, both generally and, in the case of some substances, specifically with regard to tumor control. (Basic care of the immune system is covered in Chapter 5: "Prevention 101: Immune-Boosting Basics.")

Breast cancer is a very emotional issue. It resonates with many women at a deep level, perhaps at least partly because the breast may represent sexuality, femininity, and/or beauty. For this reason, breast cancer instills a degree of terror in women that may not necessarily befit the risks. It is true that 1 in 9 women may be diagnosed with breast cancer, according to current statistics. On the other hand, cardiovascular disease is a much bigger risk for most women (1 in 3 women). More women die of cardiovascular disease each year than *all* Americans die of cancer each year. Yet you simply do not see the same kind of outrage about cardiovascular disease.

As with so many other diseases, we feel that natural remedies can play an important role in treatment as well as prevention. However, you absolutely should see a health practitioner if you suspect cancer.

We also recommend several excellent books that cover this topic in greater depth (see "Recommended Reading," pages 517–522).

URINARY TRACT INFECTIONS

One of the most annoying symptoms of my low-grade, systemic, sub-clinical lack of health in my early twenties was a never-ending series of bladder infections. As soon as the burning pain during urination would begin, off I went to the medical clinic, where I would be tested, given a prescription for amoxicillin (an antibiotic) along with pyridium for the pain, and sent on my way. I would take the drugs, the symptoms would go away, and six to twelve weeks later I would have another infection. This went on for several years.

Of course, what I learned from Karta Purkh was that I did not need to treat my urinary-tract infections per se; rather, I needed to focus on the larger issue of immune weakness, of which UTIs were only one superficial messenger. I did learn about a few things to address the infections temporarily. But I also worked on strengthening my body to fight bacteria (and other things) on its own, restoring balance to a system that had been blitzed by regular antibiotic use for over a decade. The fact was, microbes of all kinds could have a field day with me—virus, bacteria, yeast, you name it. There were many layers to work through.

Urinary tract infections are extremely common. In fact they are among the most common reasons women seek medical attention—millions of office visits annually and tens of millions of dollars for diagnosis and treatment. One-third of American women have a urinary tract infection in their lifetime, and 40 percent have recurrent infections.[18]

To short-circuit the UTI cycle, you must kill the infection if there is one currently (in a way that doesn't cripple your future disease-fighting efforts), replenish the friendly bacteria in the tract so that they can defend you next time the unfriendly ones show up, and strengthen your overall resistance to infection.

To gain the upper hand over a UTI that is currently raging, use *grapefruit seed extract* or *goldenseal* to kill the bacteria (goldenseal will also help heal the membrane). *Garlic,* the Chinese herb *isatidis,* and *myrrh gum* are also useful for the short-term eradication of these bacteria.

The polyphenols in **green tea** (called catechins) also have antibacterial action. You can drink it (up to several ounces per day, though keep in mind it does contain some caffeine) or purchase green tea capsules with concentrated extracts standardized for 15 to 50 percent polyphenols.

In addition to eradicating the "bug," you can use herbs that are specifically healing and supportive of the bladder. This can be done both for acute infection and for long-term strengthening and protection. Some of the best bladder tonics are *mullein leaf, buchu leaf, cornsilk,* and *boldo leaf*—about 1 ounce of any of these as tea daily. These are generally diuretic as well.

Uva ursi is also an excellent choice; not only does it tonify the bladder, but it also has antimicrobial action. Take 1/2 ounce of tea or 2 to 6 capsules daily for acute infection.

Other general builders include the soothing mucilaginous herb *asparagus root* (2 to 10 capsules per day), **Chinese forsythia fruit** (2 to 10 capsules per day), and *cedar/juniper berry* (5 to 10 capsules per day). Specifically diuretic herbs include *couchgrass leaf* (1/2 ounce as tea), *shavegrass* (also known as horsetail; 1 ounce as tea); and *dandelion leaf* (1/2 to 1 ounce as tea). Chinese *baical scullcap root* is both a diuretic and a bladder tonic, and it is antibacterial, making it another perfect choice in case of infection.

Asafoetida is a gum in the fennel/carrot/parsley family. It's called *hing* in Sanskrit and is high in sulfur compounds (just as garlic is) and it is often used in the Near East and South Asia as a garlic-like culinary herb. It's not a sexual tonic as garlic is. It's antibacterial and the sulfur compounds are detoxifying. One to 4 capsules per day makes a good tonic.

Cranberry juice used to be considered valuable as a urinary tract acidifier, but the truth is you'd probably have to drink more juice than is practical for that to happen. Recent studies suggest, however, a different mechanism that can be just as valuable: a compound that prevents bacteria from "sticking" well, so that they are unable to colonize. Anthocyandins are a phytochemical in cranberry that may be responsible for this; it may also prevent kidney stones. Use 4 to 8 ounces *unsweetened* juice or 4 to 8 concentrate capsules daily.

Vitamin C acidifies the urinary tract while providing an overall immune boost.

For the pain and burning, use **green vegetables**, especially juiced—they are cooling, kidney tonics, and detoxifying as a bonus. Cucumber, celery, and parsley are especially good; they are also diuretic. Try 2 to 4 ounces parsley juice, or 8 to 16 ounces celery or cucumber juice.

Drink plenty of water to keep liquids moving through the urinary tract, and avoid sugars generally.

These interventions work, and they are easier and cheaper than the drugs commonly prescribed. They are also nontoxic and are immune supportive rather than immune suppressive.

Left untreated, urinary tract infections can spread to the kidneys, which is a much more serious infection that can bring painful complications. Symptoms include low back pain, fever, or blood in the urine. If you try to get rid of a bladder infection yourself with natural medicines but the symptoms persist for more than a few days, see your doctor.

(Incidentally, men can use any of these remedies also, either for genitourinary tract infections or for long-term bladder and kidney toning and prevention.)

VAGINAL YEAST INFECTIONS

Vaginal yeast infections are as common as UTIs and just as pesky. They are also not unrelated: Women who tend to have a lot of one also tend to be troubled frequently by the other. (I was. Now, I've had neither since 1989, and I don't expect ever to again.) This cycle is exacerbated by the use of antibiotics to treat the urinary tract infections, which then encourages yeast overgrowth because the drugs upset the balance of helpful flora normally found in the vagina.

Candida albicans is a yeast that will infect any orifice of the body. The vagina is a favorite place: warm, dark and moist—just what it likes. But yeast can appear anywhere: In the mouth it is called thrush, it may be a cause of diaper rash, and the large intestine is almost as common a breeding ground as the vagina for yeast overgrowth, causing many systemic symptoms. (See Chapter 18, "Herbs for Yeast (Candida)," for more on candida-related illness.)

In serious cases yeast can spread through the body to other organs, cells, and tissues—even the blood. Yeast is one of the first health conditions to crop up in AIDS patients, because the immune system is unable to keep in check this normally harmless microorganism.

Women who have recurrent vaginal yeast infections may also have yeast overgrowth in their intestines or other parts of the body. Yeast is often a systemic issue, not just a localized infection. It is a messenger communicating weak immunity, since yeast is one of the potentially unruly troublemakers that a healthy immune system has the reserves to monitor and control. Any yeast overgrowth, vaginal or otherwise, represents the underlying problem of a depleted immune system. In addition to short-term treatment, you can and should support the immune system to handle this problem permanently.

Vaginal yeast infections are characterized by itching, burning, and sometimes a white discharge from the vagina. They are conventionally treated by over-the-counter topical creams like Gyne-Lotrimin or Monistat 7. They are messy and don't offer any long-term solution to handle the underlying health issue.

The fact is that natural medicine can knock out the infection itself so fast you don't need to suppress any symptoms or expose yourself to any drugs. The best way to get rid of the symptoms is to heal the body of the disease. Once you've gotten rid of the infection, you can take the long-term approach and never get one again!

The holistic way to handle recurrent vaginal yeast infections is with the same protocol as described above for UTIs: Kill the invader—in this case, bring the yeast population down to normal levels—while simultaneously strengthening the immune system so that your body can do the "yeast population control" work on its own.

Candida is somewhat unique in that we can't expect to kill every last bit of it completely. A yeast infection is not like a bacterial infection, such as streptococcus, in which case the pathogen is not supposed to be in your body at all, no matter what, and is only there if you have an infection. Yeast is always going to be there. We always have some on our skin and in every mucous membrane. There is no way to sterilize the world of yeast. Our bodies have to learn to live in harmony with it—and they can.

Short-term yeast suppression and immune support can be achieved effectively with the following herbs:

Celandine leaf is relatively unknown, an inexpensive treasure. For long-term work you can take 5 capsules per day; for the acute infection, 15 to 20 capsules.

Eleuthero root (Siberian ginseng) happens to be anti-yeast and immune supportive despite its primary repute as a stamina builder. For acute yeast, take 10 to 15 capsules per day, or 3 to 5 as a long-term preventive.

Oak bark can be taken at a dose of 10 capsules a day for acute infection, used as a douche, or as a mouthwash for oral thrush. It's very astringent (high in tannins).

Amur cork tree bark is a Chinese anti-yeast herb that is taken as tea in China, usually capsules here—15 to 20 for acute infection.

Gum benzoin from southeast Asia, used with black walnut hull for virus, is by itself a potent treatment for candida. Take in capsules, 10 to 15 per day acute or 2 to 3 per day long term.

Myrrh gum is a blood cleanser that also kills yeast effectively. Take 10 capsules per day for acute infection.

Pau d'arco, the bark of a South American tree, has become very popular as a yeast remedy. Since systemic yeast has become more well known, pau d'arco has gotten somewhat trendy and that's driven the price up. It's mild, so to get effective results you have to take enough that it gets expensive. It isn't bad as a tea—1 ounce per day—and is a much better choice than capsules because this fluffy herb is difficult to capsule. The tea is about one-tenth the cost of capsules. It can also be used as a douche.

Garlic is most effective for yeast in the intestine, but fairly large quantities (1 to 2 cooked bulbs daily, or 10 to 20 capsules) will help suppress vaginal yeast as well. Regular intake at a lower dose will also work preventively.

Grapefruit seed extract is not immune supportive generally, but it is a terrific anti-yeast remedy. It can be taken as liquid or in capsule form. It's quite concentrated, so 5 capsules a day should be sufficient. The capsules can also be used locally as suppositories to kill yeast on contact. You can buy the powder that's already precapsuled for this, because those capsules are very small. If you make your own, start out with half a capsule just to be sure it's comfortable and well tolerated. GSE can be irritating to mucous membranes.

Long-Term Prevention

Once the yeast has been suppressed, allowing the immune system a respite, you can concentrate on long-term support, using slower-acting, broad-spectrum tonics that have special action against yeast. *Pau d'arco* and *eleuthero* would be two good choices; for more information on immune-system tonics, see pages 133–146.

Garlic, onion, ginger, and *chilies* are good general immune-supporting foods to include in your diet on an ongoing basis as part of an anti-yeast strategy. Yogurt with live active cultures can be included in the diet almost daily, or you may wish to take an *acidophilus* supplement (look for live, active cultures in a high-potency form). These will help restore and maintain the normal bacterial balance in the vagina as well as elsewhere in the body. Acidophilus capsules can also be used as vaginal suppositories.

Limit sugar and alcohol consumption. The ideal anti-yeast diet contains *no* refined sugar. Yeast feed on sugar (alcohol included), and a high-sugar diet literally provides a large yeast overgrowth with ongoing sustenance—as it simultaneously suppresses your immune response.

Since we can't hope to eradicate all yeast in our bodies, or in our environment, we must develop a strong defense that allows us to live in dynamic synergism, or at least tolerance, with these little creatures. Support your immune system powerfully and protect your "good bacteria" and yeast won't overpopulate your system.

9

Especially for Men:
Natural Healing for a Man's Lifetime

M en, like women, also have concerns throughout their lifetimes that are unique to their physiology, and some herbs are ideal for addressing these specific concerns.

GENERAL TONICS FOR MEN

Just as for women, there are long-term tonics that work on supporting and balancing the hormone-producing system of a man's body. Some of them are among the broad restorative and immune-enhancing tonic herbs already discussed (pages 133-146) because they are also glandular, sexual, and stamina and energy tonics.

As we have discussed, *ginseng* is the premier tonic for men in Chinese medicine, considered the "king of herbs." It increases energy, stamina, and sexual functioning. It's not very "feelable" at the time you take it; it's more of a long-term builder (although in the United States it is misunderstood and often used to try for a more immediate "buzz"). Asian (Chinese or Korean) ginseng is probably the most "male-oriented" of all the ginsengs, as it tends to increase production of male hormones, although *eleuthero* (cooler in energy and more appropriate for both sexes) is good for men as a general tonic since it also regulates blood pressure and blood fats, enhances immunity, and builds stamina. Ginseng may be taken long term as capsules (1 to 2 daily) or powder (1/4 teaspoon daily).

Ashwaganda (Indian ginseng, Ayurvedic ginseng) is the Ayurvedic answer to ginseng and has some similar effects; while ginseng is energizing, however, ashwaganda is an anxiety suppressant, a "grounding" herb. It is valued by Indian culture for its specifically rejuvenating effects on glandular and sexual function, stamina, and energy, and is the main Ayurvedic lifelong tonic for men. In fact, in Sanskrit the name means "like a horse." As a tonic, 1 to 10 capsules is appropriate.

Triphala, the "three fruits" formula prized in Ayurveda for its extended range of capabilities, counts sexual and glandular tonifying among its many benefits. It is taken by almost every person in India throughout the lifetime. Two to 8 capsules is an appropriate tonic dose.

PROSTATE CONDITIONS

The prostate is a doughnut-shaped gland that sits below the male bladder and surrounds the urethra like a ring. The gland secretes fluids that lubricate the urethra and increase sperm motility.

Care of the prostate is a very serious issue for men over forty. Nearly 60 percent of men between forty and sixty years old have some benign enlargement of the prostate gland, called benign prostatic hyperplasia (BPH). Over 85 percent of men in their eighties experience this condition.

When the prostate increases in size as it does in BPH, it can begin to impinge on urine flow as it presses against the urethra. Symptoms include more frequent urination, difficulty starting urination, reduced urine flow and force, and difficulty emptying the bladder. Urine flow can become increasingly blocked, resulting in pain and inflammation; if left untreated and urine flow becomes completely blocked, urine can be retained in the blood (uremia) and death can result. Kidney inflammation is also possible.

Some theories link this condition to a decline in testosterone production that occurs in middle age. Other research identifies the increased conversion of testosterone to DHT (dihydrotestosterone), a more potent androgen, which stimulates the excessive prostate cell division that results in the gland's enlargement. (DHT is found in high concentrations in men with BPH.) Low-fiber, high-fat diets have also been implicated, possibly in part because they affect testosterone metabolism.

Saw palmetto berry is probably the premier herbal treatment for BPH and also works preventively to protect against development of this syndrome. The berry is from a little palm tree that grows in Florida. This herb is used primarily as a male tonic, although it is a long-term thyroid builder as well and can be used by men and women for that purpose. (In the stampede to use it for BPH, the fact that it is an excellent general glandular tonic is now frequently overlooked.)

One to 5 capsules daily is adequate as a BPH-preventive tonic, and may be advisable for all men over the age of forty. For existing BPH, 5 to 10 capsules daily is an appropriate dose.

Saw palmetto has proven extremely effective in halting the progression of BPH and can prevent the need for expensive, uncomfortable, and undignified surgery. According to researcher, naturopath, and author Michael T. Murray, N.D., more than twenty double-blind, placebo-controlled studies have shown that the fat-soluble extract of saw palmetto berries relieves all major symptoms of BPH.[1]

Saw palmetto also compares favorably to finasteride (Proscar), the conventional pharmaceutical drug used for this condition. Studies have shown that saw palmetto produces more improvement, and faster, than this drug. In one study, this herb helped 90 percent of the subjects after a year, and only one-third of the subjects using Proscar improved after a year.[2] Dr. Murray's review of saw palmetto studies shows that the extract is effective in nearly 90 percent of patients, usually in a period of four to six weeks. Dr. Murray also notes that Proscar must be taken for at least six months before any improvement can even be expected.[3]

Proscar works by inhibiting the activity of an enzyme that transforms testosterone to DHT. Saw palmetto extract not only blocks the formation of DHT more effectively than Proscar, it also inhibits the binding of DHT at cellular binding sites, reducing the tissue uptake of both testosterone and DHT that causes cells to overmultiply. Proscar does not do this. Saw palmetto also may prevent the synthesis of certain prostaglandins and leukotrienes, hormonal messengers that prompt inflammatory responses.

Proscar also comes with some high price tags: Besides being about four times the cost of saw palmetto, it can have very undesirable side effects. It may cause decreased libido, impotence, ejaculatory disorders, or incontinence. Perhaps most serious of all: If the drug is absorbed, via semen or a broken tablet, by a woman pregnant with a male baby, the infant could develop abnormal sex organs.

Saw palmetto is exceedingly safe. Neither the clinical trials on the extract nor detailed toxicology studies on animals have revealed any significant side effects or toxicity.

In a book review in *HerbalGram* 36, former USDA botanist James A. Duke, Ph.D., said, "I have wagered my prostate . . . that FDA-disapproved saw palmetto will do the same thing as the newly FDA-approved multimillion-dollar drug, finasteride." (Note: By "disapproved," Duke means that manufacturers are not allowed to claim in advertising or on packaging that saw palmetto is medicinal or treats BPH. Saw palmetto is a "dietary supplement.")

Dr. Murray notes:

> Unfortunately, most men with BPH will never hear about the saw palmetto berry extract. Merck has the FDA to thank for this. Despite saw palmetto extract's clear superiority over Proscar, in 1990 the FDA rejected an application to have saw palmetto approved in the treatment of BPH. The result is that even though saw palmetto extract is more effective, less expensive, and much safer than Proscar, manufacturers and distributors of the extract cannot make any claims for their product. . . . Merck, the manufacturer of Proscar, has predicted sales will soon reach one billion dollars annually.

Murray further notes that the same saw palmetto berry extracts that in the United States can be sold only as "food supplements" are widely prescribed by European physicians as medicines.[4]

It is recommended that men seek fat-soluble saw palmetto extracts in capsules or pills standardized to contain 85 to 95 percent fatty acids and sterols. The dose recommended by natural health practitioners is 160 milligrams twice daily.

Pygeum is the bark of an African tree, also highly favored for prevention and treatment of prostate disease. This herb is often used in place of or in combination with saw palmetto for treatment of BPH. It too can be used as a preventive tonic, working up to 8 capsules per day.

Other herbs and nutrients recommended for prevention and treatment of prostate disease include the following:

Zinc has been shown not only to reduce the size of the prostate but to inhibit the enzyme that converts testosterone to the potent androgen DHT that causes overproduction of prostate cells. Take 50 to 75 milligrams daily (no more except under a practitioner's care; zinc in higher doses than this may be immune suppressive) in a well-tolerated form such as lozenges.

Flax oil or *evening primrose oil*, 1 to 2 teaspoons or 4 to 6 capsules daily. The omega-3 fatty acids go into the synthesis of prostaglandins that reduce inflammation.

Bee pollen, working up to 2 teaspoons or 10 caps daily. (Clinically this is indicated, though it's not well studied. It's believed to be anti-inflammatory.)

Licorice root increases ability of the adrenals to produce cortico-steroids (anti-inflammatory hormones). One of its active compounds, gly-cyrrhizin, also prevents the formation of a testosterone by-product that may encourage the growth of prostate cancer.[5] It's a general sexual func-tion enhancer. Five capsules per day or to bowel tolerance.

Nutmeg, ground fresh and capsuled, 2 to 5 capsules daily (Caution: take 5 hours before estimated bedtime, as nutmeg has a slow-acting seda-tive effect).

Good things to include in the diet for prevention and treatment of prostate disease include *pumpkin seeds* (for their high zinc content), *ginger*, and *garlic*. Pumpkin seeds are overemphasized now, in Karta Purkh's opin-ion. They were great when it was all we had, but with saw palmetto and pygeum on the scene, pumpkin seeds are not really comparable. They are a good source of zinc as well as good fatty acids, but those can be supple-mented. One advantage of zinc from pumpkin seeds instead of supplements, however, is that it won't make you queasy. Still, the amount in pumpkin seeds lends itself better to lifelong prevention than acute treatment.

Nettle leaf and root contain *bioflavonoids* that are generally anti-inflammatory. The root also has a specific affinity for the prostate; this is less well understood. An ounce of tea a day can be beneficial, or 5 capsules per day (freeze-dried or otherwise specially processed).

Hydrangea root is traditionally considered effective (10 capsules or 1/2 ounce as tea); it is often found in commercial combination capsules for BPH. *Desert leaf* tea is also used for this condition (1 ounce per day).

Note: Prostate or urinary discomforts can have a number of causes. If you are experiencing urinary problems, see your physician to rule out other causes. BPH cannot be self-diagnosed. If you receive a diagnosis of BPH, you can then make your choice about treatment.

Preventing Prostate Cancer

For prevention of prostate cancer, the bulk of data seems to indicate that men should:

- Avoid red meat
- Eat a low-fat diet (20 percent of calories from fat)
- Eat more soy foods
- Supplement with zinc
- Avoid alcohol
- Eat plenty of tomatoes (these are rich in the antioxidant carotenoid lycopene, which has been linked to lower rates of prostate as well as colon and pancreatic cancers)
- Take a mixed-carotenoid supplement
- Avoid environmental pollutants
- Get small amounts of sunlight regularly, preferably in the morning hours to avoid burning. (The body needs UV light to synthesize vitamin D, which is believed to protect against prostate cancer. Prostate cancer prevalence is lower in the sunshine states than in northern states.)[6]

SEXUAL PERFORMANCE

General Performance

Saw palmetto berry is clinically proven to increase testosterone levels, so it's useful for increasing libido as well as for prostate care. It also increases blood flow to sex organs and acts as a tonic for the reproductive and urinary tracts. Two to 10 capsules per day is appropriate.

Damiana leaf (*Turnera aphrodisiaca*), from Mexico, is primarily used as a male tonic herb, and is a mild aphrodisiac and nerve stimulant. It works well in combination with saw palmetto berry and was used that way by Native Americans for this purpose. It's also good-tasting enough to be taken as tea (1/2 ounce herb per day). One to 5 capsules of the herb by itself can also be used.

Yohimbe bark from Africa is a very powerful aphrodisiac and should be used with care. The dosage should *never* exceed 1 to 2 capsules per day (early, with food). It's scientifically verified as an aphrodisiac, and a drug called yohimbine was purified from it.

Some herbalists are concerned about misuse of this herb because of its strength. It increases pelvic blood supply, which helps produce erections, but by doing so can also cause or aggravate irritations of the kidneys, colon, or prostate. It is also extremely energizing. Again, use caution.

Sarsaparilla root is clinically proven to stimulate production of testosterone; it also stimulates progesterone and natural cortisone. It is a blood purifier (good for arthritis) and speeds recovery after injury or hard athletic performance. It is also a good stamina-building tonic. Two to 10 capsules per day.

Muira puama root is a Brazilian herb and is called "herb of love" there. Taken as tea (1/4 ounce to 1/2 ounce herb), it's reputed to produce a dreamy, relaxed sexual experience. One to 3 capsules can be used instead of tea as a tonic.

Chinese morinda root is a mild aphrodisiac at a dose of 3 to 4 capsules per day, long term.

Impotence and Premature Ejaculation

These male complaints are *not* an inevitable function of aging. Diabetes, poor circulation, and alcohol and drug abuse (prescription or illegal) are common physical causes of impotence. Herbal restoratives that balance and stimulate deep regeneration can assist in reversing this common condition, which is now known to have physical causes in the majority of cases (although at one time it was considered to be mostly an emotional issue).

To begin with, be sure you are eating a basic healthy diet as described on pages 107–117. Almost no health condition can be said to occur independently of diet, especially if the diet is extremely devoid of nutrient-rich, live, whole, organic foods and/or if it is high in fats, sugars, and processed and packaged junk.

In addition to basic healthy eating, the diet should be supplemented with *zinc*. The prostate, which produces the fluid that accounts for about 30 percent of semen, is a zinc-rich gland. Zinc is a key nutrient for hormone metabolism, testosterone production, and sperm formation.

Garlic, onion, and **ginger**, all sexual tonics, should also be eaten regularly.

Suma, a South American herb sometimes also called Brazilian ginseng because its action is similar to Asian and American ginsengs, has a particular affinity for impotence. Try 1 to 4 capsules per day. *Asian ginseng* and *eleuthero* could also be substituted as part of an herbal treatment program for impotence. Most of the tonics that are considered general, long-term overall health-builders for men—including *ashwaganda* and *triphala*—are also useful.

Ginkgo biloba, a circulation-increasing herb, has been shown to be effective in treating impotence. Though it has been studied mostly in relationship to health conditions of the elderly, especially for its ability to increase blood and oxygen flow to the brain and to prevent or slow progression of cerebrovascular insufficiency, ginkgo is a potent antioxidant. While circulation to the brain appears to be the special forté of ginkgo, it increases blood flow to small capillaries all over the body.

Anecdotally, several people have reported that in their experience ginkgo has produced an increase in intensity and length of orgasm (in both men and women) as well as an ability in women to have more orgasms. This potential might be noted. In addition, note that in Europe the popular supplement is an extract of specific active ingredient (ginkgoflavonglycosides) in a 50:1 concentration, with the typical dose being 120 to 240 milligrams. However, about 8 capsules of the whole herb, good-quality dried and powdered, would provide the same amount of those active ingredients (plus whatever the researchers threw away)—and be more economical to boot. The individuals who reported these sexual effects were using ginkgo in this form.

Bilberry is also another powerful antioxidant and is shown clinically to improve circulation. It seems to work by increasing the flexibility of cell walls, so that capillaries can stretch farther without breaking or leaking; red blood cells can thus squeeze through tighter vessels. Its action has been especially noted regarding improved circulation around the eyes, and bilberry is often used for that purpose, but it is also a general circulatory tonic.

Gotu kola is a nerve tonic that aids healing, enhances connective tissue, and increases blood flow. A perennial plant native to Asia, Australia, the South Pacific, and southern and middle Africa, it is sometimes confused with the energizing herb kola nut, but the two are unrelated. Gotu kola is mild and works well as a tea—1/2 to 1 ounce of the herb per day, or 5 capsules.

Fo-ti root (Ho Shou Wu) is a Chinese remedy for impotence (or simply to enhance sexual functioning).

Nutmeg, at a dose of 1 to 3 capsules daily, works well as a traditional treatment for premature ejaculation. It also treats impotence. (Remember that nutmeg is sedative and should be taken about five hours in advance of bedtime.)

Chinese morinda root is a sweet, warm tonic that treats impotence, premature ejaculation, and urinary incontinence. It's also mildly aphrodisiac.

Infertility

The main way to treat infertility when no specific health problem is known to be the cause is to use the general tonics described above to fortify the system and to build and increase function, as well as the basic healthy diet and lifestyle to restore general health.

Zinc again is indicated, as deficiencies can affect sperm count and motility. Low levels of vitamin C can also impair sperm motility. Some natural health practitioners recommend the amino acids *l-arginine* and *l-carnitine* because some studies have demonstrated they can increase sperm count and motility. For example, several studies show that the lower the carnitine content of sperm, the more likely a man is infertile. In one study, 3,000 milligrams of carnitine daily for 3 months increased sperm motility in 37 out of 47 patients.[7]

Vitamin E may help enhance the ability of sperm to fertilize an egg (at least it does so in the test tube[8]). The recommended dose for the general public as an antioxidant nutrient is 400 to 800 IU; therapeutically, up to 1600 IU may be taken.

Also see "Fertility Issues" in Chapter 8: "Especially for Women," page 208, for more information.

Note: the increased use of chemicals in modern industrial society is believed to account in part for the fact that average male sperm count in the population overall has declined radically in the last 100 years. Fertilizers, pesticides, herbicides, fungicides, household products, and dyes as well as general industrial pollution all contribute to the load. Thus, we recommend that in preparation for conception, you eliminate as much toxic exposure from your environment as you can, inside and out.

Another lifestyle issue: a high-fat diet has been linked to a variety of male sexual problems from suppressed libido and decreased testosterone to impotence and sperm dysfunctions (not to mention prostate and testicular cancer). Since a high-fat diet is strongly associated with a wide range of other common and serious diseases, these are just a few more reasons to make the effort to eat low fat.

HAIR LOSS

There isn't much research on this; most of what we have is folkloric. In Ayurveda, hair loss is considered to be a *pitta* problem so useful herbs would be anti-*pitta*. These include *amla* and *bhringaraj*. B-complex and *calcium* may also help.

Hair loss can be a symptom of thyroid dysfunction; refer to Chapter 11: "Energizing Herbs," for thyroid tonics. (*Saw palmetto* is one, and may be the best choice since it has other benefits for men.)

Silicon is useful to stop hair loss. Two herbs high in soluble, digestible silicon are *horsetail* and *oatstraw*. These are synergistic with *turmeric*, so turmeric should be added to either or both to make a formula.

10

Herbs for Babies and Children

Appropriately gentle choices of herbs, foods, and other natural remedies can be effective defenders of babies' and children's health too.
You can enhance young people's immune systems to help them prevent or decrease common childhood illnesses, reduce mucus levels, minimize
the chances of developing allergies, and avoid ear infections.

Obviously, there are conditions that tend to plague children especially. Likewise, there are herbal tonics and treatments that are especially beneficial to—as well as safe for—kids.

Children are in the phase of life that is most *kapha* (earth). As we discussed in Chapter 2: "History of Ayurveda," the course of human life
moves through phases that embody the energies of the doshas. While
young adulthood and midlife are *pitta* (hot, fast, intense) and older years
are most prominently *vata* (cold, dry, crackly), childhood is most characterized by *kapha*.

Remember that *kapha* is cold and wet, and that *kapha* types suffer
more than the other two from diseases of mucus. This describes childhood
perfectly. The infant, in fact, is the epitome of *kapha*—adorable as a baby
may be, it is essentially a bag of water and mucus. Think about it: "Keeping baby dry" is the battle cry of every diaper commercial and a fundamental goal of early parenthood.

Regardless of their innate constitutions, children are most likely to
lean out of balance on the *kapha* side at this time in life, and exhibit the
most vulnerability to *kapha*-type conditions and illnesses. Excess mucus
often collects in their sinuses and lungs, leaving them open to more colds,

ear infections, bronchitis, and similar or related conditions. Preventive measures for children should focus on reducing the excess *kapha* (coldness and wetness) in their systems. This can be done both with diet and herbs.

A HEALTHY LIFESTYLE STARTS EARLY

The same kind of preventive basics discussed in earlier chapters hold true for children. That means plenty of healthy, pure food and water, limited toxic exposures, good exercise, and emotional nurturing. As with adults, ideally these basics would be a given for everyone. But many children unfortunately live in an environment as physically and emotionally stressful as that which most adults deal with.

A friend of mine recently reported after a trip to one of those discount warehouses (I cannot stand to visit them anymore because they seem to be solely designed to provide cheaper, extra-large sizes of poisonous garbage) that he was incensed at the treatment of two small children he witnessed there. Mom was leaving with several huge sacks of sugary, brightly colored breakfast cereal, several cardboard flats of doughnuts and sweet rolls, and economy-size bags of high-fat potato chips. The children were both fat and sick—coughing, sneezing, runny noses. He followed them out to their car in time to see Mom light up her cigarette the moment she got in the car—without rolling down the windows.

I see this everywhere I go. I related in my first book my continuing amazement at the lack of connection between such lifestyles and chronic illness, and I'm still aghast sometimes at the comprehension gap. There is no mystery to why those kids are lethargic and sickly. We will look at the various causes and treatments for this type of chronic childhood "sub-health," but some of the causes should be clear. If you wonder why a child in your life is "always sick," perhaps even before you look at how to support a child herbally, it would be a good idea to consider making the child's lifestyle "supportable."

Karta Purkh's four-year-old daughter, Guru Bhajan, has never had an ear infection. A pediatrician friend says that he has never in fifteen years of practice seen *one other* child of that age who has never had an ear infection. Although a child like this could probably be seen frequently in some traditional cultures, she is certainly a rare case here. Karta Purkh and Jagdish Kaur, his wife, are both yoga teachers, and have each been vege-

tarians for well over twenty years. They prepared their bodies for conception for many years with herbs and diet. They used herbal medicines to
assist the pregnancy; the baby was breast-fed and began using herbs and
other dietary supplements as an infant.

Although Guru Bhajan is seen regularly by her pediatrician, she's
never taken a drug, including antibiotics. Even though she attends
preschool with other chronically sick children, she never brings home
their colds. She's living proof of the effectiveness of raising a child naturally—and a testament to the possibility of actually being able to accomplish it—even in the fast-paced 1990s.

GETTING IT DOWN:
THE BEST HERB FORMS FOR KIDS

From about the age of seven on, most kids can learn to swallow capsules. If you want to try your child on capsules, you can have him or her
practice with empty gelcaps. Capsules come in three common sizes: "0"
(small), "00" (large), and "000" (extra large). For adults, we always recommend the "00" size. For children, use the "0" size.

Under the age of six, the lack of coordination and comprehension
makes swallowing capsules difficult, though you may be able to give smaller pills in a bite of food; hollowed-out grapes or banana chunks work particularly well for this. In general, liquids—syrups, tinctures, and teas—
serve small children better.

As we have explained, natural healing was once a highly developed
and viable presence in health care in the United States. When health-care
practitioners dispensed all of their "medicines" from their own "pharmacies" of herbal remedies, they maintained a complete selection of all major
preparations in many forms for the needs of people at different ages. Since
everyone stopped making natural remedies for kids for the period of time
that herbal medicine was languishing in the United States, herbal medicines are often difficult to find in the forms that are best suited for children. Now that herbal medicine is increasing in popularity and availabili-
ty, a good many preparations are available for adults, but there are fewer
available yet for children. It's a secondary segment of the field, and needs
some time to catch up.

One of the best ways to figure out which method of getting herbs into your kids may be to ask them. Would they like to drink some tea? Would they like flavored ice? Would they like a pill? Kids do have different likes and dislikes when it comes to this sort of thing, and you'll certainly be better off if you give them some ownership and decision-making power in the process.

As with adults, use the following basic guidelines for effective herb administering: Use enough; adequate dose is essential. Take with food. Divide your doses. Increase gradually. Continue and sustain when you have achieved the desired effect (or reduce and sustain if there is discomfort). Be more aggressive for acute problems.

Teas

Fortunately, many of the same teas that adults use for healing and prevention can be used very effectively by children, simply by giving smaller and more dilute doses. The nice thing about children and teas is that because of their smaller size, they don't need to drink nearly as much as we do to have the same effect. Brew teas as described later on pages 442–444, but use more water and less herb for a more dilute result.

A great way to get teas into kids if they are not drinking them is to freeze them to make Popsicle-like treats. These may be sweetened with a little Fruitsource or honey.

If you reduce the liquid and increase the herb (making more of a "solid extract" than a "liquid extract") you will have a much stronger solution, and will then need to give much less volume per dosage. This can be useful if you think your child will respond better to a spoonful (of something very strong) rather than a mugful (of something milder and more dilute). Some herbs are simply so strong by their nature that a spoonful is all you'd want to give in any case, but usually such strong herbs are not recommended for children anyway.

Parents have found many different ways of making teas more palatable to children. Some kids will drink anything if there is enough honey in it; while this is not something you may want to feed your child lots of every day, the benefits of getting certain teas down may be worth it under the circumstances. Apple juice is another good "mixer" to make teas more appealing. (In fact, many adults find this to be true as well.)

See pages 442–444 for general information about preparing, storing, and preserving herb teas.

Tinctures

Tinctures are herbs soaked in something other than water—usually alcohol—to make a liquid usually given in droplet form. Alcohol tinctures are generally not used with children, though in a pinch, they're probably okay—the amount of alcohol in them is minuscule and it cannot exactly be compared to giving a child beer, wine, or a mixed drink.

A way to avoid the alcohol entirely is to buy tinctures made especially for children, which are usually glycerine-based (also called glycerites). Glycerine is a clear, thick, syrupy, and naturally sweet liquid from plant sources that can be found at almost any drugstore. (It's a common ingredient in hand lotions.) Its sweetness conceals the taste of bitter herbs and it is nontoxic and emollient.

The use of glycerine to make tinctures is relatively new. It's not as good a solvent as alcohol for some herbs, but that's a tradeoff we make so that the remedy will be more appropriate for children. For example, when Karta Purkh's daughter was two, her favorite playmate of the same age came down with a cold. Karta Purkh gave her 2 to 3 teaspoons of echinacea glycerite daily for a week. She didn't catch the cold. Yes, he paid more for a less active ingredient, and alcohol is a better base for echinacea than glycerine. But for a two-year-old, the compromises were worth it— and it still worked.

Herbal glycerites can be made at home by simmering herbs in a part-water, part-glycerine mixture and then straining. There are more details about this on page 447.

There are a few companies currently making tinctures specifically for children. One, called Herbs for Kids, makes superb-quality herbal medicinals especially for kids' taste buds and bodies. You may be able to ask your natural foods store to order the products for you, or mail-order them from an herb pharmacy. Wise Woman Herbals, out of Oregon, also makes excellent glycerine-based kids' herbals. They offer larger-sized, more economical 16-ounce and 32-ounce bottles, too. Eclectic Institute, Herb Pharm, and Ancient Healing Ways also offer alcohol-free tinctures, including some remedies made especially for children. (See "Resources," page 511.)

Syrups

Syrups are another form typically used with children. A liquid preparation of an herb or tea is mixed with a thick, syrupy sweetener—for example, honey or glycerine. In addition to being palatable, such preparations have a coating action, which is helpful for soothing symptoms such as sore throat or cough.

This was the preferred way for kids to take herbs at the turn of the century, when there were hundreds of natural remedies available especially for children in this form. Today, there are very few commercial herbal syrups (though obviously there are many over-the-counter drugs that come in this form). Again, the children's herb industry is immature at this time, so you may find it easier to make your own than to try to find syrups to purchase. Eclectic Institute does make some herb syrups for kids.

Special Dosages

Sometimes herbs are chosen especially for use with children because they taste better or are easier to get down. Other times an herb is chosen for its mildness. Some of the herbs recommended specifically for children might not be as powerful for adults.

But you can also use many of the herbs and nutrients recommended for adults in Chapter 5, "Prevention 101: Immune-Boosting Basics" (pages 104–125) and in Chapter 7, "Colds and Flu: Dodging the Immune Break-down Epidemic" (pages 159–191) except if specifically indicated that the herb is not appropriate for kids. Just cut the dosage. All doses we list are per day, for one 150-pound person. When using the same herb for a child as you would for an adult, one-quarter to one-fifth or so of the dosage is a good general rule of thumb. (For our purposes, "adult" is defined as having reached puberty.)

Lauri Aesoph, N.D., a naturopath and natural medicine writer, suggests these dosages: Children up to school age should receive one-quarter of the adult dose. Kids from six to twelve years can be given half of what grown-ups take. Adolescents up to 17 should receive three-quarters of an adult dosage.[1]

The exact dosages that work for your child will vary just as they do from adult to adult. Start with the smallest dose and work up until tolerance and/or desired result.

NUTRITION

Many children these days are probably born nutrient deficient, given the dismal eating habits of their parents, in many cases—and as children begin to eat on their own, things don't get much better. In addition, many natural health practitioners believe the Recommended Dietary Allowances (RDAs) are pretty conservative. RDAs were developed as minimums required to prevent diseases like scurvy, pellagra, and beriberi that result from very extreme deficiencies that are no longer threats. The kind of deficiencies we and our children may suffer from aren't enough to cause those diseases, but they are enough to matter. They can leave us just undernourished enough to permit our immune systems to become under- or overactive. Also, there are no RDAs for many nutrients—but that doesn't mean we don't need them.

So already, by the time they are infants, many kids have subclinical nutritional deficiencies across the board. The result is a whole bunch of substandard, sick kids who may not have the overt diseases feared during their parents' childhoods—just lots of colds, ear infections, flu, and food allergies. You've seen them (they may even be your own): runny-nosed, pasty-faced, baggy-eyed, ear-infected, too-lethargic, or too-hyper kids.

Natural medicine expert Dr. Alan Gaby, M.D., coined the phrase "chronic subclinical everything syndrome" to describe this pattern. (And of course, this isn't just kids; we know all too many adults in this condition. And no wonder! "Chronic subclinical everything" kids grow into adults—adults with lots of colds, flus, and food allergies.) People feel sick, but they are superficially "normal" by conservative laboratory standards.

Nutritional deficiencies can begin prenatally, when the mother is not nutrient ready for having a child. Baby is born deficient because Mom didn't have enough to give during pregnancy. Then, all the juice gets sapped out of Mom during pregnancy, and by the time the infant is breast-feeding she is already sucked dry.

One way to ensure healthy kids is to prepare your own body for their conception and birth as we discussed earlier. The very first step in preventing allergies, hyperactivity, and "chronic subclinical everything syndrome" starts with parents before birth.

Vitamins and Minerals

A general broad-spectrum multiple vitamin and mineral supplement can create measurable health changes to start with. Get a *megapotency multiple*. Health-food-style multiples are pretty conservative in dose, so many natural pediatric nutritionists recommend doubling the label dose indicated for the child's age. Under a health practitioner's care, you might even triple the dose.

Vitamin B complex and *calcium* tend to be two nutrients really lacking in kids. The subclinical B vitamin deficiency is probably because of lack of whole grains in the diet. Stop the bleached flour and sugar and other simple carbs. In addition to a variety of whole unprocessed grains, make sure they get plenty of the B vitamins. A daily dose for kids (assuming they can swallow the tablet) is one B50 (vitamin B complex, 50 milligrams) per day. For kids under six, give half a tablet.

Because B vitamins are neurotransmitter (brain chemical messenger) precursors, they may be useful as part of natural therapy for any condition involving mood or behavior—including child hyperactivity, as some studies show.

Often children are overconsuming milk, yet not metabolizing or absorbing calcium well. Nutrients such as *zinc, boron* (found in fruits, beans, and vegetables, or supplements), and *magnesium* are needed in order for calcium actually to calcify bone. Too much protein—milk again, as well as meat—increases calcium loss. Also, phosphates (in processed foods and soft drinks, common in the average child's diet) can cause calcium loss or excretion. A well-rounded diet as described earlier and a daily multivitamin will help boost the total nutrient load to support better absorption.

Blood tests may not show a calcium deficiency, since the body maintains levels of calcium in the blood that are very narrow; a person can have borderline osteoporosis before any deficiency shows in the blood. Calcium can be given to children regularly in any form that's tolerable. It can tighten the stool, so watch for that. A 500-milligram tablet daily is appropriate for children.

According to Dr. Michael A. Schmidt in *Childhood Ear Infections*, magnesium is in short supply in American kids' diets (and there's no reason to think this is limited to kids). Interestingly, low magnesium levels are being linked to a whole slew of conditions: cancer, cardiovascular disease, hypertension, PMS, fibromyalgia, chronic fatigue syndrome, asthma, and depression—some of America's most predominant "plagues." This hardly seems coincidental when you realize that the standard diet is stripped of this important trace mineral—both through processing of grains (which removes about 85 percent of the magnesium along with important B vitamins and others) and through use of potassium fertilizers before food is even harvested.

Avoiding processed foods is one way to get more magnesium from the diet, but a supplement at half the adult dose of 250 to 500 milligrams will not hurt your child (or you).

Junk Food

The same immune-supporting dietary recommendations outlined earlier apply to children. Food is among the top health essentials throughout a person's life, if not the first priority. But food is especially important in childhood. For one thing, childhood is a time when lifelong eating habits may be formed. For another, so much growth, generation, and development is occurring at this time that the body is probably never hungrier for nutrients.

In a sense, the body is being built during this period, so think about what you want to have it made out of. Do you want your child's body built with cheap, junky materials like cake, candy, ice cream, and cookies? Or fresh whole foods that are rich in nutrients? Which "structure" is going to be more stable and sturdy and able to withstand the stresses of the environment? When the body is built in a setting of nutritional scarcity rather than abundance—when it is made out of junk instead of quality materials—problems show up not only in childhood but throughout a person's life.

So as much as possible, keep children away from the foods that weaken the immune system and displace health-promoting nutrients. These are foods that are not any better for adults, so by keeping them out of your house, you do both you and your kids a favor.

Milk

Milk is the second most common food allergy. Some sources say two-thirds of all Americans have some allergy to cow's milk.

Only a small percentage of the world's population drinks mammals' milk, but it dominates the U.S. agriculture and diet. For example, milk represents 44 percent of beverages consumed by children under 18, according to the USDA.

One possible reason for the widespread reaction to cow's milk is that it really is very different from human milk (much higher in protein and lower in sugars, for example), and we give it to kids too soon (if we should even give it to them at all). The body often reacts to milk as if it is foreign—which it is. There is growing controversy about human consumption of cow's milk.

Indeed, there is not a lot that milk has to recommend it for human consumption. Cow's milk is baby food for calves. No species on earth besides us drinks the milk of another species. Furthermore, no other species drinks milk after infancy. Milk appears to be baby food, created specifically for the needs of babies, and it has been noted that humans are the only species that is never really "weaned."

Thus it makes sense that, after weaning, a large majority of people simply don't have the enzyme that breaks down lactose (milk sugar). "Lactose intolerance" is treated as if something is wrong with the person who suffers from it. But most of the population can't digest milk properly, and it's likely that's because we're not supposed to be digesting it. If the majority of the population reacts negatively to a food, perhaps there's not something wrong with the population; perhaps there's something wrong with the food.

Giving an infant cow's milk may not only create intolerances and allergies early on, but also affects the child's immune system. Mother's milk helps to build a child's immune system by passing along antibodies.

In addition, lactose-intolerance symptoms are often misdiagnosed as much more serious bowel diseases, with great suffering and many health-care dollars spent testing and treating conditions that often disappear with the elimination of dairy products.

Milk also is responsible for a lot of the unhealthy fat in the American diet; as of 1993, only 13 percent of all milk sold was skim milk.[2] The other 87 percent of milk sold is whole milk or the misleading "2 percent fat" milk, which gets almost half of its calories from fat (it's 2 percent fat by volume). That's not including the other fatty dairy products such as cheese, butter, and ice cream.

Then there is the issue of what else is in the milk. According to nutritionist and dietitian Bob LeRoy, R.D., M.S., EdM, eighty-two drugs can legally be used on milk cows. And it is suspected that many farmers illegally use unapproved drugs in the search for even more powerful medicines.[3]

Also, in February 1994 the FDA approved the use of rBGH (recombinant bovine growth hormone) to increase milk production. The FDA refuses to implement a test for rBGH levels in all dairy products, insisting there is no need because it is safe. Not everyone is so sure, however.

Dr. George Tritsch, a cancer researcher recently retired from the Roswell Park Cancer Institute in Buffalo, New York, says that drinking milk from rBGH-supplemented cows increases insulin growth factor (IGF-1), which may enhance tumor cell growth.[4] Tritsch believes that minute levels of IGF-1 could enter the bloodstream of those who drink hormone-laced milk and create tumor cells in the breast, ovary, or prostate as people age, which would grow slowly and manifest as clinical cancer in old age. He also feels that such hormones could stimulate the progression of childhood leukemias.

Tritsch concludes that "the widespread consumption of BGH-supplemented milk is, therefore, an experiment on an unsuspecting population that could have horrendous consequences," adding that "it would be difficult to dismantle a well-entrenched BGH industry."[5]

Use of rBGH is also known to increase the amount of pus, bacteria, and antibiotic contamination in milk, since cows given rBGH are more susceptible to disease.

Finally, bovine serum albumin (BSA, a cow's milk protein) has been strongly linked to insulin-dependent diabetes mellitus in children. Studies have found, for example, that *every one* of 142 diabetic children had large amounts of antibodies to BSA,[6] that diabetic children had 8 times as many of these antibodies as nondiabetic children,[7] that insulin-dependent diabetics were 50 percent more likely to have been given cow's milk before 3 months of age,[8] and that high-risk children who drank cow's milk in the first 3 months were 11 times more likely to get diabetes than high-risk children who didn't.[9]

Note also that milk products do not contain any of the kinds of special nutrients we have discussed earlier, like the phytonutrients in fruits and vegetables that are found to have cancer-protective and immune-boosting effects. Milk doesn't even provide fiber.

In 1992, the American Academy of Pediatrics announced its recommendation that whole cow's milk not be given to infants less than one year old. This was based on the link between BSA and milk-induced iron-deficiency anemia.

Dr. Lendon Smith, M.D., pediatrician and author of *Hyper Kids, Feed Your Kids Right,* and other books, is a leading spokesperson for natural healing for kids. He believes that 90 percent of all generally sickly children will show improvement in all areas when you just take away cow's milk. He told Karta Purkh that in his clinical experience a similar percentage of ADD and learning-disability cases improve with removal of milk products. Milk is especially implicated in that commonest of childhood ailments, the middle ear infection (more on this to come).

Ayurveda considers small amounts of well-prepared dairy products to be appropriate for some people (based on body type), and in special cases for therapeutic use (some herbs are believed to be synergistic with milk or to release their active ingredient best with milk as the carrier). Ayurveda recommends that if you serve your child cow's milk, boil it first with cardamom seed, and serve it with honey. If you are preparing cheese, serve it with cumin seed for improved digestion.

We recommend you choose milk products that are certified organic. That means cows are fed organic grain and hay, never given hormones or drugs (and are more likely to be treated humanely as well). Or try some of the many excellent milk and cheese substitutes now on the shelves of your natural foods store.

Superfoods

Superfoods are foods that we can think of as being about halfway between food and medicine. They are foods with very concentrated nutrients or natural compounds known for their healing or health-promoting properties. Getting them into the diet is a great way to support your child's immune system naturally and consistently. There are superfoods that are especially helpful during childhood.

Algae, such as spirulina and chlorella, are good for kids because they have a broad spectrum of vitamins and minerals, are high in easily digestible protein (contain all eight essential amino acids) and chlorophyll (chlorella is the richest known source of chlorophyll on earth), and are easy to get down. They are both nutritive and detoxifying. They can be bought in powder form at the health-food store. They can be given in doses of a teaspoon a day, stirred into liquid. (They will turn any liquid green, which may either disturb or delight your child.) You can use an opaque cup if necessary so they can't see how weird it looks.

Rice bran syrup is a nutritious superfood for kids. Rice bran is the valuable stuff that's taken off the outside of the rice kernel when making it white. Squeezing the juice out of this bran makes a thick, brown, sweet syrup, like molasses. It's nutrient-packed, an excellent source of very digestible B vitamins, and rich in iron. The sweet taste also makes it appealing. (This is not to be confused with rice syrup, a sweetener.)

Bee pollen supports the immune system and can actually desensitize children to pollen allergies over time. It's naturally sweet, and can be stirred into juice, a blender drink, cereal, or eaten off a spoon (up to 1 teaspoon a day). The flavor depends on what plant the bee took the pollen from. You can find bee pollen at most natural foods stores.

Barley grass or other grass of grains (like wheat grass) are good for kids because they're immune supporting, nutritive, and cleansing. These grasses are a concentrated source of chlorophyll, B vitamins, vitamin K for bone metabolism, minerals, and enzymes. A teaspoon a day of the powder can be stirred into juice.

Chlorophyll can be used by itself and is an excellent blood cleanser and purifier—cooling, calming, and not extremely strong, so it's appropriate for kids. It's also a good source of magnesium. Interestingly, it's the same molecule as hemoglobin, except instead of iron, chlorophyll has magnesium, which makes chlorophyll green and hemoglobin red. This makes it something akin to "plant blood"—the plant's oxygen-transport mechanism. It comes in liquid forms and is usually concentrated from alfalfa (which is the richest land source of trace minerals).

Antioxidants: Get your kids started early on eating foods that are rich in phytonutrients, which research shows probably prevent cancer and slow aging and damaging free-radical oxidation. (Foods and their antioxidant compounds were discussed on pages 116–117.) Provide these nutrients through food as much as possible. For example, a tall glass of carrot juice every day, if you can get your child to drink it, will provide your child with extraordinary amounts of carotenoid compounds. (It's also a good source of calcium.)

If you yourself are eating these foods, and the meals you prepare are filled with them, your child will naturally be eating more of these foods.

Essential fatty acids: EFAs are important for the synthesis of "good" prostaglandins as well as healthy, normal cell membranes. The dosage for children is half the recommended adult dose. Omega-3 fatty acids (flaxseed oil, fish oils, evening primrose oil, and cod liver oil) are also important for the synthesis of helpful prostaglandins. Give one 500- or 1,000- milligram EPO capsule or a teaspoon of flax or cod liver oil daily.

KIDS' TONICS: GENERAL IMMUNE HERBS

There are two main categories of herb that are not used with children. One includes all hot, spicy, intense, and potentially irritating herbs (chilies, garlic, onion, ginger). The other is reproductive system stimulants, such as garlic, ginseng, or dong quai.

Exceptions can be made for short-term treatment in acute situations. Also, garlic and onion can be useful externally—in ear infections, for example, as we will discuss. However, these types of herbs should not be used as long-term tonics for children.

Chamomile flower is discussed in other chapters for adult use in a wide range of situations; it is an extremely versatile herb. Its apple-like flavor makes it palatable to children and it's an excellent digestive, lung, and liver tonic as well as a calming, soothing agent. Kids can take as much of it as they are willing to drink.

Calendula flower is an herb that tastes good and can be included in soups. It is antifungal, and generally immune supportive. Calendula stimulates white blood cells and lymph drainage.

Echinacea and *astragalus*, already discussed at length in other chapters, are also mild enough to be children's immune tonics. Astragalus could be used as a tea or broth, and kids like the sweet taste. Echinacea can be found in alcohol-free tinctures.

Triphala is suitable for all ages and body types and is mildly laxative, and the dose can be adjusted accordingly. The typical dose for a child would be 1 capsule per day.

Chyavanprash, an herbal tonic jam made from amla fruit, is a sweet dietary supplement for the entire family. A noted blood cleanser, the dose for a child would be 1 teaspoon per day.

Licorice root benefits children's bones. It is sweet and quite tasty, but laxative. Small amounts should be used to bowel tolerance.

Marshmallow root is a gentle herb for bones that has a bland taste. It is also a good nourishing, soothing herb for the digestive tract. Use 1/2 teaspoon as a powder stirred into food.

WHEN PREVENTION FALTERS: HERBS FOR KID PROBLEMS

Cold and Flu

While we have already devoted a whole chapter to dealing with colds and flu at any age, kids are legendary for their tendency to bring them home to you, so ways to both prevent and treat them specifically in children bear mention.

As in adults, children's vulnerability to these infections is a direct outgrowth of how nourished or depleted the immune system's protective forces are. It cannot be emphasized enough that the long-term, day-in-day-out care and replenishing of the body through a variety of different sources is the key to health. Herbs can help when your child becomes ill, but implement lifestyle changes now and you will find yourself having to use treatments—natural or otherwise—less and less.

Until you reach that point, here are some ways to make your child more comfortable when he or she is already ill, while assisting the body's efforts to clear away the invaders. All of the following herbs are excellent immune boosters, bug fighters, and/or "cleanup helpers" that support the liver and other immune-system components in the aftermath of infection.

The best form used will depend first on how they are available and then on whether your child is at capsule-taking age or must have a tea or tincture. **When using tea, *the listed dose is for a 150-pound adult*; reduce accordingly by your child's weight.**

Echinacea is especially good for bacterial infection as well as overall immune boost. Use alcohol-free tincture by the teaspoon as needed.

Cherry bark is a cough remedy; dose would be 1/2 ounce as tea or a syrup made from the tea.

Coltsfoot is an excellent respiratory tonic and cough medicine; dose would be 1/2 ounce as tea.

Yerba santa is a good respiratory tonic for extra thick, goopy congestion in either sinus or lungs. Dose is 1/2 ounce as tea per day.

Osha root is a Native American herb that is immune boosting; echinacea-like but not as well known. Dose for children is 2 capsules per day.

Astragalus is a great tonic for kids both for acute antiviral and long-term immune boosting, thanks to its mild, pleasant taste. Dose is 1 ounce per day.

Elder flower is excellent for discomfort in the head area; head colds, headaches, and sore throats respond well to this herb. One-half ounce per day as tea is the dose.

Burdock root is a liver tonic and blood cleanser that may be used with children. Tea (1/2 ounce of herb per day), capsules (1 to 3 per day), or tincture may be used.

Thyme leaf is a mild immune booster and can be made into tea, up to 1 ounce of herb per day.

Lemon grass is a mild sinus soother, up to 1 ounce of herb as tea per day.

Lemon balm (also known as melissa), is a general immune booster and digestive soother; up to 1 ounce per day as tea.

Cleavers leaf is mildly detoxifying; up to 1 ounce per day as tea.

Ribwort leaf soothes mucous membranes and is generally a good kids' tonic; 1/2 ounce per day as tea.

Slippery elm bark soothes mucous membranes and digestive distress. This can be used in the adult dose—2 to 4 heaping tablespoons made into a paste with water.

These remedies may help you avoid using OTC drugs, which do not do anything to help your child get well, are immune suppressive, and can actually inhibit healing. They can also cause harm of their own. Pediatrician Robert Mendelsohn, M.D., declares that more children are probably poisoned annually by aspirin than any other toxic substance.[10]

In October 1994, *Time* magazine reported that a *Journal of the American Medical Association* survey showed that parents use such preparations 70 percent of the time when faced with illness, "despite evidence that over-the-counter remedies such as cough and cold medicines are often ineffective and sometimes produce adverse reactions when taken by preschool children."

Ear Infection (Otitis Media)

- "For years, doctors have treated ear infections in children with a regimen of antibiotics. But pediatricians also know that if left untreated, most ear infections will clear up in a week or so anyway." (*Business Week:* November 27, 1995, "Complementary Medicine: Is It Good for What Ails You?")
- Naturopath Molly Linton notes in *Delicious!* magazine, December 1995, that some children wind up taking antibiotics continuously for up to two years because they get the infections so frequently. Yet, "the American College of Pediatrics recently admitted the probable futility of antibiotic treatment for otitis media. . . . The college has published articles indicating that routine use of antibiotics should be reserved for severe cases of ear infection."
- After a recent Dutch study on antibiotics in ear infection, the physicians conclude that 88 percent of all patients with acute otitis media never need antibiotics; and when antibiotics are begun on the first day of the disease, *the frequency of recurrence is 2.9 times higher than when no antibiotics are used.*[11]
- Dr. Andrew Weil in *Spontaneous Healing* calls ear infections "the bread and butter of pediatricians."
- One out of every three pediatric visits results in an antibiotic prescription.[12]

Despite the widespread acknowledgment of the futility of antibiotics in these cases, and the negative effects of antibiotics' overuse, childhood sometimes seems like a revolving door of kids on antibiotics. Even though their own regulating authorities admit that antibiotics are frequently ineffective and unnecessary, many doctors continue to prescribe them, and resist or dismiss natural interventions. Kids under age fifteen receive almost three times as many antibiotics during visits to doctors and HMOs as other age groups, according to 1992 data from the National Center for Health Statistics.

Antibiotics may make both doctor and patient feel like something is getting done, but whatever the drug may or may not do for the infection can backfire in spades when "friendly" bacteria in the body are destroyed along with the pathogen (if, in fact, there is a pathogen involved). As in adults, using antibiotics upsets the balance of "friendly" bacteria in the intestinal tract, making it vulnerable to yeast (candida) growth and other intestinal problems.

Killing off the "good" bacterial colonies is bad enough, but even the fact that antibiotics kill most of the "bad" bacteria can cause problems. Antibiotics may kill multiple colonies of weaker "bad" bacteria vying for food and living space, leaving the individual carrying only a few hardy strains that no longer have to compete with the others. More room and less competition means the hardy ones can take over and multiply.

In addition, prolonged use of antibiotics has been shown to weaken the immune system, lead to the development of antibiotic-resistant strains of the organism, increase susceptibility to intestinal infection, irritate the intestinal lining, and reduce absorption of nutrients.

The increased prevalence of antibiotic-resistant "superbugs" combined with the greater susceptibility to infection caused by their overuse can be a fearsome combination, especially for children. In January 1996, a Georgetown University School of Medicine study showed that kids taking a broad-spectrum antibiotic to prevent ear infection had a 100 percent chance of succumbing to a "superbug"—a fivefold increase in risk.[13]

When antibiotic treatment fails, many doctors turn not to natural remedies but to a more invasive treatment: inserting ear tubes to drain the ear or equalize pressure. General anesthesia, which burdens the liver, is required during insertion of ear tubes. According to Dr. Michael A. Schmidt, author of *Childhood Ear Infections*, eardrum scarring with membrane thickening has been found to occur in over 40 percent of children receiving tubes, compared with 0 percent in those not receiving tubes.

It should be common knowledge that ear infections are treatable without antibiotics. They are also preventable.

What Are the Alternatives to Antibiotics for Ear Infections?

Herbal treatments are highly effective at both soothing and healing middle- and inner-ear infections. Most ear infections respond marvelously to ear oils made from naturally antimicrobial herbs. *Garlic* is probably the premier antibacterial oil, and is almost always the first ingredient in commercially sold ear oils. Other common and useful ingredients are *mullein, St. John's wort, glycerine, goldenseal, onion, willow bark, calendula, usnea,* and *vitamin E.*

A home remedy taught by Karta Purkh and used very effectively by many people is the Chinese herb *ma huang* (ephedra) used externally in the ear. Brew it up very strong and apply a few drops in the ear. This opens the ear canal. This is followed by a few drops of glycerine, which pulls fluid out of the ear once the canal is open. (Note: Do *not* use ephedra for children internally.)

Pain is caused by tissue swelling against the eardrum, pressure buildup caused by the fluid, and inflammation. Heating the ear often helps ease the pain. This can be done in a way that also offers some antibacterial action: Slice an onion in half, put in hot water for one minute, wrap in a thin cloth, and apply to ear.

To make a medicine that is taken internally for ear infections, layer slices of onion and garlic with honey. When it has liquefied, strain it and use it as medicine base. (Use this only for a week or so; do not use onion or garlic for an extended period with children.)

Some good friends of ours have an ear infection story that is one of my favorites to exemplify what is possible when people take time to make a conscious choice—instead of automatically doing what everyone else does, just because it's the only choice they've ever known. Ann and Scott's three-year-old son, Jack, woke up one day after he'd had a cold, swiping at his ear and crying. They thought about taking Jack to the doctor, but they had been relying increasingly on herbal medicine for several years and were wary of the automatic dispensation of antibiotics they saw with their friends' children. They decided, for the moment, to forgo a doctor visit that would cost $100, plus the $100 worth of antibiotics, after which Ann was certain Jack would wind up with another ear infection.

So Ann went to the health-food store and purchased an ear oil that contained garlic oil, mullein oil, and St. John's wort oil. It cost $9. She put a few drops in Jack's ear. They actually didn't expect much from one application of a few drops of oil. The plan was to give it one day, and if the oil did nothing, they would go to the pediatrician.

But they didn't have to wait long. By that afternoon, Jack was smiling, laughing, running around, and playing, full of energy. The pain never recurred. No three-hour-round-trip bus ride to the doctor, no fees, no drugs, no pharmacy bill. Nice. Ann called me up to share the story, full of excitement and triumph. There was a wonderful feeling of having had the resources to provide healing for her own child, having done it naturally in a way that caused no further harm, and having saved a lot of time and money in the process.

Interestingly, Jack also hasn't had another ear infection.

What Causes Ear Infections?

The eustachian tubes go from the inner ear to the back of the soft palates in our mouths. Ear fluids backed up in these tubes are an ideal medium for bacterial growth, inflammation, and painful pressure. Why do ear fluids back up in the first place? Good question.

One assertion is that small children are so susceptible to inner-ear infections because of the shape of their ear canals—they are curved in infants and toddlers, and grow straighter as we age. Supposedly this shape fosters an environment for fluid buildup and infection. Additionally, estimates are that a child's immune system is not fully developed until anywhere between the ages of six to twelve.

Natural health practitioners often have other ideas, beyond purely structural reasons, about why kids get so many infections and ear infections in particular.

Many natural health authorities believe that kids who have chronic earaches (distinct from infection) often are suffering from food allergies, not microbial infections primarily. Indeed, notes Dr. Michael A. Schmidt in *Childhood Ear Infections*, the middle-ear fluid contains no harmful bacteria in up to 70 percent of children with middle-ear "infection" who do not respond to antibiotics. Allergies can create chronic mucous congestion, which leads to "stuffy," blocked, painfully pressurized eustachian tubes. This can also make a child more prone to bacterial ear infections secondarily, because of the wet environment and vulnerability of the tissue.

Cow's milk is the culprit most often blamed for the allergic situation that fosters this cycle. Not only Karta Purkh but also countless other natural health practitioners have observed that simply taking children off milk and milk products can result in a marked decrease—and sometimes total elimination—of ear infections. Dr. Lendon Smith, in a private communication with Karta Purkh, indicated that removing all milk products leads to improvement in 90 percent of his juvenile patients with ear infections. (See more on childhood food allergies in the next section.)

For chronic infections, whether bacterial or viral, we're back to the immune system. In this case, allergic or not, sugar can be a vicious enemy for children with recurrent infections. Sugar is a known immune suppressant, and with the amount consumed by the average American child, it's once again not shocking that infections of any kind have a heyday with their immune systems. Studies show that sugar depresses a child's white blood cell count, possibly for hours after consumption.

So, to prevent ear infections, try taking your child off all milk and milk products, and eliminate sugar from his or her diet. You may use a drop or two of garlic oil or a combination herbal ear oil once a week as a preventive measure, and follow the general dietary guidelines listed earlier. Also use vitamin C, and a tonic of yerba santa or coltsfoot tea daily.

Another thing you might try with a child whose ear infections are chronic is chiropractic or osteopathic cranial manipulation. (See "Resources," page 511, for referral organizations.) In his book *Spontaneous Healing*, Andrew Weil discusses a well-known osteopath, Dr. Robert Fulford, who was Weil's mentor in many aspects of natural healing. Dr. Fulford cured hundreds of children from chronic cycles of ear infections by restoring normal breathing patterns. The osteopath's assertion was that a restricted sacrum (five fused vertebrae forming a solid bone that fits like a wedge between the bones of the hips) impairs the whole respiratory mechanism. Restricted breathing causes inadequate lymphatic circulation, and that in turn leads to poor drainage from the head and neck. The chronic fluid buildup then provides a red carpet for bacterial breeding. Manipulation that freed sacral restrictions could end the infection cycle permanently with one session.

Last Resorts

If you do decide to use antibiotics for an ear infection (or any other illness), also have the child supplement with the "friendly" bacterial cultures *Lactobacillus acidophilus* and *Bifidobacterium bifidus*. Use high-activity "super" cultures (these are usually refrigerated and in powder form at your natural foods store). This will help restore his or her intestinal bacteria to a healthy balance.

If an ear infection does not respond to natural remedies within a few days, do consult a health practitioner promptly. Ear infections can cause hearing loss in severe cases. We must recommend that you do whatever your doctor says to do. But know this: Ear infections—and children's infections in general—*can* be managed herbally, and better yet, prevented, if you are diligent. It *is* possible to raise children who don't get ear infections at all!

Allergies

Allergies occur when you overconsume a substance at a time when your immune system is compromised. The body creates antibodies to the food as a defense to the supposed "invader." An allergy invokes an immune system response. "Sensitivities" are milder and can be outgrown; they are generally not medically diagnosed.

Food allergies are reversible. With treatment, allergies can be eliminated in about a year, and foods can be added back; it's not a matter of life-long elimination, as many people with food allergies are told. But you have to treat the problem, not just eliminate the foods. Once the offending foods are out of the system, the system itself must be nourished and balanced so that it is not overactive.

Without treatment, kids won't just "outgrow" allergies. Often childhood allergies seem to disappear, but often it's just that the symptoms change and evolve; new ones come to take their place. Once you have taught your body, albeit erroneously, that a food is something to be defended against, it will defend against it until you retrain and fortify the immune system.

Cravings are a classic sign of food allergy. Dr. William Philpott coined the term *allergic/addictive* to describe our cravings for foods that make us sick. If a child gets cranky and refuses to eat until favorite foods are given, this may be a sign that those foods are allergens. The first thing to do if you suspect a food allergy is to remove the food from the diet. Carefully monitor any changes after the removal of the food; keeping a diary is helpful.

During the period of time when the allergens are being avoided, you will need to find substitutes for the foods. This can be difficult with certain foods, such as wheat. For alternatives, consult the "Alternative Ingredients and Substitutes" list on page 506. Also remember that this is helping your child, as much as they may try to convince you that the "deprivation" of Tastykakes and Ding Dongs is destroying them.

To prevent food allergies, babies should ideally be breast-fed for at least one year. Breast milk contains the ideal nutrient composition for infants. In addition, it has the advantages of passing on immunity and facilitating emotional bonding. There is really no adequate substitute even close to the perfection of breast milk for human infants, though fortified soy- and cow's-milk formulas are used widely by mothers who logistically or physically cannot manage breast-feeding. Cow's milk is the most common food allergy in babies under one year old.[14] Soy also becomes a common allergen in young children.

For more on food allergies generally, see Chapter 16, "Herbs for Allergies."

Hyperactivity, Learning Disorders, and the Allergy Connection

Childhood should be a time of exploration, growth, and security. For an increasing number of children, however, it has become an emotional nightmare, complete with academic failure, depression, fatigue, frustration, and physical pain. Many natural health therapists have noticed a trend in this generation of young people toward a broad syndrome that includes behavior problems, attention deficit disorder (ADD), and moodiness, in addition to frequent infections.

Karta Purkh's conclusion after two decades of clinical experience with these especially sickly children is that their condition is the result of a general spiral of degeneration that starts at birth. As stated earlier, mothers become less well nourished with each decade, so their children have less chance of getting a good start, and often fail to develop the basics of strong immune and glandular systems. Karta Purkh's experience of children with the most pronounced cases of this syndrome are that they are typically younger siblings who were at the mercy of the mother's depletion from previous pregnancies.

Many of these children also have systemic yeast infections, often the result of prolonged antibiotic use. The weakened immune system, sugar abuse, and the decline in friendly bacteria all foster yeast overgrowth. The yeast further weakens the immune system, allowing more infections, which are then treated with more antibiotics.

Multiple food allergies frequently affect the nervous system and hormone levels, making thinking unclear or slow. Ear congestion will inhibit normal hearing. This causes difficulty at school, as well as delay in language development. Scholastic difficulties may be further exacerbated by many missed classes due to illness. All of this, in turn, may cause aggression and frustration.

These children can be saved. Without therapy, they are headed for a long, slow, difficult path through school, often branded as "learning disabled," "hyperactive," or "slow." Natural interventions, on the other hand, can produce very rapid results. Complete success can be achieved in one to two years.

Usually, a general nutritional tune-up will work wonders right away. Children respond quickly to nutritional therapy. They have had less time to degenerate than adults, and their small bodies fill up rapidly.

The first task is to eliminate all problem-causing foods temporarily. At a minimum, milk and wheat, especially all refined (white) flour, and sugar should be removed. Some practitioners believe that 40 to 50 percent of hyperactive children are sensitive to artificial food colors, flavors, and preservatives; and the consensus of natural healing practitioners is that children do better with as little exposure to these artificial additives as possible.

A megapotency multiple vitamin/mineral, at substantial doses (two to three times the dosage recommended on the packaging, with your practitioner's guidance), usually produces instant reduction in symptoms. Additional B vitamins in liquid form, vitamin A, and high-dose chewable calcium are also part of therapy for these children (calcium deficiency can lead to hyperactive behavior and is common in kids with milk sensitivities). The "superfoods" listed earlier are also added to the diet. For treatment of yeast infection in children, caprylic acid, essential fatty acids, and evening primrose oil can be given. Ear infections are treated as described earlier.

During Karta Purkh's years of personal experience with these children, he was gratified to see many, many young lives completely turned around through nutritional and herbal intervention. One three-year-old girl Karta Purkh met twelve years ago had been diagnosed as learning disabled, and was on her way to the "special education" track. When tested, she had thirty-five food allergies, including wheat, milk, and corn. When the parents immediately removed all allergic foods (a big job, but worth the effort), all ear infections ceased, never to return. They noticed that one corn chip would cause a runny nose. Only one year later, the child was nominated for the "gifted program" at school, and continues to be an honor roll student to this day.

Another child Karta Purkh knew personally would zoom around like an animal and bounce off walls screaming so loud that an adult conversation was impossible with him in the room. His parents followed the recommendations above, and the next time Karta Purkh saw him, two months later, even he was astonished at the results—he hardly recognized the child. He was sweet, nice, and relaxed. He sat quietly in his father's lap. The change was the talk of the child's neighborhood.

OTHER CHILDHOOD ILLS, SYMPTOMS, AND DISCOMFORTS

While infections and allergies are chief among childhood health concerns, there are a handful of other health disturbances that can be distressing to both child and parents. Here are some gentle, effective ways to deal with these typical issues.

Colic

Colic is a buildup of trapped gas in the baby's colon. It is extremely treatable. It is also believed to be—once again—the result of milk allergy in a large percentage of babies. Milk is the most common culprit in colic by a wide margin. In studies all over the world, removing cow's milk consistently cures colic in approximately 70 percent of the test samples, returning in every single subject when the milk is returned to their diets. (Note: Removing cow's milk means not drinking any if you're nursing.)

Dill seed tea or tea from *fennel* or *cumin* seeds—any seeds from that family—will work to relieve colic when it occurs. *Cardamom* is also an excellent choice. Microwave a cup of water with a teaspoon of seed, strain, put in an ice cube to cool it, and give it to the baby in a bottle. The child will suck it down, and the effect will be dramatic and instantaneous.

Other remedies include *chamomile* as an herbal bath, or 15 drops of *lavender oil* in a tablespoon of *almond oil* rubbed over the abdomen.

A baby with colic needs to have its whole digestive function investigated. Acidophilus can be used to reestablish and maintain a colony of good bacteria in the gut. Original gut bacteria comes from breast milk—this is the first "inoculation" of these bacteria, because a child is born with a sterile gut. Bifidus are the first bacteria to establish, and then between the ages of one and two, acidophilus becomes the predominant intestinal bacteria.

Fever

A high fever in a small child is one of the most frightening health conditions a parent may ever deal with. However, natural health practitioners today agree that a "fever paranoia" is needlessly promoted by pediatricians at least as much as parents, according to pediatrician Robert Mendelsohn, M.D.

The persistence of the myth that fevers commonly cause brain damage keeps many parents medicating small children with suppressive over-the-counter drugs in efforts to deal with a symptom that is really a healing response of the body. A fever doesn't mean the child's body is doing something wrong; it means the immune system is doing its job. By suppressing that healing mechanism, you prolong the illness.

As we have discussed, invading organisms evolved with us, their hosts, to thrive in a very narrow temperature range. Raising the temperature makes the host less hospitable in numerous ways. The growth rate of certain microbes is impaired at specific temperatures, and the death rate for various microbes at specific temperatures has also been determined. The immune system also responds to the increase in body heat by increasing white cell activity and mobility.

It may be the heat itself, increased immune function, and/or corresponding changes in blood chemistry that kills the invader or reduces its replication rate. The body, in its wisdom, has a biochemical interaction between brain and immune system that raises the thermostat when these responses would be beneficial.

But what about very high fevers? A fever above 106° can cause death, so it is important to reduce fever if it approaches 105°. But 95 percent of childhood fevers never get that high.[15] Other than that, a fever will not hurt your child. Except under very rare and unusual circumstances (poisoning, heatstroke, severe toxic exposure, or encephalitis), the body will not cook itself to the point of injury. Dr. Mendelsohn explains that fevers caused by common viral and bacterial infections will not exceed 105°.

Most cases of brain damage with fever have resulted from meningitis and encephalitis, both of which can cause brain damage independent of fever. Even in the small number of children who have seizures with high fevers, the seizures themselves are apparently usually harmless (and the cause unknown). They are also extremely rare and, contrary to popular belief, they occur due to the speed of temperature rise, not the temperature itself. The height of the fever is not necessarily an indication of the severity of illness.

If a fever gets near 105°, an attempt should be made to bring it down (and you should contact your physician). Other than that, try to let your child's body do its job. Treat the child and the illness, not the fever. We list natural remedies to reduce fever only because so many parents find it almost irresistible to bring fever down, so strong is the paradigm. If you must do it, it's better to use natural methods than drugs.

All of these herbs will reduce fever:

Isatidis root—If the child can swallow capsules, this energetically "cold" Chinese herb is an excellent fever reducer and, handily, is also antimicrobial. (It's too bitter for use as tea.) Give 1 capsule every two hours as needed.

Yarrow—Causes sweating. Use 1/3 ounce as tea.

Catnip—Cooling and relaxing. Use 1/4 ounce as tea.

Borage—Cooling. Use 1/4 ounce as tea.

Elder Flower—Cooling, also respiratory tonic (especially sinus) and good for sore throat. Use 1/3 ounce as tea.

Tulsi—This Ayurvedic herb, also known as holy basil, promotes sweating and is tasty, so 1/3 ounce as tea or powder mixed into food will work. The capsule dose for adults would be 2 to 10.

Chinese chrysanthemum flower—Sweet, cooling, relieves headache, clears sinus, reduces inflammation. Use 1/3 ounce as tea.

Honeysuckle flower—Cooling, calming, reduces swelling and inflammation. Use 1/3 ounce as tea or a couple of capsules.

We disagree with the old saw that Jell-O, Popsicles, and soda pop are good things to give a child when he or she has a fever. All of these are likely to contain sugar, which impairs immune function. Homemade herbal "Popsicles" are fine. Plenty of water is always a good idea to avoid dehydration.

Note: Infants under three months old who have any fever should receive medical attention, as should any child with a fever lasting more than three days. If your child is having trouble breathing, repeatedly vomiting, twitching, or otherwise acting in an alarming manner, seek medical help.

Note: Children should avoid aspirin, since it has been linked with Reye's syndrome, a potentially deadly (though extremely rare) disorder in children who have flu or chicken pox, both of which may initially resemble a cold. For this reason we also do not recommend willow bark (an herb whose active ingredient is a salicylate, like aspirin) to be used with children, even though no case of Reye's syndrome is known to have been caused by willow bark.

Digestive

These are general digestive tonics appropriate for children who are having garden-variety indigestion. Use beverage-strength tea throughout the day as tolerated.

Catnip—Increases digestive secretions
Peppermint—Increases digestive secretions, reduces gas, speeds digestion
Chamomile—Soothes digestive membranes, antigas
Orange Peel—Increases digestive secretions
Ginger—Warms the intestinal tract, reduces gas

In addition, *papaya* fruit or a *papain* (papaya enzyme) supplement will assist in protein digestion.

Constipation

An Italian study showed that 21 out of 27 children under the age of 3 had a significant increase in bowel function (number of stools, softening, and lack of discomfort and anal fissures, among other factors) within 3 days of having cow's milk removed from the diet. A "cow's milk challenge" caused rapid return of symptoms.[16] If your child is constipated, eliminate cow's milk in the diet as the first step, say these investigators.

If the removal of cow's milk alone does not help, any of the remedies for constipation listed on pages 328–330 for adults may be used with children, in proportional doses, with the exception of senna and buckthorn bark, which purge too harshly for children. The mildest choices would be *rhubarb root, rose petal, licorice root*, and *butternut bark*.

Diarrhea

Diarrhea is common in childhood. The cause of any diarrhea that is especially severe or lasts more than one day should be evaluated medically.

An excellent remedy is *carob powder*, perhaps stirred into plain yogurt, 1 to 2 tablespoons per day. Alternatively, you can use *blackberry root syrup* or a gruel made from *slippery elm bark* and water.

Loose stool may be caused by lack of proper large intestine bacteria (acidophilus, etc.), which may be killed by antibiotic use. Acidophilus powders, available in the refrigerator at the health-food store, can restore the proper intestinal flora.

Roo was a two-year-old who stopped growing at age one, at which time she had also been given high doses of antibiotics for a lung infection. The lung infection cleared up, but Roo developed constant diarrhea—up to twenty liquid bowel movements per day. When her parents questioned their medical personnel, they were informed that there was no connection between the antibiotics and the diarrhea. Eventually, after a year of no growth, injections of growth hormone were suggested. No treatment was indicated for the chronic diarrhea, unless it worsened.

That was the final straw for the parents. They brought Roo to a nutritionist, who concluded immediately that the antibiotics had killed the beneficial bacteria in her colon, and suggested large doses of potent acidophilus. The diarrhea immediately ceased, never to return, and Roo began to grow rapidly, normalizing in size over a few months.

Teething

For infants' and children's gum pain due to first teeth coming in, there are several effective natural remedies.

Almond oil—Rub on gums.

Chamomile—Taken internally it soothes structural-type tissue; a strong brew can also be rubbed on or made in a frozen "pop."

Clove oil—This can be rubbed on gums, but should be used only as a commercially made preparation from a natural products store. *Do not use undiluted clove oil on an infant's gums—it is way too hot and strong.*

Vitamin E—Rubbed on gums, it is a tissue healer and irritation reliever.

Goldenseal—A common secondary use of goldenseal, after its antibacterial application, is as a soother of mucous membranes and irritated tissues. It has an anti-inflammatory and strengthening effect on these tissues. Also, many bitter herbs are good at reducing pain. Goldenseal powder can be mixed with olive oil and applied directly to the gums.

Bed-wetting

Bed-wetting can be a chronic problem starting at around age three or four and continuing right on up to middle school age. The nervous system and bladder develop at different rates in different children, so the main strategy with bed-wetting is to support the nervous system and gain control of the sphincter muscle of the bladder. Concentrated wastes in urine, either because there is not enough liquid intake to dilute it or due to a buildup in the body, can irritate the bladder as well.

You can try these remedies:

Vitamin E—Clinically, this works, though the mechanism is unclear. 200 IU daily for a child is acceptable.

Plantain leaf—This is a general urinary tissue tonic. It can be given as a beverage-strength tea throughout the day (but of course avoid giving liquids right before bed).

Calcium/magnesium—These nutrients are essential for proper nerve and muscle function. Deficiencies cause muscles to cramp more easily. If the muscles relax, the bladder can hold more urine; if they cramp up, urine is forced out. Up to 1,000 milligrams of calcium before bed is appropriate, with 500 milligrams magnesium.

Trace minerals—Broad-spectrum mineral deficiencies tend to be involved in bed-wetting. These include zinc, selenium, and copper. A balanced diet as described earlier, plus a good multivitamin and mineral supplement, should suffice for this part of the program.

Sesame seed—One reason these may be effective is that they are high in calcium. The child can eat sesame butter or tahini or have seeds sprinkled in cereal.

Vinegar—Acidifying the urine slightly before bedtime can help with bed-wetting. A teaspoon or two of apple cider vinegar in juice can accomplish this; vitamin C or cranberry juice (diluted plain, not sweetened) are alternatives.

Nosebleed

Ayurvedic medicine offers preventive ideas as well as numerous treatments for this classic childhood condition. (These remedies work fine for adults, too!)

To treat chronic nosebleed preventively:

Vitamin C—Crucial for the function of collagen, the main structural tissue in the body. Vitamin C deficiency causes bleeding generally; that's one of the symptoms of scurvy.

Vitamin K—this is crucial for proper blood clotting. One good source is pith, the white part of citrus fruits (that thin membrane that usually shreds off when you peel it). Supplements are also available.

Acidophilus—The theory about why this works is that it assists bacteria in producing vitamin K in the intestine.

Bioflavonoids—The first bioflavonoid was called vitamin P for "permeability factor"; these blue and red pigments from fruits are needed along with vitamin C to prevent bleeding problems. Supplements of mixed bioflavonoids are available in the health-food store. Eating plenty of berries and grapes will help, too.

To treat an acute nosebleed immediately (basically, to keep it from going on and on) any of the following can be inhaled or sniffed, or dropped into the nose with an eyedropper.

Ice water
Alum powder (good astringent)
Camphor powder
Ginger juice (This is hot; use just *1 drop!*)

Sandalwood oil (This is the miracle treatment, in Karta Purkh's experience. It can be smeared up into the nose by the child using a finger saturated with the oil.)

Diaper Rash

Topically, the following are effective:

Yarrow oil
Calendula cream
Paste of powdered *acidophilus* with water

Internally, give 1 teaspoon per day acidophilus powder.

THEY ARE WHAT THEY TAKE

A last word on natural medicine and your children: The substances you give them today not only affect their health now and later, but the attitude you take with them regarding wellness and healing will help shape the attitudes of the next generation. The pharmaceutical mentality—which encourages reliance on quick fixes and "a pill for an ill," and downplays the connection between self-care and sickness—trickles down quickly from adult to child. This perpetuates a society that is highly tolerant of self-abuse, punctuated by last-minute, high-tech attempts to mitigate the abuse. The first year my best friend's younger sister, Emily, went off to college, she sent both of us an E-mail that I saved because it was such a painful example of this:

> I do have a cold but I don't think I need any medicine. The people here go to the Wellness Center daily. Get up in the morning and drink some coffee, go to the doctor and get medication, take medication, take a mid-morning coffee break, eat lunch at McDonald's, take an afternoon coffee break and a second dose of medication, eat dinner and throw in an *extra* (un-prescribed) shot of asthma medication, and then go to bed so you can get up in the middle of the night when you're not sleeping well and take a sleeping pill. :-) What a life!

11

Energizing Herbs

The energizing or stimulating properties of specific herbs can be
tapped to help build stamina and endurance, increase alertness,
and even warm the body. These are useful at a time when "slow,
tired, and cold" seems to be the human condition, at least in the United
States. Fatigue, or lack of energy, may be the most common chronic symptom anyone experiences in our culture. At home and at work, think about
how often you hear someone (or yourself) say, "Oh, I'm so tired!"

ADRENAL DEPLETION

Obviously, fatigue can have many different causes, but primarily, it's
adrenal gland depletion. Noted women's physician Kaaren Nichols, M.D.,
believes that adrenal insufficiency—the result of the mental and physical
stresses of the American lifestyle—is so widespread in our culture that it's
probably come to be regarded as "normal" by physicians and the public
alike.

The adrenal glands give us our moment-to-moment energy and mastermind our response to stress. Our stress-response mechanism—what we
sometimes call the "flight-or-fight" response—is wired into us from ances-
tral times.

Think of it this way: A million years ago, the survivor was a being who
could respond to immediate stress very quickly. Those who survived had a
mechanism for that response: adrenaline. So if an angry, hungry animal
jumped out of the bushes at you, your body would provide the "juice" to

let you either stab it with a spear or run away. Five minutes later, the whole thing would be handled, and you could relax, your heart would stop pounding, and you could go eat some berries.

Today, we don't have animals jumping out at us from the bushes—but our stress isn't over in five minutes. You have things like your boss is bugging you, and you'd *like* to be able to stab him or her with a spear or run away, but you can't do that, so you sit there and take it for eight hours. Then you sit in rush-hour traffic for an hour and a half each way, five days a week. Then there's family, errands, and endless other sources of chronic, unremitting low-grade stress. Physical assaults such as toxic exposure, overexercising, not enough sleep, trauma, injury, and illness can all stress the adrenals, too.

So we often remain in a constant state of agitation, bathing in our own stress hormones. Our bodies were not intended to work like that. The immediate response—instantly alert, attention drawn, muscles strong, breathing fast—is supposed to happen. What's not supposed to happen is the low-grade, constant arousal. Naturally, it's wearing for us to be cranking out these hormones constantly; overuse can wear anything out eventually.

The main goal with adrenal depletion is to support the glands and give them the raw materials they need to produce the hormones. It also helps, of course, to remove as many of the stressful environmental factors as possible. This means relaxing, learning to handle stressful situations psychologically, and adjusting our lives as much as possible to limit exposure to the pressures and tensions of our modern world.

THYROID DEPLETION

Low thyroid activity is another nearly epidemic condition in our country. It's estimated that 6 to 7 million Americans produce insufficient amounts of T4 (thyroxine) and T3 (triiodothyronine) hormones—and this estimate may be conservative, because many natural health practitioners feel that the condition is underdiagnosed. This can result in a variety of symptoms so common that, sadly, they are often accepted as an inevitable function of everyday life or, as we explained above, "normal." These symptoms include headaches, lethargy, a tendency to be cold, puffy eyes and dark circles under eyes, depression, dry hair and skin, thinning hair, unprecipitated body-fat gain, and menstrual irregularities.

Many Americans have such low standards for health and are so resigned to feeling lousy most of the time—or are even unaware of what feeling good feels like—that many don't even pay attention to such symptoms or consider them significant, let alone connected. Unfortunately, doctors often agree: They may chalk these signs up to aging, menopause, or even mental problems.

Worse, even when underactive thyroid is diagnosed conventionally, the only treatment generally offered is hormone replacement therapy. This does nothing to improve the condition; it simply fills in for the missing hormone. It does not address the underlying problem, or even question what that problem is.

Why did the gland get that way in the first place? Again, poor eating habits and other physical stresses, as well as mental stress, are likely factors. We would do well to look at our lifestyles rather than simply to crutch the gland.

Since thyroid hormones regulate metabolism, the rate at which food is broken down and converted into energy, they are without a doubt affected by the misguided epidemic of purposeful dieting and unwitting low-grade starvation in this country, which I discussed in *BodyFueling*® and which goes on to this day in mind-boggling proportions. A depressed metabolism is a common outcome of a very low calorie diet, in which insufficient fuel is provided to run the body. People experiencing this are most likely suffering from other symptoms of depressed thyroid function (also known as hypothyroidism). Some antidepressants, asthma drugs, and cancer treatments also have the side effect of lowering thyroid activity.

Another cause of hypothyroidism, believe it or not, is treatment for hyperthyroidism, or overactive thyroid. This is a prime example of iatrogenic disease (a condition resulting from medical intervention). The standard treatment for hyperthyroidism is typical of the sledgehammer mentality: drugs literally to "knock out" the hormone-producing tissue. These are given knowing that the long-term outcome will be a need to switch to replacement hormones. This seesaw from a drug that pushes in one direction to one that pushes in the other can be avoided.

Left untreated, low thyroid activity can increase blood pressure and cholesterol levels, increasing the risk of heart disease, and may also be linked to infertility and miscarriages, in addition to the daily difficulties caused by lack of energy and other symptoms.

Low thyroid hormone production can be detected by a relatively simple blood test called a TSH assay. This is a very sensitive test that can detect deficient hormone production well in advance of symptoms. Endocrinologists may perform even more sophisticated tests. Basal body temperature is widely believed to be the most consistent measure.

If you find out that you do have low T3 and/or T4 levels, however, it will probably be suggested that you begin to take synthetic thyroid hormone, probably in the form of Synthroid or Levoxine. Be aware that once you crutch your thyroid in this way, nothing will happen to stimulate the gland to do its own work. In fact, the problem may be worse if you try to stop taking the hormone later on, because the thyroid senses no need to keep producing anything at all if all of the work is being done for it. Most people are told that once they begin this treatment, they will be on synthetic hormone for the rest of their lives. (Actually, using natural therapies, most people can gradually wean off synthetic hormones over a year or so.)

During that period of time in my early twenties when I was so tired and sickly, riddled with food allergies, intestinal candida, menstrual irregularity, and poor immune function, I was also diagnosed with low thyroid. Again, no surprise; as I have said before, my lifestyle at that time provided the perfect setting for both depressed adrenal and thyroid function. I was an underfueled, nutrient-deficient chronic dieter and overexerciser; overworked, underrested, and under extreme emotional stress. But no one asked about or looked at my lifestyle. I was simply given a prescription for Synthroid.

Fortunately, I never filled that prescription. I tried natural hormone replacement through a naturopath, but this was an intermediate step; I was still dissatisfied because it was a glandular "prop-up." It was through education from Karta Purkh and the use of herbs that I went from icy cold (my boyfriend at the time complained that "only someone dead could have feet that cold") to naturally warm, and from being lethargic to being a powerhouse of energy. Healthy eating went a long way toward this change, but I didn't feel 100 percent better until I had nourished my glands herbally for about a year. I used some of the herbs that will be discussed next.

CASE STUDY:
FROM EXHAUSTED TO EXHILARATED

Massage therapist Maurice Collins, LMP, showed up in Karta Purkh's "Energizing Herbs" class looking for information about dealing with her exhaustion as well as a number of other garden-variety health complaints. She had been diagnosed with low thyroid and placed on hormone replacement therapy. She did in fact exhibit many of the classic symptoms of hypothyroidism. She tells her story:

"I had begun taking Thyroxine (now called Levoxine) for my exhaustion, prescribed by my doctor, about a month before I first met Karta Purkh. I had seen absolutely no difference in the way I felt, and I didn't really want to be taking the stuff anyway. Within five days of taking the herbs I learned about in Karta Purkh's class, I literally had so much energy that I must have been running on fumes previously. I felt wonderful. I immediately decided to stop taking the synthetic hormones, even though I was told I should reduce them slowly. Periodically I adjusted the dosages and types of herbs and I have continued to feel wonderful."

ONE GOOD GLAND SERVES ANOTHER

The hormone-secreting glands are arranged from the bottom of your body to the top in order of priority. At the low end are the gonads—the ovaries or testicles. Moving up the body you have the pancreas, adrenals, thyroid and parathyroids, pituitary and pineal, in ascending order. The farther up the body you go, the higher priority and more powerful the hormones.

The glandular system functions cooperatively; the glands support one another and give one another signals. If one gets worn out, the others are headed that way eventually if the problem isn't corrected, because they will have to work extra hard to compensate for the loss of the first.

Therefore, it is not coincidental that both adrenals and thyroid are involved in the low-energy syndrome. When the adrenals are depleted, the thyroid senses the loss of adrenal hormone and secretes more hormones, urging the adrenal glands to get with the program. Then the thyroid gets depleted. All of the glands get involved when there is an imbalance. If you can take a load off one, you're supporting the others.

General glandular tonics that support the whole system are an excellent way to manage this. If one gland is a problem, it will be nourished by the general tonic, and improving its function will enhance the function of the whole system. Some of the general tonics we recommended earlier are phytosterols, which provide the body "food" to make hormones. The body can turn some of these plant sterols into a wide variety of hormones as needed, so the herb does not necessarily need to be specific to one gland.

Among the remedies that follow, the shorter-acting ones tend to work more on the adrenals, and the longer-acting more on the thyroid. This reflects the nature of the roles these glands play: Adrenals are responsible for moment-to-moment activity and so they respond very rapidly to substances that affect them. Thyroid function is more of a long-term, ongoing regulation, and so herbs that work on thyroid function generally match that activity level.

CAFFEINE AND OTHER SHORT-ACTING STIMULANTS

Most of the things people use in day-to-day life to increase energy are actually contributing to the overall low-energy problem in the long run. That's because those things work by overstimulating the adrenals. They provide a short-term boost, but at the long-term expense of the glands whose overwork is part of the problem in the first place.

Caffeine works by mimicking a hormone that tells the adrenal glands to crank out more adrenaline. The adrenal glands think there is a stressful situation and that they are supposed to be making more adrenal hormone.

But with caffeine, we don't provide the glands anything to make that hormone out of—we just cry "emergency" and force them to figure it out, one way or another. So the body reaches down into its reserves and makes more hormone because it thinks it is the right thing to do. Caffeine forces your glands to secrete when they don't have much left to give, and they have to keep digging deeper and deeper, making you more and more tired over time. And over the years, it takes more and more coffee to get the same result. Some people reach the point of drinking half a dozen or more cups a day and it's barely keeping them awake. That's severe adrenal depletion.

Therefore, powerful stimulants tend to deplete energy rather than build it. Herbs, on the other hand, can provide gentle stimulation for short-term energy—and, more importantly, building blocks and long-term strengthening for the increased self-sufficiency of your glands. Herb Research Foundation president Rob McCaleb describes a fitting analogy: "The Chinese characterize the use of chi tonics as 'feeding a tired horse' and the use of a powerful stimulant as 'beating a tired horse.'"[1]

This "beating a tired horse" can go to serious lengths. One individual came to an associate of Karta Purkh's, a psychologist, because he thought he was having a nervous breakdown. He was having uncontrollable crying fits, shaking, and couldn't sleep. The psychologist began interviewing him, and was surprised to find nothing so stressful in his life as to cause this sort of extreme reaction. The client was asked about sugar: Did he consume a lot of cookies, candy, cake, pie, soda? The client kept denying it was anything in his diet until the subject of caffeine came up. It turned out the man was drinking seventeen cups of coffee a day with three teaspoons of sugar in each cup. He might have been institutionalized if he had gone to someone else. All he needed was to stop pounding on his adrenals.

Another problem with caffeine is that for most people, it is addictive and causes side effects. Some people who do not get their morning cup(s) become extremely irritable and experience headaches and nervousness. Others experience physical responses such as hot flushes and excessive sweating when they drink coffee. Such strong reactions suggest a powerful drug.

SO WHAT CAN YOU DO TO NOURISH YOUR ADRENALS?

Herbs energize calmly. This may sound like a contradiction in terms, but if you think about it, perhaps you can recall a time when you had all the energy you needed without being nervous. (By the same token, you can be exhausted, yet nervous—like when you stay up all night and drink coffee.) Herbs simply can provide sustained energy without overstimulation.

Some herbs are useful only as a short-term crutch, acting in ways similar to caffeine, but without the addiction and the excessive hammering effect. Others are long acting, used to get you off of all crutches eventually so that your body is doing a balanced job on its own.

Needless to say, in addition to using herbs, be sure to eat a healthy diet and take good basic care of yourself as we outlined earlier. Poor diet, cigarettes, alcohol, caffeine, and drugs all stress adrenals, and do not potentiate healing.

Short-Term Energy

Many people with fatigue, by the time they seek help, are crawling on their hands and knees begging for something to get through the day. They can't always wait the weeks or months it may take to build the body back to the point where it is providing enough energy on its own. These short-term herbals help hour by hour, till the long-term building takes effect.

Guarana seed is a good short-term adrenal builder. This herb from South America supplies raw material the adrenals need to make hormone, rather than simply signaling your adrenals to make more hormone. It provides food and nourishment instead of a mere command, so it's a good initial step to treat fatigue instead of coffee or other stimulants. It doesn't do much long-term building, though, so if you don't rejuvenate the adrenals in some long-term way, you will just wind up taking guarana seed your whole life for the daily supply of hormone food.

Guarana is sometimes misunderstood because it contains a small amount of compound that is in the same chemical family (methyl xanthenes) as caffeine. However, the whole seed with all of its complementary components doesn't have the harsh effect of caffeine with its potential for addiction, fast "rush," nervousness, irritability, and so on. Tannins and saponins in the seeds slow down the rate at which guaranine (a group of alkaloids) is dissolved and absorbed; this slow release provides a sustained long-term energizing effect. Indeed, a daily 1-gram dose contains less than 20 percent of the caffeine in a regular cappuccino.[2]

Guarana seed can be taken in capsules, not late in the day, 1 to 5 per day.

Kola nut is an herb from Africa and is interchangeable with guarana seed as a shorter-term adrenal herb. Guarana appears to work more quickly in some people, so for people who are more severely depleted, it may be a better option. Kola nut is mellower and its action a little slower. Kola nut was in original Coca-Cola (which also had cocaine, but now contains neither).

Like guarana, kola nut is essentially still a crutch. It's a better crutch, and won't hurt, but still a crutch. Kola nut is taken powdered in capsules, not late in the day, 1 to 5 per day.

Yohimbe is an African herb that should be used with care. It is one of the very few herbs in which getting enough of a dosage is not a problem, and you would *not* want to take as many as you could. In fact, it may be the most powerful of all the herbs we discuss in this book. As an energizer it's about five times as strong as guarana seed, for example. The dosage should be small—1 capsule or tablet a day is plenty for most people, and we recommend you don't exceed a maximum of 2 per day. Yohimbe should be taken early in the day, with food.

Yohimbe is a broader glandular tonic that works on several glands: adrenals, gonads, thyroid, and pituitary. It's a good short-term energy booster. It's also the only herb or natural substance scientifically verified to be an aphrodisiac by orthodox medical studies. Yohimbe increases energy, elevates mood and . . . draw your own conclusions about the aphrodisiac effect. (Basically, it increases blood flow to the pelvis.)

As an herbalist, Karta Purkh remembers that there was a three-year period in the 1980s when no one could get any yohimbe and the story in the market was that the world pharmaceutical industry bought up the entire supply to develop patentable aphrodisiac drugs. (There is one now, called yohimbine.) Now yohimbe is widely available again.

Yohimbe is never taken as a tea. It would taste unbelievably bad, and since it's so powerful that one capsule produces results, there is no motivation for making it into tea.

Yerba mate is a good short-term energizer that can be taken as tea (1/2 ounce dry herb in water) or in capsules (1 to 5 per day).

Ma huang, also known as ephedra, is a Chinese herb; there is also some that grows in American Southwest desert regions ("desert tea") that is not as powerful. It is the world's oldest known cultivated plant. Ephedrine is the plant compound that most closely resembles our own natural stimulant, epinephrine (adrenaline). It is also the compound from which the active ingredients of the OTC bronchial dilator Primatene (ephedrine) and the nasal decongestant Sudafed (pseudoephedrine) were synthesized.

Ma huang as a tea, or ground up in capsules, is excellent for dilating bronchial pathways—it does the job as well as or better than the pharmaceutical copies. The herb is used widely for sinus problems and asthma. The tea is not great tasting (very astringent), but it's drinkable.

The consensus among most herbalists is to be conservative with ma huang. It has been the subject of some negative attention from the media and local government-regulatory agencies because of its potential for side effects if used inappropriately. It is energizing, but it is safe in moderate amounts for most healthy people. Anyone who has a condition that requires they abstain from caffeine consumption should treat ma huang the same way.

Ma huang is, unfortunately, abused by dieters for its adrenaline-mimicking effects in hopes of stimulating "weight" loss. Some "herbal dieter" teas and capsules combine ma huang with caffeine, which should not be done unless recommended for medicinal purposes by your practitioner. This misuse has created an unfortunate image problem for ma huang, which can be a very effective botanical medicine for people who use it appropriately in the interest of healing.

I had excellent results with ma huang during my first year of herbal work. It was energizing and warming at a time when my body had wound down to a "slow and cold" state due to the long-term wear and tear my lifestyle had created. After about six months of daily use—about 1 cup of tea a day, brewed not too strong—I no longer needed it, because the long-term builders had produced a substantial, permanent effect. I didn't use it again until five years later, when I developed my first cold symptoms since that time. With two ma huang capsules, I was able to perform in a three-hour musical, singing nine songs, without any nasal congestion.

For best results, use plain ma huang in capsules starting with 1 or 2 and working up only as needed, or up to 3 tablespoons of crushed herb in water as tea. For a complete discussion of the politics and issues surrounding both real and exaggerated safety concerns about ma huang, see pages 483–487.

Medium-Term Energizers/Builders

Licorice root is valued by the Chinese as a general tonic and is excellent as a mild energizer while it performs longer-acting work on the adrenals. Licorice root actually contains compounds that are similar to the adrenal cortical hormones. It is also excellent for many other purposes in immune building, cold and flu treatment, and detoxification, as discussed in those relative chapters. Two to 5 capsules a day is appropriate for long-term building.

> Note: As discussed on page 481, European licorice root (*Glycyrrhiza glabra*) should be used with caution by people with existing hypertension (high blood pressure). DGL (deglycyrrhizined) licorice is missing the active ingredient that raises blood pressure, and can be used for liver and ulcer treatment. But DGL will be useless for adrenal building because the glycyrrhizin is what works on the adrenals. In fact, that's why it theoretically could raise blood pressure: Too much of the active ingredient could get adrenal hormones pumping excessively.

Cubeb berry is discussed in detail on page 175 with regard to its immune-building and antiviral capabilities. This warming, spicy, and aromatic black pepper relative also has an affinity for the lung tissue, making it an excellent tonic for adrenal insufficiency while also targeting the bronchial symptoms of adrenal weakness. It is very effective used daily as a tea, 1 to 2 strong cups a day. Five to 10 capsules per day may be used instead of tea.

Herbs that treat lung conditions such as asthma in the short term as well as adrenal insufficiency over the long term are very efficient "multitaskers." Practitioners of healing in the East have long recognized that asthma is basically an adrenal disease manifesting through the lungs—a symptom of weakened, tired adrenals. (Note that symptomatic treatment for severe asthma attacks always involves stimulating adrenaline.) Long-term asthma treatment, in herbal healing, always involves adrenal support.

Garlic, onion, and **ginger** are warming, energizing herbs that act as glandular tonics in the long term. These herbs have already been discussed in great detail. Ginger is mildly energizing short term, and garlic is especially good as an endocrine tonic. (The endocrine system is that which includes all ductless, hormone-producing glands.) Garlic and onion are mildly sexually stimulating as well. All three are enhanced synergistically when used together. Use to maximum tolerance in food.

Long-Term Builders

Fo-ti root (Ho Shou Wu), a Chinese herb, is somewhat like ginseng in action, but is much slower and more broad spectrum. It's primarily a thyroid tonic, builder, and strengthener, but also works well for PMS, especially in combination with other herbs. (See Chapter 8, "Especially for Women: Natural Healing for a Woman's Lifetime.") Secondarily, it's also a reproductive tonic, liver tonic, and kidney tonic.

Since this herb addresses the deficit underlying the energy shortage, it's not something you can take a bunch of today and feel a quick energy boost. You take it over a period of weeks or months and build the foundation of energy in the body. Eventually you will find yourself naturally having more energy all the time. The nice thing about this is that it's your energy, created by your body, not by the herb. The slumps you may have experienced will go away, even without the day-to-day short-term boosters.

In this building mode, the typical dose is 4 capsules per day; up to 10 may be used.

Astragalus root is a Chinese tonic herb described in detail in our discussion of immune building (pages 134–136). It is particularly valued for immune support, but as a Chinese *qi* tonic it is also used to restore energy overall. It is one of the most valued of all herbs by the Chinese for its ability to nourish and boost almost every system of the body, and it's an excellent long-term energy builder that can also provide more immediate, though mild, energy increases. It can be taken as tea (1 ounce of herb per day is a fine long-term dose) or capsules.

Eleuthero root (also known as Siberian ginseng) is another excellent energy and stamina builder. It is an exceptional overall long-term tonic for health, immunity, and strength. In the context of addressing energy problems it works specifically on the thyroid and is especially useful for those diagnosed with low thyroid activity. Four to 10 capsules per day is a reasonable dose. Eleuthero is discussed in detail on pages 142 and 232.

Saw palmetto berry, from a little palm tree that grows in Florida, is currently best known for its use as a tonic for men over age 40 to 50 because of its impressive performance in prevention of and treatment for prostate disease (See Chapter 9, "Especially for Men: Natural Healing for a Man's Lifetime"). However, it is also useful as a thyroid tonic and long-term builder. It also increases production of sex hormones. Two to 8 capsules a day is an average dose.

Triphala ("three fruits") is the revered Ayurvedic herbal tonic preparation made from amla, bibitaki, and haritaki. You may recall that it's legendary in India for its prodigiously broad range of action in promoting health and healing for virtually every body organ and system. It also has an extremely high vitamin C content. One of its chief uses is as a glandular tonic, very long term. Two capsules a day, every day of your life, can only help you. See pages 139–140 for more on triphala.

Black cohosh root is a Native American herb from Appalachia, used widely in midwifery to prepare the body for pregnancy (not during pregnancy, however). *Cohosh* in Native American languages means "root." (Black cohosh and blue cohosh are two completely different herbs; they're just both roots. Blue cohosh is not a tonic.) Black cohosh is a good long-term glandular tonic that can be used by men and women. Two to 5 capsules a day may be used for this purpose.

Prickly ash bark is grown around Ontario, Canada. It's a good general tonic, although it may work especially on the adrenals. It happens to be well known traditionally for benefits to the teeth. The glandular system does regulate mineral metabolism, including calcium, which obviously affects the teeth. Two to 5 capsules a day can be used indefinitely to maintain glandular balance.

Muira puama root is from Brazil, where it's known as the "herb of love." It's a relaxing general glandular, although in larger doses can increase libido. (Actually, all of these in large ongoing doses would increase libido and sexual function somewhat, because they regulate hormonal secretions generally, including those of the sex hormones.) Try 1/2 ounce as tea or 1 to 3 capsules.

Sarsaparilla root grows in Mexico, India, China, and Central America. It was formerly used to flavor root beer. It is a general tonic, believed to work on the adrenals because it has anti-inflammatory action and probably stimulates adrenal anti-inflammatory hormone. This makes it a good joint remedy, especially for arthritis. (Thanks to that root-beer taste, tea works well for the large amounts required for arthritis relief.) As a tonic, 1 or 2 capsules a day is sufficient.

Bladderwrack is a source of iodine; 1 to 10 capsules a day.

STAMINA AND ENDURANCE HERBS

Another use for energizing herbs, in addition to therapeutic treatment for low energy, is to stimulate and maximize energy, stamina, and endurance for sports and athletics. This is not a new concept: athletes around the world have been using stamina-promoting herbs to improve athletic performance for decades.

Herbs can also help replenish what is lost to extremely demanding athletic regimens. Without conscious, diligent supplementation to meet the body's increased need for support, the stresses of athletic training and competition can deplete energy reserves, lower immunity, and increase the risk of injury as well as infection. But it doesn't have to be that way. Heavy exercise may be an extra burden to the body, but the body can handle it as long as you match the output with extra sustenance.

Sometimes athletes use stimulants like caffeine to provide a "jolt" before competition, but these can backfire, causing nervousness and jitteriness. Caffeine may stimulate the desired physical response in the muscles but make you mentally less competitive. For this reason, ma huang is also probably not the best choice. Many of the herbal adaptogens favored by athletes have the opposite effect—they actually enhance mental focus rather than fracturing it.

Panax (Asian) ginseng, prized for millennia by the Chinese as an overall energy (*qi*) tonic, is used to increase strength and athletic performance as well as immunity, sexual vitality, concentration, mental acuity, and energy. Thousands of studies worldwide confirm these uses. It may be especially valuable to athletes because of its versatility: As an adaptogen it can help buffer the effects of stress, trauma, and the "shock" of extreme training, and speed recovery from injury and inflammation. Ginseng's blood-sugar-regulating effect would also be useful in a heavy athletic training schedule.

Eleuthero is an increasingly popular adaptogen that was used extensively by Russian athletes and was first scientifically studied there. It's now become very popular in the United States. It has been shown to increase mental alertness and adaptation to environmental stress as well as increase physical endurance, immunity, and adaptability to a wide range of conditions. It is also considered to be a thyroid tonic.

The Chinese *qi* tonic herbs discussed on pages 144–146, such as *astra-*

galus, ligusticum (best paired with astragalus), *fo-ti, codonopsis,* and *atracty-lus,* are all useful for athletes who want long-term energy building. Most of these will not provide an immediate energy burst but will "feed" the body's energy-making apparatus over time and prevent depletion.

Circulatory stimulants may also be useful to athletes. Maximizing blood circulation and oxygenation can enhance athletic performance. *Cayenne pepper, ginger, ginkgo,* and *bilberry* concentrate would all be appropriate for this purpose.

Triphala, Ayurveda's premier tonic remedy, is a gold mine for athletes. Its ability to rejuvenate virtually every part of the body, speed healing, balance glandular function, and enhance immunity makes it a terrific all-around "athletic supporter."

Most of these herbs are discussed in more detail in the "Noteworthy Tonics" section on pages 133–146.

12

Herbs for Depression, Addictions, Anxiety, and Insomnia

Herbs can enhance mental as well as physical health. Some herbs and foods have properties that help calm anxiety, promote clear-headedness, assist with depression, relieve tension and insomnia, and improve sleep.

DEPRESSION

Most everyone has the occasional attack of "the blues" or a "down in the dumps" funk, short periods when things don't seem to go well and life isn't looking too rosy. Clinical depression is different. It is a medical disorder characterized by persistent and sometimes severe feelings of worthlessness, guilt, sadness, helplessness, and hopelessness.

Some 25 percent of the population may suffer from a depression over the course of a lifetime. Depression strikes men and women of all ages, across all socioeconomic lines, but most studies indicate that women are more often afflicted. Women are also more likely to seek help, however, which may mean that depression in men is merely underreported.

Karta Purkh's observations as a teacher suggest that depression is on the rise. Many of our colleagues corroborate this alarming rise in the proportion of clients with diagnoses of depression, and the observation bears out national statistics (more than 15 million Americans diagnosed with depression annually). Karta Purkh notes, "I have met more people with depression in the last two years than in the entire twenty years prior."

There are probably numerous reasons for this increase, from people reaching their limit in an increasingly complicated and stressful world to the physical imbalances caused by daily lifestyle abuses, including poor diet and lack of exercise. Another reason is improved detection and diagnosis by skilled clinicians, and a further reason is the push by pharmaceutical companies to market prescription antidepressants.

The specifics of depression can be as unique as the person experiencing it, but generally it seems to be triggered by one of two types of catalysts: a tragic or traumatic event, or a neurochemical imbalance of brain messenger hormones. Both catalysts may also be present in a patient. Depression resulting from circumstances, such as the death of a loved one, is typically shorter and can often be helped by counseling or psychotherapy. Those with a biochemical basis for the condition, on the other hand, feel depressed regardless of circumstances. These sufferers are often prescribed drugs to balance the neurotransmitters in the brain.

It's important for anyone with serious symptoms of depression to be evaluated medically. In addition, we do not want to recommend that anyone simply stop taking medication that has been prescribed for them. But you should be aware that many people with long-term chronic depression have been able to reduce or eliminate antidepressant medication and begin to function well and feel good using natural remedies. Herbs and nutrients can also provide transitional support when it's time to "wean off" medication.

People suffering from depression often have sleep disruption and a complicating lack of energy. With fatigue during the day and insomnia at night, it becomes impossible ever to feel comfortable and relaxed. Therefore, part of the long-term strategy also includes rebuilding the endocrine and nervous systems. Energizing tonics are taken earlier in the day, so that the adrenal glands can be nourished during waking hours, and to avoid further sleep disruption. Natural remedies to support sleep are taken late in the day, so that the natural hormonal rhythm can be reestablished.

Depression can be a very complicated issue. With insight and careful application, many people have success with self-treatment. Most cases, however, are multifaceted, and do better with the assistance of an experienced practitioner. Herbs and nutrients are extremely important in a natural healing program for depression, but professional counseling, exercise, diet, and stress management can be equally important. Patients should ask their health professionals how much experience they have in treating depression. A practitioner who simply prescribes Prozac (fluoxetine) and does not consider the wide range of other alternatives may not be your best choice. There are definitely safe and effective natural alternatives to these drugs.

The Ayurvedic View

Interestingly, from the Ayurvedic point of view, in many instances depression is simply another possible outcome of imbalance in the doshas—in this case, *vata* or *kapha*. Many milder cases represent a typical expression of excess *vata* or *kapha*—much more likely to affect those constitutional body types, but possible in any type.

A slow, sad, lethargic type of depression is notoriously *kapha*. Recent changes in depression diagnosis also include anxiety, nervousness, moodiness, and fearfulness as symptoms; these are more characteristic of the jittery, changeable *vata* energy. The Ayurvedic point of view is empowering: such a person is not "depressed" at all; he or she is simply manifesting *vata*. Rather than be saddled with the stigmatizing label of depression as a disease requiring drugs, such conditions simply represent tendencies that are predictable for certain bodies. Just as with any body type, the challenge is to manage these tendencies and maintain proper balance. This does not necessarily mean "treating a mental illness"—it may mean treating *vata* (or *kapha*).

Herbal Depression Treatment

The standout remedy for depression in the herb world is the leaf of **St. John's wort** (*Hypericum perforatum*). This herb is used as an antiviral (particularly with AIDS), antibacterial, and possible anti-cancer agent, but it's been in the spotlight for its antidepressant properties. Particularly for depression that is mild to moderate, St. John's wort has proven extremely effective.

The compound in St. John's wort that has been isolated and was believed to be the main active ingredient is hypericin. However, hypericin is no longer believed to act alone. As is the case with most herbs, the complex interplay of many compounds is believed to be responsible for the beneficial effects.

St. John's wort inhibits the enzyme monoamine oxidase (MAO), just as Prozac and other serotonin-selective reuptake inhibitors (SSRIs) do, but it does so more weakly. It also modulates and balances the brain chemicals serotonin and norepinephrine, much as tricyclic and tetracyclic drugs (used for the most common form of serious depression) do. It may also increase endorphin levels.

According to Dr. Michael Murray, N.D., St. John's wort consistently achieves a greater than 50 percent reduction in the Hamilton Depression Scale (a series of measurements used to quantify depression) in a large percentage of patients, and does better than tricyclic antidepressants, without the side effects.[1]

Research studies typically use standardized extracts containing 125 percent hypericin. Capsules of this extract can be found in most health-food stores. The recommended dose of the extract is 300 milligrams 3 times a day. St. John's wort can also be taken as a tea (1/2 ounce of dried herb per day) or tincture. Capsules of the whole herb can also be taken, about 10 to 12 capsules daily. It is widely available at herb stores in many forms.

It can take a month or more for the effects of hypericum to kick in. However, the same is true for the prescription drugs used to treat depression. And at the recommended dosage, St. John's wort doesn't cause the mouth dryness, anxiety, oversedation, headaches, nausea, insomnia, digestive problems, heart problems, or other side effects of many common antidepressants. Prescription MAO inhibitors also interact with tyramine, an amino acid found in cheese, beer, wine, and other foods, and can cause severe hypertension in patients who eat these foods.

In the United States many health practitioners are advising that you do not take this herb with Prozac or other antidepressants, theorizing that the herb will be "additive"—that is, intensify the effects of the drug and/or the herb. However, this is purely supposition. In Germany (where half of all prescriptions for depression are for St. John's wort), the herb is specifically used concurrently or transitionally with antidepressant drugs to help patients taper off the drug, according to David Overton, PA-C, R.N., a physician's assistant and expert in brain biochemistry (on the clinical faculties of the University of Washington and Pacific Lutheran University). Overton, who practices in the area of mood disorders, suggests that the two can be used safely together in this manner if your practitioner has experience handling both prescription drugs and herbal medicine.

There are some considerations and contraindications for the use of St. John's wort. This herb should be taken with food to avoid stomach upset. Also, a small number of people experience extreme photosensitivity and must avoid prolonged sun exposure at extremely high doses of St. John's wort (such doses should, in any case, only be taken under the supervision of a health practitioner).

Actually, until recently this reaction had only been observed in pasture cows who grazed on enormous amounts of the plant; there were no documented cases of photosensitivity in humans before practitioners began recommending it in high doses to AIDS patients. In fact, research shows that sunlight exposure may expedite the effects of St. John's wort. People using high doses of St. John's wort long term are advised to avoid prolonged exposure to direct sunlight, but to maintain consistently shorter exposures to indirect, low-level sunlight.

Another herbal remedy showing some promise with depression is *ginkgo*. This circulatory tonic is used widely in Europe to prevent and treat disorders involving decreased blood supply to the brain (cerebrovascular inefficiency), and numerous double-blind, controlled studies have shown it to be effective in this regard. Most studies have initially dealt specifically with potential improvements in common cerebrovascular conditions of the elderly, such as senility and Alzheimer's. Ginkgo apparently can retard the progress of, or even reverse, these conditions.

However, ginkgo is also believed to increase the rate at which information is transmitted at the nerve cell level. This could affect depression, which is influenced by these neurotransmissions. Indeed, research on depression and *Ginkgo biloba* extract has been a secondary offshoot of research on its effects on cerebrovascular efficiency. Subjects in double-blind studies noticed mood improvements along with improvements in areas being studied, such as memory and other markers of mental performance. Still, ginkgo may be most useful for older patients.

The effective daily antidepressant dose in one of the studies was 240 milligrams daily—twice the 120-milligram daily dose usually recommended for GBE. This dose may cause headaches or dizziness initially in elderly people. Starting at the lower dose of 120 milligrams daily and then increasing to the 240-milligram level over a period of 6 to 8 weeks will usually handle this problem.

The Ayurvedic herb *coleus* (or an extract of its chief active ingredient, *forskolin*) shows antidepressant activity in animal studies.[2] Typical dose is 50 milligrams of the extract 2 to 3 times per day, or 4 to 8 capsules of the whole herb daily.

Nutrients

B-complex vitamins are also extremely important for normal formation and function of brain neurotransmitters, which are the chemical messengers of the nervous system. The B vitamins are sometimes thought of as brain nutrients. Again, we must distinguish between acute deficiencies (the kind that caused pellagra and beri-beri in the 1920s) and the levels of B-vitamin deficiencies found commonly today. Almost no one is so acutely deficient anymore as to be at risk for these diseases, but recent research has spawned newer thinking about the significance of marginal deficiencies that create neurological changes. These subtle shifts in brain chemistry can cause behavioral and emotional changes that are definitely noticeable.

Some of the B vitamins are synergistic, and deficiencies in one can drag down the others. That's why B vitamins are most often sold as a "B-complex" so that you get a balanced quantity of all of them at once. However, sometimes supplementation in one—B_6 or B_{12}, for example—is indicated for a particular condition. A health practitioner can test B-vitamin levels to detect deficiencies.

B complex has been a popular part of nutritional treatment for the emotional symptoms of PMS for many years. Vitamin B_6 in particular has been effective for this purpose and is probably the most effective principle in the B complex for depression. Vitamin B_6 (also called pyridoxine) is key to the synthesis of all major neurotransmitters. Natural medicine author, researcher, and professor of botanical medicine (at Bastyr University) Michael T. Murray, N.D., thinks that there may be millions of people on Prozac who merely have a B_6 deficiency.[3] Other research has shown deficiencies of B_{12} and folic acid consistently in depressed people.

An increase in serotonin, one of the key mood-regulating neurotransmitters, has been observed in various studies when subjects are given B complex.

The processing of food destroys B vitamins, so the typical highly processed diet may well be a factor in the ever-increasing spiral of depression in our culture. Some drugs decrease B absorption—antihistamines, tranquilizers, and sleeping pills, not to mention many recreational drugs. Another cultural and lifestyle factor may be the use of coffee, alcohol, and cigarettes, all of which deplete the B vitamins, and can deplete vitamin C as well. (Vitamin C deficiencies can cause depression, according to Dr. Murray.)[4] Cigarette smoking especially causes vitamin C to be used more heavily and rapidly, probably for detoxification.

Inositol, considered by some nutritionists to be part of the B-vitamin group, can be helpful in treating depression, especially when tricyclic antidepressants have been prescribed. Low levels of this nutrient have been found in patients with depression. One double-blind placebo-controlled study found therapeutic results from inositol similar to that provided by tricyclic antidepressants, but without side effects.[5]

Amino acids are believed to play an important role in moderating the activity of nerve cells and the transmission of their impulses. Certain essential amino acids are precursors for brain chemicals that are calming and mood-boosting. *L-phenylalanine* (best if a tricyclic has been prescribed) and *l-tyrosine* (best if Prozac or another SSRI has been prescribed) are two amino acids that are recommended as supplements for depression and lethargy. Use one or the other. They can be purchased at most health-food stores. (Note: Obtain the L-forms, not the DL-forms. The DL-forms are part synthetic and not useful for depression—although DL-phenylalanine is useful for pain.)

These amino acids may raise blood pressure (one of the neurotransmitters they help synthesize is epinephrine, or adrenaline) so increase the dose slowly if you have high blood pressure. They also should not be used by pregnant or nursing women. Check the label for drug contraindications.

Calcium and *magnesium* are muscle relaxants and play a role in proper nerve and muscle function. They modulate brain chemicals that stabilize nerve cell membranes and assist in proper neurotransmission. They can be taken individually or together in a 2:1 ratio of calcium to magnesium.

GABA (gamma-aminobutyric acid) is a neurotransmitter and amino acid in the glutamine family. It is the most widely distributed neurotransmitter in the brain and plays a specific role in regulating anxiety. It inhibits excitation of brain cells receiving anxiety messages. If GABA stores are depleted (such as from long-term stress or anxiety), the flood of anxiety messages is no longer buffered. It is available as a supplement.

Special Foods

Using *chilies* for depression originated in Ayurveda, and Karta Purkh originally learned about them from his mentor and teacher Yogi Bhajan. The "chili eater's high" may come when the ingestion of hot food boosts brain levels of endorphins, the mood-modulating chemical that also regulates sleep, appetite, cognition, and some aspects of the immune system. The capsaicin in chilies is also known to deaden or deplete substance P, a neuropeptide that transmits pain signals.

Celery, especially the juice, is relaxing (studies also show it lowers blood pressure)—more useful for anxiety than depression, though it can help with sleep. High in vitamin A and vitamin B_1, celery also contains potassium, sodium, and magnesium.[6]

Essential fatty acids (*EFAs*) from evening primrose, borage, or black currant oils (or flaxseed taken as oil by the tablespoon, in capsules, or as ground seeds) are important to the synthesis of "friendly" prostaglandins (hormonelike messengers that give cells instruction). Low levels of EFAs have been linked to depression (as well as child hyperactivity, alcohol abuse, and premenstrual syndrome). Anti-stress hormones are made out of EFAs.

In addition, EFAs go into the manufacture of cell membranes, and cells need these and other healthy fats discussed earlier to maintain optimal function. If these "good fats" are deficient in the diet, the body has to make cell membranes out of "bad fats" (saturated, trans-fats, animal fatty acids, and cholesterol) which can lead to "faulty," makeshift cell membranes. This can affect the brain because membrane fluidity is crucial to nerve cell function. Less-fluid membranes made out of poor-choice fats may interfere with neurotransmitter synthesis, transmission, uptake, and binding, among other factors.

Interestingly, heart disease and depression share some of the same links to nutritional deficiencies as well as to lifestyle and dietary habits. Heart disease and depression seem to occur together frequently (one reason Dr. Dean Ornish's program has yoga, meditation, and support group elements). Low levels of folic acid are linked to both conditions; low levels of EFAs in the diet, along with high intake of omega-6 and animal fats, are also associated with both conditions.

Natural Depression Therapy

Here are some ideas for a sample program to treat depression using the above herbs and nutrients. Some of the herbs listed below have been discussed in other chapters or later in this chapter for their specific properties (such as valerian as sedative, or kola nut and guarana for short-term energizing). Do not take all of these remedies simultaneously; choose a few to start and substitute or add others if you are not satisfied with the results of your first choices:

	Daytime remedies	*Night remedies*
Herbs	Kola nut, guarana seed, ephedra (ma huang) or yohimbe Ginseng, fo-ti root, or licorice root Gotu kola, ginkgo	Valerian root, hops leaf, or scullcap leaf
Vitamins & Minerals	B₁ 100 mg.; B₆ 100 mg. B complex 50 mg.	Calcium 1,000 mg. and/or Magnesium 500 mg.
Amino acids	l-phenylalanine 1,500 mg. or l-tyrosine 1,500 mg.	GABA (gamma-aminobutyric acid)
Foods, Other	Chilies (especially red, e.g., cayenne), Flaxseed oil (cold pressed)	Celery (especially juice)

Diet, Exercise, and Lifestyle for Depression

An unhealthy lifestyle is no less a factor in depression than it is in most other disorders from which Americans suffer. Lifestyle changes are really the long-term treatment for most depression; supplements just provide a natural, nontoxic transition. If depression arises as frequently from nutrient deficiencies as is suspected, triggered by harmful substances we use and healthy things we neglect, then both prevention and treatment must eliminate unhealthy influences and incorporate health-promoting ones.

In addition to the above-described supplementation, healthy diet and exercise habits should be cultivated, both because they are therapeutic by themselves and because they provide a foundation for the effectiveness of supplements. The program outlined above is excellent for short-term crisis management. For general health, energy, and particularly adrenal rebuilding, some of the foods and tonics outlined earlier in the book for those purposes should be used on a long-term basis. These would include astragalus root, schizandra berry, licorice root, fo-ti root, saw palmetto berry, eleuthero root, triphala, and cubeb berry, as well as garlic, onion, and ginger.

Metabolic processes in the brain depend on a steady supply of glucose and oxygen carried by the blood. Therefore, it makes sense that diet and exercise, which help stabilize blood sugar and maintain cardiovascular fitness, could prevent or improve conditions of depression.

An antidepressive diet, not surprisingly, doesn't look that much different from the diet presented as generally healthy and immune supportive on pages 107–117. Again and again the same dietary recommendations apply no matter what condition or disease we are discussing, and whether we are looking at mind or body, prevention or treatment.

In particular, alcohol (which is a nervous system depressant and can interfere with B-vitamin absorption and the neurotransmitter GABA) should be avoided. So should simple sugars, which cause blood sugar irregularities that create mood problems of their own and can aggravate existing ones. There seems to be a definite relationship between sugar abuse/cravings, mood, and a brain chemical called serotonin, which among many other tasks is involved in the regulation of insulin.

Deficiency of complex carbohydrates has been linked to low levels of serotonin. This calming "feel-good" neurohormone appears to be connected in numerous ways to how well we sleep, eat, relax, and handle stress. Low serotonin levels are associated with depression. They are also associated with cravings for carbohydrate (which, as I explain at length in *Bodyfueling*,® are quite normal and predictable if you are consistently deprived of carbohydrate through either dieting or "hapless eating"). Carbohydrate foods trigger the release of serotonin, so starving the body of carbohydrates could certainly reduce levels of serotonin. This can contribute to depression directly, and also can set up a cycle of sugar craving that aggravates the condition and causes a vicious cycle.

For people who are depressed, this is just one more good reason to emphasize whole grains, fruits, vegetables, and legumes.

Regular aerobic exercise has been recommended for many years as part of prevention and treatment for depression. Some researchers and health practitioners have observed that it's simply very difficult to find a clinically depressed person who is a regular exerciser. Exercise has also proven useful in treating mood disorders specifically associated with PMS, and it's interesting to note that many of the basic lifestyle factors that seem to improve premenstrual depression and irritability—a higher-complex-carbohydrate diet, reduction in simple sugars and dietary fats, and regular aerobic exercise—are indicated for clinical depression as well.

One of the chief reasons that may make exercise beneficial for treating depression is its ability to regulate norepinephrine, or "brain adrenaline," and increase endorphin levels. Endorphins are brain chemicals sometimes likened to "natural heroin." They are associated with a "high" that many people experience with regular, moderately strenuous aerobic exercise; it has been called "runner's high," but you don't have to run to get the benefit. Any regular aerobic activity that raises the heart rate and makes you sweat and breathe faster than normal should do the job. (*BodyFueling*® has a chapter on exercise that discusses these and other benefits of various types of exercise.) Again, chilies and some herbs (such as St. John's wort, kava-kava root, nutmeg, and borage leaf) also boost endorphins.

Exercise may also be useful for many other reasons: It improves overall health and well-being, often results in a body that feels and looks more culturally acceptable, may involve social activity or contact, and provides a feeling of *doing* something—taking action and taking control. These factors may also play a role in the antidepressive effects of exercise.

Cigarettes, alcohol, caffeine, and refined sugar should be eliminated, as discussed above. The connections of addictions to these substances is convoluted—depression may cause people to begin using them, or using them may cause depression (or both). Trying to stop using them may also create chemical imbalances that affect mood; dealing with those issues is the subject of the following section.

ADDICTIONS

Those recovering from addictions and eating disorders can benefit from physical as well as psychological therapies. Addiction recovery treatment often overlooks the physical aftermath of addictions (and sometimes an initial physical trigger as well). Herbal and nutritional therapies can help restore proper brain chemistry, eliminate allergies, and shore up immune systems that have been depleted by health-robbing addictive behaviors and substances.

The right herbs and foods used properly can also greatly assist with efforts to eliminate drugs, alcohol, and cigarettes from your life, easing withdrawal symptoms and providing safe, natural, and positive ways to experience well-being and vitality.

It is probably not possible to separate this discussion completely from the discussion of depression above. The imbalances that may cause depression are often indirectly responsible for addiction to mood-altering substances, which may be sought in an attempt to mask the depression.

In addition, many of the mood-regulating brain chemicals discussed earlier have been shown through research to modulate a variety of behaviors. Biochemical behavior regulation in the brain is complex enough to involve many different behavioral cause-and-effect situations. A "which came first" relationship is often difficult to establish. Abusing the body with addictive substances may cause imbalances, or imbalances may trigger addictive cravings in the first place. Drugs, alcohol, and sugar may be craved due to deficiencies in serotonin or norepinephrine, for example. However, drugs, alcohol, and sugar obviously don't solve the problem; in fact they aggravate the deficiencies.

The bilevel work that is characteristic of herbal therapy—relieving the symptoms while working on balancing or healing the underlying issues— holds true in addiction recovery. Skilled clinicians recognize this bilevel approach and in fact sometimes call mood disorders and addictions a dual diagnosis. If you have a dual diagnosis, be sure to find a practitioner who is experienced at treating both illnesses, and who will work on long-term rebuilding and replenishment as well as the immediate concerns of cravings or withdrawal symptoms. A counselor who only works on the addiction or a doctor who only works on the depression may not be sufficient.

Just as with depression, diet and exercise should be used to build and maintain a general base of health. In addition, herbs and nutrients can be used to restore specific body systems and organs that may be exhausted, as well as provide comfort as the body adjusts to its "new life."

As mentioned earlier, amino acids are believed to play key roles in maintaining proper brain chemistry, nerve cell activity, and the transmission of nerve impulses. Amino acid supplementation can be an important part of addiction recovery because many abusive behaviors can result in low levels of the amino acids that nourish the brain. Abuse of alcohol or drugs, anorexia, and bulimia all deprive or deplete the body of these essential substances, and the resulting imbalances in brain chemistry disable the work of the "feel-good" neurotransmitters. Naturally, this makes it difficult to stay away from the addictive substances or behaviors, since those were the original "solutions" of choice for pain and unrest.

In a way, brain chemicals are our natural drugs—natural speed, sedatives, and opiates—and perhaps if they were all present in adequate levels, people would not feel the need to seek outside sources for their effects.

Sample Addiction Recovery "Bridge" Program

Short-term Energizing	• Kola nut, guarana seed, or yohimbe • l-phenylalanine 1,500 mg. *or* l-tyrosine 1,500 mg.
Calming/ Relaxing	• Valerian root, hops leaf, scullcap leaf, or chamomile • Taurine, glutamine, B$_6$, manganese • GABA (gamma-aminobutyric acid), glutamic acid • Calcium 1,000 mg., magnesium 500 mg.
Long-term Rebuilding	• B$_1$ 100 mg., B$_6$ 100 mg., B complex 50 mg. • Vitamin C two to 5 grams daily or to bowel tolerance • Fo-ti root, licorice root, ginseng, or astragalus

Special Foods	• Celery juice—up to two quarts daily (late in day for relaxing/sleep)
	• Chilies (for endorphin boost plus immune boost)
	• Onion, garlic, ginger (for general health rebuilding, glandular balance, immune boost)
	• Root vegetables (for liver cleansing; use small amounts [two ounces juice maximum per day])
	• Essential fatty acids (EFAs):
	    Linoleic acid (LA) and gamma-linolenic acid (GLA)
	      from evening primrose, flaxseed, hemp, borage, or black currant oils

Again, don't take every single herb and supplement listed above. Try one or two from each category.

Herbal "Stop Smoking" Program

Kola nut—A mild stimulant to elevate mood and feel energized (2 to 10 capsules per day, not late)

Vervain leaf or *cubeb berry*—Lung rejuvenative (5 to 10 capsules per day or tea)

Saw palmetto berry—For stamina, adrenal/thyroid nourishment (2 to 5 capsules per day)

Ginger—For circulation and detoxification (2 to 5 capsules per day)

Prickly ash bark—Adrenal builder (2 to 5 capsules per day)

Start the above program two to three weeks before stopping the cigarettes. Then reduce or stop the cigarettes and continue with the above program, lowering doses progressively until cravings are gone.

Post-Recovery Healing for Specific Addictions

Specific addictions can leave particular kinds of damage in their wake, and you can give your body an added edge in healing the affected areas by supplementing with herbs and foods that have an affinity for those areas. For example, the liver is a focus of concern for recovering alcoholics; former smokers may want to accelerate and enhance the healing of lung tissue.

If you are trying to or have successfully gotten off barbiturates ("downers," such as Seconal, Amytal, or Nembutal), calming and relaxing herbs and nutrients may be useful in transition. If you have weaned away from amphetamines ("uppers," such as diet pills, Ritalin, or cocaine), more stimulating herbs may be helpful in maintaining energy and stamina in the transition.

If You Have Stopped Smoking

Oat (*Avena sativa*) can be used as a cigarette withdrawal aid (it is recommended by German physicians for exactly that purpose). Extracts can be made from the fruits of *Avena sativa*; these contain an alkaloid called gramine. The mature stem of *Avena sativa* (*oatstraw*) does not appear to contain the gramine but is high in silica, which increases absorption of calcium, an important neurotransmitter mineral. Even oat cereal can produce a sedative effect.

Passionflower is also useful for smoking withdrawal, but, like oat, this is not very strong medicine; both need to be used in consistent high doses over a longer period of time to see results.

Lung tonics for ex-smokers include **elecampane root, yerba santa leaf, nettle leaf,** or **mullein leaf.** Any of these would be brewed with 1 ounce of herb by dry weight and taken daily for 1 year. **Cubeb berry** is another lung tonic and could be taken in capsules (2 to 10 per day) or tea.

If You Have Stopped Drinking Alcohol

Valerian, folic acid, thiamine, evening primrose, and *flaxseed*

Milk thistle seed, borage, boldo, or *turmeric* with *dandelion root* for liver

If You Have Stopped Taking Amphetamines (Under a Doctor's Supervision)

Tyrosine or *l-phenylalanine* (500 to 3,000 milligrams) for fatigue; *folic acid, thiamine*

Eleuthero (stamina), *fo-ti root* (stamina), *gotu kola* (nervous system rejuvenation), *ginseng* (stamina, antifatigue)

Milk thistle seed, borage, or *turmeric* with *dandelion root* for liver

If You Have Stopped Taking Barbiturates (Under a Doctor's Supervision)

Taurine, glutamine, B_6, *manganese*

Willow and *cinchona bark combo* (2 to 15 capsules per day)

Calcium and *magnesium* (calming)

Milk thistle seed, borage, boldo, or *turmeric* with *dandelion root* for liver

If You Are Recovering from Anorexia or Bulimia (Under a Doctor's Supervision)

EFAs (as described earlier)

Herbs: *khella* (tincture), *nettles, turmeric*

Calcium, magnesium, zinc, vitamin C

Chromium (best taken as chromium picolinate or nicotinate) and **vanadium** (best taken as vanadyl sulfate) are two minerals that may assist in balancing blood sugar regulation and help to control cravings. Chromium can be taken up to 800 micrograms daily, and vanadyl sulfate can be taken at 15 to 30 milligrams daily (they usually come in 7.5-milligram tablets).

Potassium is an electrolyte, and electrolyte imbalances caused by potassium shortage can cause sometimes fatal heartbeat irregularities in cases of extreme dieting, anorexia, and bulimia.

Zinc, up to 50 milligrams daily. Zinc deficiency is a suspected contributor to anorexia nervosa and reportedly some cases respond dramatically to zinc supplementation.

Astragalus root, schizandra berry, licorice root, fo-ti root, saw palmetto berry, eleuthero root, triphala, cubeb berry, garlic, onion, and *ginger* for immune and glandular rebuilding.

Milk thistle seed, borage leaf, boldo leaf, or *turmeric* with *dandelion root* for liver repair and protection.

ANXIETY AND INSOMNIA

Many relaxant herbs work for simple anxiety as well as insomnia (both for falling asleep and staying asleep). Also, anxiety and insomnia are often related. Therefore, we will look in this section at relaxant and sedative herbs that work for both types of conditions.

Relaxant herbs, for the most part, treat symptoms. They cannot and should not be used to mask or ignore a systemic problem, which may be either physical or emotional in nature. There is nothing wrong with using herbal relaxants as natural, nontoxic ways to relieve tension, anxiety, and nervousness during times of occasional stress—say, before exams or speaking engagements, during travel, or to ease the way after a traumatic event.

But if stress is such a way of life for you that you need relaxant herbs night and day just to function, there is obviously a larger problem to be handled. Additionally, if you experience anxiety or insomnia on a long-term basis and cannot determine the source, you should see a health professional experienced with anxiety evaluation and treatment.

Valerian Root

Valerian is a relaxant herb that has a calming effect on the autonomic nervous system. It is a good short-term sedative that works quickly, offering a healthy, nontoxic alternative to strong prescription drugs.

For insomnia, valerian is taken right at bedtime to help induce sleep quickly. Valerian is best for insomniacs who have trouble falling asleep, because it decreases the amount of time it takes to fall asleep, but doesn't necessarily work on the quality of sleep. (If your trouble is staying asleep, there are longer-acting herbs that will work better.) Valerian is also useful as an interim remedy to withdraw from an addiction to sleeping pills.

Valerian's sedative properties are in the root. It can be used as a tea made by brewing dried and cut root, but most people find the intense, acrid smell (stench is perhaps a better way to put it) of the dried root off-putting. I have found that the entire home can smell of this herb for weeks after brewing the tea, and that's not to mention the issue of actually drink-ing it. So, practically speaking, you may well find the best way to use valer-ian root is in a capsule, tablet, or tincture; all are widely available.

Because this is a mild herb, you may need 5 to 10 capsules to get the desired result; valerian cannot be thought of like a "sleeping pill," which is generally much stronger and just requires 1 or 2 tablets. One or 2 valerian capsules or tablets may work simply for calming nerves, but more may be required as a sleep aid. Start with a lower number and work up till you get the desired result. (I've found that 5 is the magic number for me to fall asleep if I'm "wired.")

Valium and valerian both affect the same neurotransmitter (they both modulate GABA). GABA receptors are present in 40 percent of the brain's cells, and overactivation is thought to cause excitation or nervous-ness. These are the sites of action for the benzodiazepine drugs like Vali-um, but valerian balances those same receptors without side effects. Stud-ies comparing valerian with Valium and Xanax, another tranquilizer, show that it stacks up favorably in treating mild to moderate cases of anxiety.

Not only is valerian at least as effective as these drugs, it is not habit forming and does not interact with alcohol and other drugs the way the prescription tranquilizers do. While excess valerian may cause a headache, taking too much Valium (or taking it with alcohol) can cause death. Valer-ian doesn't cause death even when someone wants it to, as in the recent case of a woman who attempted suicide by taking a bottle of valerian but succeeded only in causing some muscle tremors and (obviously) fatigue, which were resolved in twenty-four hours.[7]

Valerian is used widely in Europe, and many of the studies showing its effectiveness have been conducted there. In the past 35 years, more than 200 scientific studies have been done on valerian. In much of Europe, physicians are more likely to recommend valerian instead of pharmaceuticals. Valerian is an active ingredient in about 150 over-the-counter medicines in Germany, including some preparations for children. (In fact, studies have shown positive effects on hyperactive children.) Valerian is also one of England's best-selling herbal medicines.

Valerian is yet another good example of why herbs are more valuable as a whole rather than as isolated extracts of compounds. Three major groups of active components in valerian have been identified: alkaloids, essential oils, and valepotriates. Valerenic acid and a volatile oil were believed by many researchers to be the components with sedative effects, but at least one study shows that these weren't as effective when used individually.

One reason for this is that the third class of compounds, valepotriates, are not present in extracts of valerian. Valepotriates develop during the body's processing of valerian, supporting the traditional herbalist view that in most cases the whole herb is more balancing and therapeutic.

Valepotriates balance GABA neuroreceptors. Valepotriates are technically not "sedative," but rather are relaxing to the whole autonomic nervous system. Valepotriates make valerian a tonic, as defined earlier; it both pushes and pulls, exerting a multidirectional effect. Several valepotriates have been isolated, and one is suppressant while another is stimulating, thus exerting a balancing effect on neuroreceptors.

Valerian is a versatile herb with many other uses. It has been valued and used by all major healing systems for thousands of years as a pain reliever, fever reducer, antispasmodic, and smooth muscle relaxant. It was used as an insomnia remedy and tranquilizer until the 1940s, when herbal medicine went into decline and pharmaceuticals were introduced for this purpose.

In the United States, it's recommended that valerian not be used by children, pregnant women, or nursing women, except on the advice of a health practitioner.

Nutmeg

Nutmeg is an excellent alternative to valerian for inducing sleep. It may even be more powerful. Its action is delayed, however, so it's not as convenient to use. It takes effect four to five hours after ingestion, so you'll need to know at least that far in advance when you plan to go to sleep. Once it takes effect, it lasts about eight hours; it is more effective than valerian to help you stay asleep.

Nutmeg used medicinally must be ground fresh because it loses potency quickly. A coffee grinder works well for grinding whole nutmeg. You can grind enough to make your own capsules to last you up to a week; then fresh capsules should be made. Unlike valerian, it is powerful enough that it is possible to become overly sedated on just a few capsules. Start with 1 capsule four to five hours before bedtime, see what happens, and try 2 if you don't get the desired effect. Work up one by one. (One capsule taken in the morning will act as a relaxant for most people rather than a sleep aid throughout the day.)

The exact mechanism for nutmeg's sedative properties is not established, although German studies suggest that nutmeg affects endorphin neurotransmitters.

Like valerian, nutmeg is a versatile herb with many other benefits. It has been used in Ayurveda throughout the history of that healing system, for a diverse range of conditions. It's a warming agent, a good cardiovascular tonic, helps lower blood pressure, increases circulation, and enhances digestion. It's also a useful tonic for men, recommended as part of treatment for benign prostatic hyperplasia (BPH), infertility, impotence, and premature ejaculation. It has been used as an aphrodisiac.

Kava-Kava Root

For an anti-anxiety effect without drowsiness, the dried roots of this Polynesian herb offer an option. It can be used for insomnia, but in smaller doses may be more calming than sleep inducing. Kava-kava is a central nervous system depressant and skeletal muscle relaxant. It may also modulate endorphins.

There are over 800 scientific references on this herb. Six major active ingredients, called kavalactones, have been identified in this herb. As usual, while many attempts have been made to synthesize drugs out of a single derivative, the activity depends on the combination. Some of the kavalactones also provide pain relief and others may reduce the side effects of amphetamines.

In the South Pacific, chronic overusers of this herb (20 to 30 capsules daily for over 6 months) developed a scaly skin condition that suggested niacin depletion. The condition disappeared when use was discontinued. The *British Journal of Phytotherapy* suggests long-term use not exceed 400 milligrams or more of kavalactones per day to avoid the skin rash. A study reported in that journal did not result in adverse effects after 8 weeks of continuous use.[8] A dose of 1 ounce of herb in tea or 5 to 8 capsules should be perfectly safe as needed.

German Commission E (the German government health agency that publishes monographs on herbs) contraindicates use of kava-kava during pregnancy and lactation or in cases of depression.

Chamomile

Chamomile is a much milder herb than valerian and is generally better for daytime relaxing, calming, and soothing than as a nighttime sleep aid. Chamomile is frequently taken as a tea because it is such a pleasant-tasting beverage, but the herb is so mild that commercial-packaged teas are of little value therapeutically. A *medicinal* tea must be made using one ounce of the herb (medicinal quality from an herb pharmacy) per pint of water. Tinctures and capsules are also available, but chamomile is so mild that it's simply not practical to get a sleep-inducing dose with those forms.

Studies of chamomile to isolate its active compounds have revealed several components responsible for its beneficial effects. The essential oil azulene may be responsible for chamomile's anti-inflammatory properties and may also inhibit the release of histamine, making chamomile additionally useful for allergies. The coumarins and flavonoids are antispasmodic.

Other Relaxant Herbs

A variety of other herbs also have some mild sedative effects, although some are less well known and less studied than herbs like valerian and chamomile. Some are used in combination formulas or teas along with chamomile or valerian. Any of these can be taken as tea with about 1/2 to 1 ounce of the herb daily.

Hops leaf contains volatile oils and acids that convert into isovaleric acid.

Catnip leaf, with a minty flavor, is one of the best very mild relaxants.

Scullcap leaf is more of a nervine relaxant than a sleep aid, and it is also an antispasmodic. It's a little more powerful than others on this list, but overall is considered mild. Up to 10 capsules may be taken.

Passionflower leaf is a nervine relaxant, very mild.

California poppy leaf is similar to the opium poppy but its constituents are far less potent, so that its action is gently balancing rather than narcotic. The Native Americans used it as a sedative. In Germany, an herbal formula that is 80 percent California poppy and 20 percent *corydalis root* is used to treat nervousness, anxiety, and insomnia, as well as depression. (Corydalis was originally used in Europe as an antispasmodic.) Poppy is shown to inhibit adrenaline and monoamine oxidase, and corydalis enhances adrenaline destruction.

Lemon balm calms and sedates, and is mild enough for children to use.

Ashwaganda is the Ayurvedic tonic generally used by men, but it has a special ability to ease anxiety, especially when used on a long-term basis. It's not a remedy to be taken at the moment you feel anxiety, but used day-to-day, the effects will kick in within a week. Several women told Karta Purkh they were able to discontinue use of Valium by taking 10 to 15 capsules of ashwaganda daily on an ongoing basis.

Shankapushpi is an Ayurvedic relaxant similar to valerian; it's especially good for *vata* (air) types.

Teas made from *lavender flower, linden flower, blue vervain leaf*, and *woodruff leaf* are less common and the mildest of all—use of these teas throughout the day will just take the edge off anxiety. The Chinese herbs *fo-ti root* (Ho Shou Wu) and *mimosa bark* are also mildly sedative. Five capsules of either would be an average effective dose.

Piscidia (also called Jamaican dogwood bark) from the West Indies and South America is a very potent relaxant. It can be hard to find and is more expensive than the others listed here, but 1/4 to 1/2 ounce as tea before bed does the trick for just about anybody.

Other Supplements for Insomnia or Anxiety

Melatonin is not an herb, nor is it a nutrient. It is a hormone produced by your pineal gland, a natural product of the body that appears to be manufactured in decreasing amounts as you get older. Melatonin is now being sold and heralded as a wonder drug, although its primary use is as a sleep aid. Already almost as many books have been written about melatonin as have been written about Prozac, and magazines from *Newsweek* to *Natural Health* have been publishing long articles on the explosion of interest.

We have mixed feelings about melatonin. On one hand, it's a crutch that doesn't solve whatever problem is causing the insomnia. Philosophically, we have reservations about use of a hormone that powerful, in doses so much larger than those seen in the body, to obtain a druglike action (even though, as a hormone, melatonin is not technically a drug). And it's currently being overhyped for every condition under the sun.

On the other hand, the reality is that some people are going to take something for insomnia, and if they insist on taking an over-the-counter drug, there is a lot to recommend melatonin. It works rapidly with no known side effects, it's inexpensive, the dose is reasonable, and the form is convenient. There have been no reports of toxicity despite widespread use. So synthetic melatonin supplementation may be useful short term, to treat jet lag or temporary sleep disturbances. However, we do not recommend ongoing, indefinite "hormone replacement" using synthetic copies of body hormones.

I personally would not take melatonin because I think there is logically more of a potential long-term risk than there is with the many botanicals that are known to be useful for this condition. While the botanicals can be less convenient, and they can be extremely mild and slow to act in some cases, it is precisely their mildness and slowness that appeals to me. I'm willing to wait. The long history of use of these botanicals and nutrients is also reassuring; melatonin "replacement" is still so new that we really don't know what the long-term effects might be of suddenly having very high levels of the hormone in the bloodstream.

Russel Reiter, Ph.D., a leading melatonin researcher and co-author with Jo Robinson of *Melatonin: Your Body's Natural Wonder Drug*, notes that even a small dose of only 1 to 2 milligrams can cause the blood concentrations to be hundreds or even thousands of times greater than normal—and people often take more. The pills have up to 10 times the amount of melatonin needed for sleep. Says Reiter, "You should have a specific, well-informed reason for taking melatonin, not just because you heard it's good stuff."[9]

Besides, there are ways to get your body to increase its supply naturally. In fact, the consensus of leading melatonin experts is that—surprise again!—lifestyle habits play the biggest role in supporting melatonin production and preserving the function of your pineal gland. And most of those supportive health habits are an exact match for the diet and supplementation basics that have everything else going for them.

The vast majority of melatonin supplements on the market are derived from beans and grains.[10] Complex-carbohydrate food will help your body to produce more melatonin, since insulin (produced when you eat carbos) removes from the blood substances that compete with tryptophan. Tryptophan is an amino acid the brain uses to make melatonin. Too much protein will interfere with melatonin, because the protein's other amino acids will be present in the blood to compete with tryptophan for entry into the brain.

B vitamins, calcium, and magnesium (whose roles in brain chemistry we discussed earlier) can all contribute to increased melatonin production. And to help prevent free-radical damage to the gland itself, eat your antioxidants—both vegetables and supplements—as covered in earlier chapters.

A University of Massachusetts Medical Center study showed that women who meditated had significantly higher levels of melatonin than those who didn't.

Avoid coffee, cigarettes, and alcohol (we've already offered dozens of other reasons that make this a healthful choice) and drugs, as much as possible—Prozac, for example, appears to suppress melatonin.

Calcium and *magnesium* at the doses suggested earlier can assist in sleeptime relaxation. Calcium is a known, natural histamine antagonist; many OTC sleep aids are antihistamines. Of magnesium, which also reduces the histamine response, anxiety disorder specialist Dr. Billie Jay Sahley, Ph.D., says, "I have never yet found a person with an anxiety disorder who was not magnesium-deficient."[11]

Diet and Exercise for Insomnia

Once again, the high-complex-carbohydrate, low-to-moderate-protein, low-fat diet emphasizing whole, fresh, organic foods provides the best basis for health. In addition, if insomnia is a problem, all stimulants should absolutely be avoided, including but not limited to caffeine and sugar.

Celery (best juiced) and banana are two good foods to include daily.

Regular aerobic exercise can be helpful. Exercise should be fairly strenuous for at least 30 minutes, 5 times a week or more.

As you can see, the herbal kingdom is a rich supply of ways to relieve and heal mood disorders. A diagnosis of such a disorder does not have to mean life on drugs.

13

Keeping Your Head (and Your Body): Herbs for Longevity

It's important to give life to years, not just years to life.

—Ron Anderson, M.D.
Chairman of the Texas Department of Health and CEO of Parkland Hospital in Dallas, in *Healing and the Mind* with Bill Moyers

Taking care of yourself is a continuum, so that there is really no definitive place where the strategies for staying well and feeling terrific on a daily basis leave off, and strategies to slow aging and its negative effects pick up. Natural, preventive self-care is for now *and* later. Generally, what it takes to feel, look, and be great today is also what it takes for tomorrow, ten years from now, and fifty years from now. Taking great care of yourself is a lifelong process that need not change all that much from birth to death.

In most cases, the basic suggestions made throughout this book for use of herbs, foods, spices, and complementary lifestyle factors hold true for preventing illness and promoting exceptional health and well-being at any age. Anti-aging—staying healthy, vibrant, energetic, and strong in advanced years—is just one of multiple benefits offered by many different herbs and foods we've discussed. Therefore, we don't have an extensive separate program or system for anti-aging that is especially distinct from what we have presented all along. Healthier, more graceful aging is a payoff to be expected from virtually every self-care investment.

Still there are some herbs and foods that are especially appropriate as we get older and for addressing health conditions most commonly associated with aging in this country. In this chapter we will provide an overview of those strategies most relevant to preventing age-related dysfunctions, including a review of the herbs and foods that help maintain the positive qualities we associate with youth.

POSSIBILITIES AND ATTITUDES IN AGING

What Do We Mean by Anti-Aging?

We must distinguish clearly what we mean when we use the term *anti-aging*. It is a common abbreviation for a concept, but the concept should be clarified. Anti-aging sounds as if it means to counteract aging itself, to interfere somehow with the very passage of time. Of course, that is impossible; we cannot control the advancement of years. So we don't suggest that anything can stop aging in the literal sense.

When people say they want to "fight aging," we think what they really mean is they want to counteract the degeneration, deterioration, and decay of body and mind that our culture has almost inextricably linked to aging. But avoiding those conditions does not have to mean avoiding aging itself. This is a crucial distinction.

The problem is that aging itself—the simple adding of years to life—is assumed to be synonymous with that type of breakdown, and this association is considered to be necessary and inevitable. But aging really just means getting older; we're the ones who superimposed those undesirable images over it. We have an unfortunate picture of what "older" looks like. We lump the inevitability of reaching the age of seventy-five in with a bunch of diseases, discomforts, and distresses that are *not inherent* in being seventy-five years old. We should expect changes, yes; but not a radically reduced quality of life.

Most of us are unaware that there are many other cultures in which people simply don't experience the same kind of impairments that we typically do at older ages. There is no evidence that our bodies are designed to degenerate severely after a certain age. There is certainly no evidence that heart disease, cancer, and stroke are inevitable results of wear and tear no matter what we do. The American life span is in large part determined by the likelihood of those conditions, but the life span that is intrinsic to the human design may be much higher—possibly almost double the American average.

Thus, what we really mean—though it's too cumbersome to say it—is not "anti-aging," but rather "anti-conditions-usually-associated-with-aging." Anti-aging should not be confused with resisting the inevitable. In fact, we might wish to call it something more positive and empowering, such as "pro-aging," because what we really want to do is go *for* the healthiest, fittest, richest-quality life at any age—not against infirmity. Aging itself is not a tragedy to be endured if you live it in a body that's been nourished, nurtured, and well preserved.

Letting Go of Chronology

One of the hardest things for our culture to relinquish is our obsession with chronological age. There is such a thing as *biological age*, the actual degree to which the years and life habits have physically impacted on the body. However, we have such limiting images of what different ages "mean" that we have a hard time seeing the difference. In our culture's simplistic views, young is healthy; old is unhealthy. Age twenty-five is pretty, fifty-five isn't. Age sixty-eight is sick, age eighteen isn't. Age twenty is agile and athletic; age sixty is fat and unfit.

In reality, this is a terrific example of the mindless assumptions that surround health in our culture. I have known twenty-five-year-olds who eat fast food every day, are sedentary, drink and take drugs, and are supremely unhealthy. (The same goes for twelve-year-olds, eighteen-year-olds, and forty-two-year-olds.) I know vital and athletic sixty-year-olds who eat smart, exercise, use herbs, and never even get colds, let alone experience extreme physical incapacitation or decline.

The twenty-somethings who *are* wonderfully healthy are that way because they do the kinds of nurturing things we discuss in this book, not merely because they're twenty. Their peers may be "aged" and degenerated, despite their "youth." I have two forty-year-old female friends—modest athletes, fuelers, and herb users—who both have been genuinely mistaken for college students. Yet another friend's sixty-two-year-old stepmother is an Ironman triathlete—while other peoples' moms at the same age can't walk up a flight of stairs. *Such debility is not a function of being sixty. It is a function of what's been done to the body over sixty years.*

Chronologically, based on cultural assumptions, I was supposed to be healthier at eighteen than I am now at thirty-one, simply because I had put in less time on earth. But at twenty-five I was much better off than at twenty, and at thirty better still. I more easily pass for twenty now than I did when I was actually that age. Ironically, once when I was twenty, someone guessed my age at forty. At the time it was devastating, but it was an important wake-up call for me.

The numbers lie or mislead us. They take us astray from the goal of health because they make us fearful about consequences that we don't have to dread, or all too complacent about an illusory protection of sheer youth. The sixty-year-old shouldn't have to worry that the very fact of being sixty is dangerous to her health, and the twenty-year-old endangers himself by assuming that merely being twenty guarantees impunity.

Getting Older, Getting Better

It is possible to actually *improve* with the years, not just to resist cracking and fraying. Five years ago many people told me I would soon reach the point where I would start to see a general decline, where things would begin to "fall apart." But in that five years I treated myself better than I ever had previously, and better than I think many people ever take the time or energy to do throughout their lives. As a result I have gotten stronger, healthier, and more vigorous, energetic, and outgoing. My skin is clearer, my muscle mass is bigger, my body fat is lower, my immune resistance is vastly superior, and my incidence of illness has dropped to nearly nonexistent. I've actually reversed the trend; I'm not just treading water.

It's true that I'm not forty, fifty, or sixty yet, but the people who point that out are the same people who told me to expect a decline at thirty. When I hit forty, those people no doubt will slide the ruler up another ten years and tell me, "Just wait till you're fifty." The fact is I don't need to wait, because I'm not the only yardstick for the power and flexibility we have to determine how we age. I have friends and acquaintances of every age all around me who are wonderful role models for the potential of real health care and an ageless attitude.

My friend Chris, a beautiful, fit, and radiantly healthy woman soon to turn forty, says she has been hearing "wait till you turn forty" for a decade. As she approaches that supposedly dreadful milestone, still very much intact, agile, and pain-free, she laughs, "Well, here I am—what are they going to say now?"

Of course I may be proven wrong, and only time will tell. What I know now is that since I began caring for myself in a purposeful and proactive way, there isn't a year that's passed that I have not been significantly more vibrant, powerful, and attractive than the year before. And I have watched those around me who care for themselves in the same way enjoy the same upward trend. Isn't that a more exciting way to live than the aging sentence our culture has slapped on us?

The Luck of the Draw?

Evidence for the influence of personal choices on our health is abundant. Simply, most data show that who stays healthy and who gets sick is for the most part fairly predictable. Degeneration is not a mystery!

The healthy fifty-something referred to above, the sixty-year-old triathlete—these are not "lucky" people. In every instance they are simply doing the same things that keep the twenty-year-old healthy. The difference between the triathlete and the woman who can't walk up stairs is not "good genes." Uniformly, the sixty-year-old triathletes live one way, and the ones who can't climb stairs live another way. The difference involves effort.

People often seem willing to put a lot of energy into agitation and worry about illness, while simultaneously putting no effort into preventing it (or actively engaging in behavior that causes it). People seem to be addicted to what they can't do, not to what they can. For example, I know a man who is so afraid of dying he has refused to go to the funerals of his friends—but he chain-smokes, eats poorly, is a workaholic, and gets no exercise.

There are people who are defying our notions of what it's like to age, our conceptions about what our bodies, minds, and lives "have to" be like when we get older. We just don't see them or hear about them as often. Find yourself some ageless role models to offset the scarcity of positive images. (I'm fortunate to have some extremely active, athletic, outgoing older people in my circle of friends and community. Or you can choose a well-known figure. One of my favorites is Paul Newman—seventy-something, gorgeous, fit, and regularly victorious in auto racing against people less than a third his age.)

THE BASICS

First, let's review the basic lifestyle factors and choices (all of which have been explored fully earlier) that lay the smoothest and strongest foundation for an ageless body and mind.

Fuel smart. Don't starve yourself and don't gorge yourself. Get enough fuel to run your body, consistently, with calories broken down as follows: 50 to 65 percent complex carbs, 20 to 30 percent protein, and 15 to 30 percent fat. (See pages 107–117 for more.)

Consume little or no refined sugar, trans fats, damaged oils, and saturated fat. (See pages 108–109 on sugar and 152–158 on fats for more.)

Go as vegetarian as you can. Beyond the fat, there may be other aspects of meat consumption that increase cancer and heart disease risk, as well as senility. Paul Giem, M.D., a clinical instructor at the Loma Linda University School of Medicine in California, studied vegetarians and meat eaters and concluded, "If you stopped eating meat today, in ten years you would have half the risk of dementia of a heavy meat-eater."[1] Meat consumption can also cause high homocysteine levels, which has been linked to increased risk of heart attack as well as dementia.[2] And high protein consumption, especially animal protein, can increase osteoporosis risk because bone releases calcium to compensate for the acid imbalance caused by meat eating. Finally, red meat in particular is implicated in some cancers in which total fat or fish and poultry fat are not.[3]

When you do eat fat, use healthy oils. Choose healing omega-3s and monounsaturates such as olive, almond, flaxseed, and fish oils. Essential fatty acids can be supplemented with flaxseed oil and hemp oil, or capsules of evening primrose, borage, black currant, or flaxseed oils. (See pages 152–158 for more on fats.)

Max out on fruits and veggies for phytonutrients. Cabbage, broccoli, brussels sprouts, kale, cauliflower, deep yellow and orange vegetables, dark leafy greens, soybeans, tomatoes, citrus, melon, red grapes and berries are especially loaded—eat as many of these as possible. Don't forget your garlic, onions, ginger, and chilies, too. (See pages 112–119 for more on phytonutrients.)

Take vitamin and mineral supplements wisely. The antioxidant vitamins and minerals are especially important.

Drink plenty of water. We recommend at minimum 8 to 10, preferably 12 to 15 glasses of water a day (I manage 20 plus).

Bust stress. Consciously seek to arrange your life so that there is as little physical and emotional wear and strain as possible.

Reduce toxicity. Take measures to reduce your exposures to environmental pollutants. Pay attention to drinking water (filter it), electromagnetic frequencies (EMFs), and air (even an air purifier in the home may be wise if you live in a smoggy area). Choose organically grown food to avoid chemical fertilizers, pesticides, herbicides, fungicides, and hormones and drugs whenever possible.

Don't smoke or drink heavily. There is a great deal of confusing research about the benefits and risks of alcohol consumption, but after much examination we think it boils down to this: one, *maybe* two drinks a day maximum is okay and possibly healthful for some people. (See pages 121–123 for more on this issue.)

Generally follow the constitutional diet. Ascertain your Ayurvedic constitution and try to emphasize the foods and spices that support it, at least 80 percent of the time. (See Chapter 2, "History of Ayurveda: Ancient Healing Wisdom," for more.)

Sleep and rest. You may not need ten hours a night, but if you're consistently getting four hours and waking up exhausted, maybe you should reexamine your daily routine. When you feel especially drained or susceptible to illness, rest—don't push through it.

Exercise. Both aerobic activity and weight-bearing, muscle-building activities offer huge benefits against disease and, more important, for youth, strength, vigor, and maintenance of metabolism. It doesn't need to be maniacal or even competitive—just consistent.

Use herbal tonics. Choose at least a couple of tonics, possibly by the organs or systems that may be most vulnerable based on your individual constitution or history, and use them regularly. (See pages 133–146 for more.)

Use herbs for specific conditions. Manage and heal existing health conditions naturally, without toxicity or side effects. Deal with and eliminate the underlying issues rather than symptoms alone.

Make drugs and surgery last resorts. Steer clear of toxic and invasive medical therapies except in cases where those are the only options for your condition or where they are clearly the most effective solution.

Express yourself, have meaningful work, engage fully with life, love, give, and be at peace. It may sound simplistic or trite, but there is a mammoth amount of evidence that these are relevant to health, especially immunity.

THE TOP ANTI-AGING HERBS AND NUTRIENTS

Culling from the vast array of health-preserving herbs around the world, including some that have been presented elsewhere in the book for various conditions and purposes, here is a review of herbs, nutrients, spices, and special foods that are particularly relevant in the context of aging. If forms and doses are not detailed here, you will find them elsewhere in the book.

Amla fruit or triphala. Amla fruit from India has twenty to thirty times more vitamin C than oranges, pound for pound, and is more bioactive and heat stable. It is a superlative antioxidant. Chyavaprash—amla fruit jelly, containing amla fruit along with about forty other herbs—is a mainstay of herbal medicine in South Asia, used as a rejuvenating tonic for the whole family from birth to death. The jelly can be purchased here in health-food stores and eaten from a spoon or spread on toast.

Triphala is the most basic, highly prized tonic of Ayurvedic medicine, and contains "three fruits" (the meaning of its name)—amla, bibitaki, and haritaki—which are dried and powdered. Triphala stabilizes all three doshas, contains a perfect balance of all six tastes, restores every system and organ, and you can take 2 capsules a day, every day, throughout your life. (See pages 139, 230, and 286 for more.)

Arjuna. Karta Purkh considers the bark of the arjuna tree from India to be the top cardiotonic in the world—even more so than hawthorn, the very popular European heart tonic. It is just becoming popular with American herbalists. Arjuna does it all: slows and regulates the heartbeat (treating irregular or fast heartbeat), lowers cholesterol and blood pressure, boosts circulation, and eases angina. In India, arjuna is used as tea (up to an ounce of herb a day); in America capsules are preferred. As a tonic take 2 capsules per day.

Ginkgo. The brain, like the heart, needs healthy arteries to supply it with blood carrying oxygen and nutrients. It is also a capillary-rich organ. Ginkgo is a circulatory tonic herb that strengthens capillaries, making them more flexible and allowing more red blood cells to squeeze through to the capillary-rich brain and eyes without the capillaries bursting. Hundreds of studies worldwide show that ginkgo improves circulation, protects the nervous system, and fights oxidation. Its effect on circulation to the brain and extremities in particular has been studied extensively—about fifty double-blind controlled clinical trials show that ginkgo improves cognitive function and reduces cerebrovascular insufficiency (decreased blood supply to the brain associated with aging).

This herb both prevents and treats senile dementia and related cognitive conditions of the elderly better than many drugs—so effectively, in fact, that ginkgo is the best-selling herbal medicine in Europe and one of the most commonly prescribed botanicals in the world (over 100,000 physicians worldwide wrote over 10 million prescriptions for Ginkgo biloba extract in 1989 alone). It works preventively for cerebrovascular insufficiency as well, and treats impotence, inner-ear dysfunctions such as tinnitus (ringing in the ears) and vertigo (dizziness), degenerative eye diseases such as macular degeneration and diabetic retinopathy, and headache. It may also speed recovery from head injury, treat depression, and facilitate communication between nerve cells.

According to Rob McCaleb, president of the Herb Research Foundation, the British medical journal The Lancet conducted an extensive review of studies and concluded side effects from GBE are rare and not serious, and there are no known drug interactions.[4] The recommended dose is usually 120 to 240 milligrams daily.

Bilberry. Another circulatory-enhancing antioxidant, bilberry has an affinity for the capillary-rich area of the eye, improving vision and reducing degenerative eye disease. Bilberry's antioxidant compounds, anthocyanosides, also improve blood flow to the heart and extremities. Stronger, more flexible cell walls and capillaries resist free-radical damage and squeeze more red blood cells through tight spaces. Studies also show that bilberry can reduce plaque deposits on blood vessel walls, increase heartbeat strength, and thin the blood, reducing clotting. (See page 415 for more.) The usual dose is 60 to 120 milligrams daily.

Hawthorn berry. This cardiotonic and circulatory herb acts directly on the heart muscle, slowing and strengthening the heartbeat, increasing blood flow, and preventing irregular heartbeats (arrythmias), which can increase with age and lead to heart attacks. Hawthorn berry is a Chinese remedy (used by them as a sour digestive tonic) as well as a European remedy, and has garnered much attention in Europe as a heart and circulatory medicine. Like bilberry and ginkgo, this antioxidant supports the cardio-vascular system by neutralizing free-radical damage to cells and capillaries. Hawthorn berry is effective in reducing angina pain, and unlike the heart drug digitalis, is not toxic or dangerous. (See pages 414–415 for more.)

Gotu kola. This tissue-rejuvenating and -healing and nerve-tonic herb is called Brahmi in Ayurveda, meaning "godlike." It has been used for cen-turies as a medicine in India, China, and the islands of Indonesia to delay aging, accelerate wound repair, and enhance all central nervous functions. Its active compounds are triterpenes, which demonstrate tranquilizing and anti-anxiety effects.

Gotu kola also works in ways similar to *ginkgo* to improve blood flow to limbs in cases of venous insufficiency. Because of this ability as well as its regenerative effect on connective tissue and nerves, it is another good "brain tonic" for long-term prevention of age-related mental decline. Additionally, gotu kola helps improve the function and integrity of con-nective tissue by increasing blood supply to the tissue and actually increas-ing the formation of the tissue's structural components. It acts similarly for skin and the support structure of the skin. (See page 346 for more.)

Ginseng. The Chinese call this tonic "the King of Herbs" and value it as a lifelong rejuvenator, primarily for men. It's used to restore overall *qi* (vital energy) and has an affinity for the lungs and digestive system. It also helps the body adapt to stress, shock, inflammation, and trauma, and builds stamina, enhances the immune system, and balances or regulates body processes. (See pages 141–142 for more.)

Dong quai. The "Queen of Herbs" in Chinese medicine, dong quai is is beneficial tonic for both men and women, though it is particularly valued as a female tonic. It is warming and balances the entire female reproductive system. It is also useful for menopausal discomforts. (See Chapter 8, "Espe-cially for Women: Natural Healing for a Woman's Lifetime," for more). The Ayurvedic herb *shatavari* is a worthy—and probably less expensive—stand-in for these effects. Either can be taken as capsules, 1 to 4 daily.

Astragalus. This very mild yet powerfully health-enhancing tradition-al Chinese herb is used both as a long-term tonic and to assist healing and recovery in chronic illness or infection. It boosts energy, increases adapta-tion to stress, is especially antiviral, and heightens the efficiency of virtu-ally every type of immune-system activity. It can also mitigate the effects of toxic medical therapies. (See pages 134–136 for more.)

Ahswaganda. This ginsenglike adaptogenic herb is popular in Ayurveda for its rejuvenative effects in practically any situation. It's used in that culture for arthritis, cancer, colds, asthma, digestive problems, cystitis, skin problems, hemorrhoids, high blood pressure, mental decline, and wound healing. It's also anti-anxiety and an aphrodisiac. As a tonic, it is treasured for its anti-aging properties. Studies have indeed confirmed that ashwaganda can inhibit tumors, protect the liver, stimulate immunity, and enhance learning and memory retention. As a tonic, take 2 to 5 capsules per day.

Ho Shou Wu (fo-ti root). In China, fo-ti is specifically regarded as a longevity herb, the most renowned of all the herbs for this purpose. The translation of the name Ho Shou Wu is something like "Mr. Ho has black hair" because it is said to preserve hair color. It's regarded as a reproductive tonic—a sperm increaser for men and fertility enhancer in women. It's also an excellent long-term energy builder, working through the thyroid, and is anti-inflammatory, anti-tumor, and detoxifying. It calms the nervous system and is very mildly sedative, so it can be used for mild insomnia. Finally, it is tonifying to the kidneys and liver. As a tonic, take 2 to 4 capsules per day.

Schizandra. Another Chinese herb, schizandra has been discussed already as a general tonic, especially a women's glandular tonic, and for use with coughs and other lung issues. In China it is valued as a youth preserver and sexual tonic that increases sexual energy and "staying power." The dried berries make a tart red tea.

Lycium. Also called lycii or lycii fruit, this Chinese herb (actually red berries) has been used for longevity since a famous user, Li Ch'ing Yuen, reportedly lived to be 250 years old. It's also designated as a liver and blood tonic, calming, circulation-enhancing, and vision-improving. A tonic dose would be 3 to 5 capsules per day.

Turmeric. This versatile herb is a lifetime rejuvenator and is especially helpful for many conditions associated with aging. It's a superlative anti-inflammatory, antioxidant, tissue healer, and joint rejuvenative—all valuable for fending off, soothing, or healing age-related conditions, especially arthritis. Up to 1 ounce daily can be taken as a tonic.

Red jujube date. Yet another Chinese longevity herb, these dates are generally strengthening as well as life extending and are used widely in Chinese medicine to purify all twelve organ meridians and clear blocked *qi.*

They are considered especially to increase sexual vitality and vigor, tonify the sex organs and glands, improve digestion, and moderate mood swings. Five to 10 dates can be eaten daily.

CoQ10. Coenzyme Q, also called CoQ10, is a heart-protective antioxidant nutrient found in especially high concentrations in the heart and liver. The body's supply of CoQ10 appears to decline with age as well as from a poor diet, stress, and during infection. When the body fails to manufacture adequate levels of CoQ10, oxygenation of the heart and tissue and cell repair may be impaired. Low levels are found in the majority of people with heart disease (as one of many factors), and may also be one of a number of elements involved in aging and the discomforts often associated with it. CoQ10 is available in capsules as a dietary supplement.

Antioxidant vitamins. Vitamin E and selenium (synergistic together), vitamin C, vitamin A, and beta-carotene are all free-radical scavengers that help block or repair oxidative damage blamed for unhealthy aging. Individually, they also support or stimulate the immune system in various ways—some against infection, others against cancer and degenerative disease. Doses for each are discussed in other parts of the book.

B complex, including choline and folic acid. The B vitamins are brain and nervous-system food, and as such these nutrients might help ward off the mental decline associated with aging. Investigators at the U.S. Department of Agriculture Human Nutrition Research Center on Aging suggest that age-related cognitive decline may be preventable or reversible with adequate doses of vitamin B_{12}, vitamin B_6 and folate.[5] Choline is a building block for the neurotransmitter acetylcholine, which enables neuron-to-neuron communication. Low acetylcholine levels lead to breakdown of one important brain chemical that in turn allows creation of a damaging one, which causes the neuron damage we know as Alzheimer's.[6] Daily B-complex doses can range from 50 to 100 milligrams.

14

Herbal Renewal:
Cleanse, Detox, Rebuild

At the most basic level, health maintenance is relatively simple: Provide the body with what it needs, don't give it much of what it doesn't need, and the body will run itself. Failing that, imbalances occur, and toxins to which you are exposed may not get eliminated quickly or efficiently enough. Cleaning out toxins that build up in the body—safely, naturally, and effectively—can result in renewed strength and vitality.

The body is certainly made to do its cleansing and elimination on its own. So why might we have to intervene? One of the reasons we may need to support the process is that our environment is increasingly toxic, and our lifestyles don't give our bodies everything they need to handle the increasing burden. It's sort of an American standard not to give the body what it needs, and give it plenty of what it doesn't need. Such burdens can include: stress, overwork, sugar and fat; pollutants in the air and water; pesticides and herbicides, preservatives, additives, and colorings in food; forceful synthetic drugs that we take to mask our discomforts. All of these pollutants and toxins can gunk up the machinery inside.

Internally, nutritional imbalances and insufficiencies can interfere with the body's normal cleansing pathways, and externally, more chemicals are being introduced into our environment every year. For example, the Environmental Protection Agency estimates that in 1989 more than 5.7 billion pounds of chemical pollutants were released into the environment—and that was just one year.

Cleansing and detoxifying is something that, in fact, is taking place in your body all the time, and many organs have some responsibility for these tasks. The liver is the chief orchestrator of detox. The kidneys, skin, lungs, blood, and intestines also play roles in eliminating unnecessary and possibly damaging wastes from cells and tissues. These systems all work hard to keep toxins and wastes from affecting our health.

In addition, the body uses certain nutrients to detoxify or block the actions of toxic molecules. Many of the common vitamins and minerals demonstrated to have anti-cancer properties and other health benefits do so by mitigating chemical and other environmental exposures. Such nutrients are depleted (used up) in the face of toxic exposure, and if they aren't replenished, you're left "naked" in the face of future exposures. Unfortunately, the standard American diet doesn't do a good job of replacing these nutrients, leaving deficiencies that decrease your detoxifying ability at a time of unprecedented chemical exposure.

Considering all this, the fact that we have more cancer and chronic illness than any other generation does not seem coincidental. The burdens of modern living create processing and elimination jobs that are bigger than the organs, systems, and nutrients assigned to handle them. When we fall behind handling the "garbage flow," opportunistic diseases both chronic and acute can gain the upper hand.

Some doctors and scientists blame high levels of accumulated toxins in the body for conditions ranging from allergies to Alzheimer's disease. Toxic overload can make the immune system weak or overreactive, or cause pain, mental symptoms, or cancer. Toxic bodies are also more likely to experience less serious—but nevertheless aggravating—symptoms such as headaches, gas and poor digestion, muscle aches, joint pain, and skin problems. Autoimmune diseases and pain and fatigue syndromes like chronic fatigue and fibromyalgia may be on the rise because we are a poisoned planet and people, paying the price for our carelessness with both medical and environmental chemicals.

Sherry A. Rogers, M.D., a specialist in environmental and nutritional medicine, says, "Actually, if you have any symptoms at all, don't feel peppy most of the time, or require any medications, you most likely have biochemical abnormalities that can be identified."[1]

It certainly is common sense that buildups of substances not meant to be stored in the body could cause havoc in you, and that dealing with a constant barrage of such material can tire the body out. If a car wash was built to handle 100 dirty cars in every eight-hour period, and 500 dirty cars started forcing their way through the line rapidly in each eight-hour period, there would probably be breakdowns in the machinery, and some of the cars would also probably not get as clean as they should.

KEEPING IT CLEAN

The first line of defense against toxins is prevention—same as for most conditions.

Not surprisingly, a nontoxic lifestyle does not differ from the lifestyle basics recommended for so many other purposes. Healthful habit recommendations were detailed on pages 107–125 and recapped on pages 318–320.

SWEEPING IT CLEAN

When a health condition rears its head, it's probably not too far off the mark to think that part of the problem may be that something in your body wants to come out. That's why cleansing and detoxifying are successful as part of treatment for many conditions.

Cleansing/detoxifying is not a magic bullet, however, just as no one herb or vitamin can clear up all problems. You can rid your body of toxins that are causing irritation, inflammation, overload, or exhaustion, but if you do not make changes that eliminate the source of the toxin from your life, you will wind up having to cleanse yourself again and again. This is not a natural state to be in.

Also, some people get fanatical about cleansing, and keep the body in a constant eliminative mode instead of restoring and rebuilding. Constant, ongoing cleansing is not necessary! Once you're clean, you're clean; you don't need to keep scouring yourself raw. "Extra" cleaning can be harmful. "More is better" does not necessarily apply here.

Herbal cleansing and detoxification can be done in a number of ways. Some herbs (or foods or nutrients) do the cleanup directly themselves, sometimes in a specific part of the body. Others stimulate or support one or more of the key organs or systems to do the work themselves. Following we will discuss the best herbs and foods for each toxin-eliminating part of the body.

COLON HEALTH

This may not be what you talk about with your friends over coffee, but it is important. Conventional medicine doesn't pay much attention to this—when was the last time your doctor asked you about your bowel movements? But most natural health practitioners include this in the list of detailed concerns about your health and history.

Many conventional health practitioners also don't consider anything amiss if the bowels are moved only a few times a week, and on the whole we are not encouraged to expect regularity or consistency in our bowel movements.

However, if you think about it, isn't it strange to consume three meals a day plus possibly snacks for three or four days and not eliminate anything? Talk about wastes and toxins building up! Many holistic health practitioners suggest that a minimum one daily evacuation is healthy and that two or three is much better—and best of all would be to have those on a predictable schedule.

Constipation

Thirty million Americans suffer from constipation. Americans spend more than half a billion dollars each year on over-the-counter laxatives! Constipation is an American epidemic that, like hemorrhoids, doesn't get talked about much. Lack of fiber is a key cause of constipation, so the epidemic is not surprising because the standard American diet is low in fiber. In addition, it's important to drink enough water (at least ten glasses daily) and exercise—simple but usually very effective advice.

There are several ways to handle constipation.

1. Increase peristalsis. Muscular contractions must be sufficient to "squeeze" out the waste.

Herbs that are bowel stimulants induce peristalsis. They include:

Triphala—This Ayurvedic preparation, which we have already discussed elsewhere, is a mild peristalsis enhancer. It can be used at a dose of 6 to 8 capsules a day as necessary; this will stimulate a bowel movement in about 8 hours. It's extremely gentle and can be used by anyone, from infants to the elderly.

Senna leaf—This herb from India is widely used in Europe as a laxative; in Switzerland it is mixed with other herbs and sold commercially as "Swiss Kriss," now available here as well. Senna makes a pretty decent-tasting tea, but can be used in capsules, 1 or 2 a day.

Cascara bark—Found in the Pacific Northwest, the bark must be cured for one to two years to reduce the potency. It tastes bitter and is generally only practical in capsules, 1 or 2 a day. Properly cured, it's about equal in strength to senna.

Rhubarb root—Also called Asian rhubarb or turkey rhubarb, this is milder than senna or cascara and 2 to 10 capsules a day would be appropriate.

Aloe vera can be taken as juice (2 tablespoons) or 6 to 8 capsules per day.

Rose petal—This Ayurvedic remedy is also very mild; 1 to 5 capsules per day.

Licorice root—Still another mild option; 1 to 5 capsules per day.

Butternut bark—And yet another very gentle laxative; 1 to 5 capsules per day.

Buckthorn bark—This one is purging, more like senna or cascara; 1 to 5 capsules per day.

Senna, cascara, rhubarb, and aloe vera all contain anthraquinones, compounds which cause contractions of the bowels. In higher doses or stronger preparations, this can cause cramping or "griping." For this reason they are often mixed with carminative herbs (those that prevent gas or soothe the digestive tract). These herbs should not be used long term or if you have abdominal pain or diarrhea.

2. Increase moisture. To give stools their necessary moisture and "slipperiness," *magnesium* may be used at 1,500 milligrams per day.

Slippery elm bark and *marshmallow root* are similar in action and can be used together or by themselves. Both are mucilaginous agents (demulcents). They create a slimy, gelatinous mass that is nourishing and healing to mucous membranes, including those of the digestive tract. Two to 4 heaping tablespoons of powder a day, mixed with water (or yogurt, oatmeal, applesauce, or maple syrup) to make a paste will increase stool motility.

Castor oil (1 to 2 tablespoons) is also a good way to moisten the stool.

Aloe vera juice offers a soothing effect on membranes and a liquefying effect on intestinal contents, along with bowel stimulation, as noted above.

3. Increase bulk. Insoluble fiber (cellulose) creates bulk so the large intestine has something to grip on and squeeze. In addition to bulk, insoluble fiber (such as wheat bran), provides a "scraping action" to clean the intestine. Some studies show that *rice bran* is even better than *wheat bran* for this, though wheat bran has been shown to reduce bile acids and bacterial enzymes (which reduces colon cancer risk). Work up from 1/4 teaspoon per day. *Flaxseed* is also a good choice, as it provides bulk *and* exerts a laxative effect. Try 1 to 2 tablespoons ground into cereal, salad, or yogurt.

Soluble fiber cleanses by absorbing toxins in the intestinal tract rather than physically sweeping them out. A common source of soluble fiber is pectins from fruits and vegetables, such as *apples, citrus, bananas,* and *carrots.* Other soluble fibers include gums and mucilages.

Psyllium seed is considered to be soluble fiber, but has also received attention for its "broom-sweep" effect on the colon. *Chia seed* is another good choice in this category. Start slow with psyllium and chia seed—1/4 teaspoon daily, increasing to maximum tolerance until stool is normalized.

Bacterial Enzymes

High amounts of certain bacterial enzymes present in the intestinal tract are associated with cancer. Meat and fat in the diet increase this activity. Friendly bacteria that create beneficial flora in the intestine can help keep the upper hand over the unfriendly ones that create these enzymes. A daily supplementation with **L. acidophilus** can help maintain this intestinal bacterial balance.

LIVER

The liver is a powerful organ. It is the ringleader of the toxin-processing and -elimination system and is able to field all kinds of "garbage," ranging from dead blood cells to the litter aftermath of infection (especially viral), to synthetic chemical exposures.

Too much going on at once—whether a series of infections, drug and alcohol abuse, or ongoing toxic environmental exposure—gives the liver more work than one organ can handle. When the liver is overworked, weakened, and overwhelmed, toxins build up and outward signs begin to show elsewhere in our bodies. Eruptions on the outside of us often reflect some failure to control the waste on the inside.

Many symptoms are noted by natural health practitioners and other cultures' healing systems as being specifically liver related, even though in conventional medicine they are not generally associated with the liver. Skin problems, particularly acne, are considered in natural healing to be a liver toxicity issue. Certain kinds of headaches, particularly those around the top of the head, are considered "liver headaches" in the major alternative healing systems. Hemorrhoids are a classic liver toxicity symptom, as are nausea, difficulty digesting fats, yellow skin or eyes, dry skin, and constipation (the liver's secretion of bile from the gallbladder—the "bile-holding bag"—into the small intestine provokes bowel movements).

As mentioned earlier, "liver herbs" typically cross-treat other conditions that benefit from cold, bitter herbs. Like liver inflammation, fever is a *pitta* (fire) excess, so liver herbs tend to be fever herbs. Virus usually calls for liver support as well, because the liver is so burdened by the post-battle cleanup. Immune support and liver support are not mutually exclusive. To support a crucial "cog" in the immune system, such as the liver, is to support the whole system.

Liver Herbs

With all of these herbs, start with the lowest dose and work up as necessary. Liver herbs can cause queasiness as they begin the work of flushing wastes that will temporarily circulate in the blood before excretion.

Boldo leaf—This South American herb, from Chile and Peru, was very popular at the turn of the century as a kidney tonic, useful for kidney infection. It still is a good kidney herb, but is also now known to be a superlative liver herb—according to Karta Purkh, one of the top five liver herbs in the world. Research shows that boldo leaf is liver protective and antioxidant. It can be taken as a tea or in capsule form, 1 to 10 a day.

My experience with boldo leaf has been phenomenal. One summer day I mentioned in casual conversation how bothered I was by the tiny, hard red bumps covering the backs of my upper arms, which had been there for about fifteen years. Karta Purkh noted that in natural healing this is considered a classic sign of vitamin A deficiency, but that given how I eat, a dietary deficiency was virtually impossible. In that case, he said, it's a sign that the liver is not efficiently converting vitamin A precursors (carotenoids) to vitamin A. He suggested four capsules daily of boldo leaf. Within two months, the bumps were one hundred percent gone. I had absolutely smooth upper arms for the first time in fifteen years! (This is also a good example of a health issue—some possible weakness in the liver—that would never have been detected or treated by standard medicine now, yet down the road might have progressed beyond "bumpy skin" to a more serious condition.)

Barberry root—Found growing on the East Coast of the United States, this classic liver herb was the first discovered source of the alkaloid compound berberine (a compound also significant to goldthread and goldenseal). Barberry is bitter and astringent and thus controls both *kapha* and *pitta* well; it's also a mild antibacterial. One to 5 capsules per day.

Bayberry root—Pungent, astringent, and hot, this mild builder is a perfect *kapha*-controlling herb (it dries and warms). It is especially effective in combination with turmeric. Two to 8 capsules per day.

Dandelion root—Common, well known, the quintessential liver herb. It's good with turmeric and well tolerated by most people. It can be obtained roasted for use as a tea, or the fresh root can be made into a tea or juiced. In capsules, average dose would be 1 to 10 capsules per day.

Yellow dock root—All of the "dock" plants are liver cleansing. This one is a little milder than boldo or barberry. One to 10 capsules a day.

Phyllanthus leaf ("bhumy amalaki")—This ancient Ayurvedic herb for the liver can be used as a long-term, slow-acting nonflushing (i.e., doesn't cause all accumulated toxins to be dumped quickly) treatment for all liver-related conditions, including skin conditions like eczema and acne, and eye problems. It's liver protective and exceptionally good for hepatitis; it makes liver tissue less vulnerable to disease and damage. (Some people have used it as a supportive adjunct to conventional hepatitis treatment; others have successfully used it alone as part of a natural healing protocol under a health practitioner's care.) Five capsules per day.

Milk thistle seed—Possibly the most trendy liver herb currently, certainly the most researched, with more focus on protective than cleansing qualities. Used extensively in Europe, milk thistle is usually sold as an extract containing three flavonoid compounds collectively known as silymarin (silybin, silydianin, silychristin). Karta Purkh notes that because it's an extract and because it comes from Europe, it's expensive. He suggests getting the seed in bulk (it's about 4 to 5 dollars a pound) and taking 2 to 4 tablespoons of seed (ground as a powder into cereal, or with water, or soaked whole and eaten in granola). Also, because it's trendy, people are using it as a tonic when it is really much more appropriate as a remedy or antidote.

Milk thistle appears to be particularly useful in cases of poisoning. The liver fields food, drug, and hormone substances between the gastrointestinal system and the blood. Milk thistle interrupts this cycling between the liver and gastrointestinal system—called the enterohepatic circuit—and prevents reabsorption of poisons. A treatment called silybinin made from milk thistle extract is even used intravenously or as an injectable in European emergency rooms, saving the lives of poison victims if used soon enough after exposure.[2] In addition to treatment after the fact, milk thistle can actually prevent adverse liver reactions if taken prior to exposure to poisonous mushrooms.[3]

In the United States, herbs aren't given a place in the emergency room of a hospital (although milk thistle is available as a dietary supplement). Herb Research Foundation president Rob McCaleb, who lists milk thistle among his ten most valued herbs and takes it anytime he has a few glasses of wine or over-the-counter painkillers, including acetaminophen and aspirin (known to be liver toxic), writes, "Instead of being illegal as a liver-protective medicine, perhaps milk thistle should be a mandatory addition to liver-toxic drugs."[4]

Turmeric root—Bitter herbs are generally known to promote bile flow. Turmeric is one of the premier Ayurvedic herbs for the liver. Classically in Ayurveda it's used mixed with bayberry. It can increase bile acid output by over 100 percent. Curcumin, the most-researched compound in turmeric, also increases bile solubility, supporting its historical use in the treatment of gallstones. These same qualities indicate the use of turmeric for the treatment of alcohol abuse. As a potent antioxidant, curcumin has hepatoprotective effects comparable to silybin from milk thistle.[5]

Baical scullcap root—A Chinese remedy and another one of the leading liver tonics, especially for inflammation and jaundice; like many liver herbs it also treats fever. It also happens to be a good remedy for cough or headache, and as an anti-inflammatory it is a valuable part of arthritis and allergy treatments. Five capsules per day.

Borage leaf—A mild, cooling liver cleanser. Also a good blood cleanser, borage is indicated for arthritis or arterial cleansing. Three to 10 capsules per day.

Stone root—Provides a powerful flush through the liver and relieves congestion; especially good for hemorrhoids. Two capsules per day.

Chinese bupleurum root—Yet another classic liver herb that's excellent for hemorrhoids, bupleurum also lowers fever, increases sweating, and is anti-gas. Two to 5 capsules per day.

Chinese rhubarb root—A bitter, cold remedy for constipation, hemorrhoids or congested *qi* in general. Also reduces fever and is indicated in Traditional Chinese Medicine (TCM) for hot, swollen eyes. Two to 5 capsules per day.

Isatidis root—This Chinese antiviral discussed earlier is an excellent choice for viral hepatitis because it is antiviral and reduces liver inflammation.

Schizandra berry—This Chinese tonic herb, which has many other uses (as discussed elsewhere) and is especially good for women, is liver supportive. Three to 8 capsules per day or tea.

Black walnut bark—An astringent liver herb that's especially good for hemorrhoids and any condition of prolapse, leaking, or protruding (3 capsules per day).

Culver's root—This liver herb is especially good for jaundice and has an affinity for the gallbladder. Five to 10 capsules per day or 1 ounce as tea.

Guduchi leaf—An Ayurvedic herb that's good for short-term treatment of acute liver congestion or weakness. Ten to 20 capsules per day.

Kutki—This Ayurvedic herb is liver protective and balancing. It also stimulates the pancreas and is immune supportive. One to 5 capsules per day.

Neem leaf—One of the most cooling and bitter herbs, neem also improves digestion, is antimicrobial, and stimulates the pancreas to produce insulin, thus lowering blood sugar. One to 5 capsules per day.

Wood betony—A European herb with the unique taste and energetic combo of being pungent and cold (it is also bitter). Five capsules per day.

Licorice root—Another Chinese tonic herb with outstanding versatility, this herb counts liver detoxification among its many healing qualities. It's relatively mild in this regard, but since it's also antiviral, a good choice to support yourself during and after infection. It's a preferred hepatitis treatment in Japan.

Fringetree bark—This general cleanser is known for its ability to promote bile flow. Two to 4 capsules per day.

Black radish—Below we discuss the root vegetables' role in liver cleansing. This one is strong enough to be used in capsules rather than simply eaten. One to 5 capsules a day.

Chamomile flower—This extremely mild herb is known for a wide range of benefits, probably chiefly as a relaxant for its calming properties. It's less well known for its ability to support the liver, but it is in fact an excellent liver tonic and has a long history of traditional use as such. Don't try to use beverage tea bags for this purpose—get medicinal-quality chamomile from an herb pharmacy and brew it up strong to make a potent liver remedy. Karta Purkh knew a man who was diagnosed with a serious case of hepatitis and was told he would be out of work and in bed for six months. He stayed in bed for two weeks and drank a *gallon* of strong chamomile tea a day. He was back to work after two weeks. Brewed more mildly, it's ideal for kids.

Hyssop leaf—Another extremely mild herb, this can be taken up to 10 capsules a day or as tea.

Some other general, very mild liver-building herbs are **hibiscus flower** (tea), **lemon balm** (tea), **agrimony leaf** (5 to 10 capsules per day), and **nutgrass root** (5 capsules per day).

Note: If you take too much of any liver-detoxifying substance too rapidly (either the herbs above or the foods below), you may experience symptoms such as headaches, acne, hemorrhoids, or diarrhea as elimination is stimulated and wastes are dumped into the blood. These symptoms are temporary, but it's better to start slowly and work up to higher doses. Less "aggressive," slower-acting liver herbs will work more gradually over time, so that less sudden and overwhelming action is created. The herbs noted above for producing powerful liver "flushes" will significantly boost circulation through the liver and unblock restricted bile flow so that wastes are rapidly flushed through the ducts into the gallbladder and out through the small intestine. This will not hurt you, but symptoms such as acne can temporarily get worse before they get better when you use these more aggressive herbs. Be assured you are still moving in the right direction.

Root Vegetables

The root vegetables are unparalleled for liver support and detox. Beets, carrots, and radishes are the best for this job—raw, cooked, or juiced. Their properties in this regard have not been studied to our knowledge, but they have a long history of traditional use in other cultures for this purpose.

Beet juice is the king of liver detoxifying root vegetables; in fact, it's so powerful that it must be used carefully. It detoxifies the liver so quickly that it must be mixed with other juices so that excess toxins don't get blasted into your bloodstream all at once.

Karta Purkh remembers one time he happened to bump into someone who wasn't aware of this. In the checkout line in an Asian grocery, a young woman was chatting with the checkout clerk. She was wielding an empty container and proudly announcing, "I just drank sixteen ounces of beet juice!" Karta Purkh turned to the clerk and asked, "Do you have a bed or couch somewhere in this store?" The clerk responded, bewildered, "Sure, why?" Karta Purkh explained, indicating the woman, "Because she's going to faint." Right then, the woman slumped to the floor, caught just in time by the clerk. She slept for an hour in a back room of the grocery. The problem was that such a large quantity of pure beet juice stimulated her liver to dump accumulated toxins and wastes into her bloodstream that couldn't be eliminated all at once.

Another personal experience of Karta Purkh's, when he tested the efficacy of these vegetables on his own health, attests to this. Along with about fifty other people, Karta Purkh was exposed to hepatitis at a picnic. Most of the attendees received shots of gamma globulin (an antiviral immune system protein fractionated from other peoples' blood that cannot be produced in sufficient quantities fast enough by the body to ward off hepatitis). Karta Purkh opted instead to drink one pint of daikon radish juice daily for six weeks. He was the only person exposed who didn't receive a shot who also did not contract hepatitis.

Used properly, these foods in therapeutic doses are obviously potent medicines.

I once developed several classic symptoms of liver stress, all in one week, for no reason I ever could figure out (I hadn't been sick). Who knows what life stress or exposure may have put my liver a little behind on the job at that particular time? But knowing that all of the symptoms were linked to the liver, according to natural healing, I embarked on a mild liver detox program: namely, beet soup ("Preparation B"). This root-vegetable extravaganza is a detox borscht with beets and carrots in a tomato base, along with lots of onions, garlic, red cabbage, and celery. This violently pink, red, and purple soup was absolutely delicious and we ate it for four nights with fresh whole-grain bread. By the fourth night, all symptoms were gone (i.e., my skin was totally clear, the headache was gone, etc.) and have never come back.

(This soup is a great food-as-medicine way to get your beets, especially if you don't like beets that well, as I don't. It's better for you than Clearasil, Preparation H, and Advil. The recipe is included on page 502.)

BLOOD

There are many herbs in natural healing known as blood cleansers or blood purifiers (a more modern term in herbal medicine is *alterative*). Conventional science-oriented practitioners often don't recognize this as a valid function, because there is no specific scientific mechanism to describe it. It's a natural healing term that describes a concept—namely, that waste materials can accumulate in the blood and certain substances naturally tend to assist the body in clearing them out. One mechanism by which some herbs do this may be a chelating action—bonding to the waste and creating insoluble molecules, which are then eliminated instead of reabsorbed.

Regardless of the mechanism, this is an old and traditional concept that draws our attention to the fact that the blood is a sewer system as well as a delivery system, and must be kept free of excess wastes for best health.

The following herbs have been used traditionally in other cultures as blood cleansers and have been observed by their practitioners as effective; that experience is echoed by modern herbalists and natural healing practitioners today. These herbs will reduce symptoms of toxicity because they reduce the toxicity itself. (Many of these herbs also have other functions and have been discussed at length elsewhere in the book.)

Blood Cleansers

Garlic	Onion	Guggul
Turmeric	Yucca root	Hawthorn berry
Echinacea	Thyme	Alfalfa
Amla	Black pepper	Pipali (long pepper)

Oregon grape root	Cayenne	Nettles
Triphala (Ayurvedic formula containing amla fruit, haritaki fruit, and bibitaki fruit)	Trikatu (Ayurvedic formula containing ginger, black pepper, and long pepper)	Shilajit (a mineral pitch found on rock cliffs in the Himalayas)
Chaparral	Echinacea	Dong quai
Chlorophyll	Cilantro	Ligusticum
Borage leaf	Gentian root	Myrrh gum
Licorice root	Cloves	Sarsaparilla
Burdock root	Mahasudarshan (Ayurvedic formula containing chiretta, guduchi, trikatu, triphala)	Karaya gum
Pau d'arco bark		Prickly ash bark

Foods that Produce or Assist Detoxification

Onion, Garlic, Ginger (Sulfur containing, circulation enhancing)

Watermelon (Antioxidant compounds)

Chilies (Increase circulation)

Pineapple (Proteases reduce excess protein accumulation and toxic by-products of protein breakdown.)

Yogurt (Good bacteria keep toxin-producing "bad" bacteria at bay.)

Papaya (Proteases reduce excess protein accumulation and toxic by-products of protein breakdown.)

Crucifer family (Cabbage, kale, and broccoli, among others, contain sulfur compounds; also antioxidant compounds.)

Turmeric (Antioxidant compounds)

Green vegetables (Especially raw, are considered the most overall detoxifying vegetables available.)

Citrus (Antioxidant compounds, including vitamins, minerals, and phytonutrients)

CLEANSING EXTREMES

Fasting

I'm personally not enthused about total fasting. Modified fasts in which you can have juice or other thin liquids, providing at least some sustenance, make more sense to me. I think it is important to consider that in the case of fasting, there is a price paid for whatever cleansing is accomplished. There is a loss when you consume no "body fuel" for periods of days at a time—a loss of lean muscle tissue that will, after a certain amount of time, be converted to glucose to fill the gap—and it seems to me that such a loss is unnecessary when there are other ways to cleanse the body more gently and safely. Also, conversion of body protein to glucose itself leaves toxic by-products.

Karta Purkh notes that total fasting is not recommended much by ancient holistic healing systems of the world, except occasionally for very short periods. These systems are much more inclined to recommend monodiets of short duration. In a monodiet, the diet is limited to specifically therapeutic foods for a short period of time to reduce the stress on the digestive system while keeping fuel coming in for the health and comfort of the person. Monodiets should be individualized to the person and/or condition, and are best undertaken with the advice and supervision of a trusted and experienced natural health practitioner.

Colonics

A key point of herbal and nutritional cleansing is that it can be done slowly and gently, without invasive physical procedures. Laxative herbs, liver-protecting and -stimulating herbs and foods, the use of fiber, and the introduction of friendly bacteria into the digestive tract can all very effectively cleanse the intestines (and other organs and systems) without something this radical, although they may have their place in individual circumstances. Dr. Ralph Golan, M.D., author of *Optimal Wellness*, notes that colonics can deplete friendly bacteria in the intestines as well as electrolytes, and says, "It's advisable to improve dietary and lifestyle factors that would render such future interventions unnecessary."[6]

Hydrotherapy

Saunas and/or steam baths can be cleansing by promoting circulation and encouraging the elimination of toxins through the pores.

Herbal baths are also good. A bath is actually a reasonable way to get herb material into the body that would be difficult to get through the digestive tract. For example, baths with epsom salts are a way to get magnesium sulfate through the skin in amounts that could not practically be consumed, and they can be very calming. Chamomile can be put in the bath by brewing half a pound of the herb, making a very strong pot of tea, and pouring it into the bath. A few tablespoons of ginger powder can be put in a bath. Essential oils are useful, not so much for the aroma (though that can be relaxing or energizing) but because the volatile oil compounds are activated and can be inhaled in the steam.

HERBS TO COUNTER DRUG EFFECTS

In the event that you do need to take drugs for a health problem, it's advisable to support your liver as it cleanses your blood of the wastes and breakdown products of the drugs. Drugs are absorbed through the intestinal tract into the blood, and the blood goes to the liver to be detoxified. The presence of a drug definitely places an excessive burden on the liver, so you would do well to use one of the milder liver-supportive or -protective herbs listed above, and/or one of the blood-cleansing herbs listed on page 337.

15

Herbs for Skin

The skin is the body's largest organ and an important part of the immune system. Its condition reflects the health of the body underneath it.

In our culture, when our skin gets pimply, itchy, scaly, or otherwise inflamed, we typically take suppressive prescription drugs (the antibiotic tetracycline for acne, as an example, or antihistamines and steroids like cortisone for inflammatory dermatitis) or douse it with over-the-counter medications.

But from a natural healing point of view, skin disease is an accumulation of waste at the cellular level causing inflammation. Eczema, psoriasis, acne, and general dermatitis are all inflammatory skin diseases. They have different names and symptoms, and infection or hormonal factors may be involved, but all are considered to be idiosyncratic expressions of the same fundamental toxicity problem and are treated with cleansing and detoxification as discussed in Chapter 14, "Herbal Renewal: Cleanse, Detox, Rebuild."

A classic example of skin healing through detoxification instead of topical suppression was described in the public broadcasting radio documentary *The Medicine Garden*, a well-researched herbal medicine program produced by David Freudberg for public radio. A young man named Jerry appeared in the documentary, describing his terrible acne problem. His doctor told him it was the worst acne he had ever seen; Jerry was on antibiotics for two years, with absolutely no result. At the end of two years, the doctor said he was sorry but he had nothing more to offer. Jerry began to read about herbs and started taking blood-purifying botanicals. Within four days, his pimples started shrinking. His skin is now completely clear.

Another example: Drs. Murray and Pizzorno in *Textbook of Natural Medicine* note that psoriasis has been linked to high levels of circulating endotoxins—toxins normally found in the cell walls of intestinal bacteria. If the liver is overwhelmed by the size of the toxic burden or is functionally too weak to filter and detoxify as needed, psoriasis can result and/or worsen.

Skin can be treated topically for inflammation—say, with turmeric and gota kola—and for infection if it exists. We can control symptoms naturally, but detoxification is the real work of skin healing. The blood, liver, and large intestine are all worked on to get the waste out.

TREATING THE INFLAMMATION

Green vegetables are widely regarded in natural medicine as the most cooling, anti-inflammatory treatments for skin. They also happen to be detoxifying, so they work for healing and to treat symptoms. Wheat grass is especially good, but broccoli, cucumber, celery, and dark, leafy greens will do the trick. Juice is the best way to get enough green vegetables into you—after all, how many cucumbers or celery stalks can you eat? If you can drink a quart of vegetable juice a day, you will rapidly de-inflame skin.

If infection is present, use immune support and antimicrobial herbs (you can refer back to the appropriate chapters for information on these).

If you just stop at the skin, however, you have to use the green vegetables for the rest of your life. A person with severe skin disease who eats a 50 percent green vegetable diet can clear up acne, psoriasis, or dermatitis in a matter of days or weeks—Karta Purkh has seen it happen countless times. But if those individuals did not also work on the deeper issue—toxic overload—the problem came right back as soon as the green vegetables were decreased.

Turmeric, the world's best anti-inflammatory in Karta Purkh's experience, works as well to de-inflame skin as it does for joints and acute injury conditions. It can be taken internally to soothe inflammation from the inside out. Turmeric is a major skin-treatment herb in Asia, with a wide variety of uses, both oral and topical. In fact, turmeric is a good general treatment for all connective tissue. Being a polyphenol, the compound curcumin stabilizes collagen.[1] It is used to enhance healing after surgery, reducing adhesions and scarring.

Turmeric is particularly appropriate in treating inflammatory skin diseases, such as psoriasis and eczema since it reduces heat and cleanses the liver. One individual Karta Purkh met, Mrs. S., had such bad eczema that blood soaked through the bandages in which she was forced to wrap her arms. She had endured chronic eczema since childhood, and over the decades it had worsened until it covered every inch of her body below the neck.

Though Mrs. S. was generally conscious about her heath, she had never been able to control the eczema, despite numerous programs from various practitioners. The dose of steroid drugs necessary to control the condition produced intolerable side effects. She was miserable.

When she was forty, a friend led Mrs. S. to herbal medicine. She began a rigorous program of herbs and special diet, the centerpiece of which was one ounce of turmeric per day. Within days, her skin began to respond. She faithfully continued to take her turmeric. By the end of six weeks, she had a patch the size of a dime on one hand. The entire rest of her body was covered with fresh new skin. Five years later, Mrs. S. has not had a speck of eczema since and manages her skin with diet and two capsules of turmeric per day.

The cooling properties of turmeric also make it a perfect internal and external treatment for all herpes diseases (oral, genital, shingles).

Turmeric both kills insects and heals skin lesions. In one study, a combination of turmeric and **neem,** another Ayurvedic insecticidal herb, applied topically, eradicated scabies within 3 to 15 days in 97 percent of subjects treated. This formula is also traditional for ringworm.[2] Neem is a classic skin and anti-inflammatory herb.

Berberine-containing herbs such as **Oregon grape root** have historically been used as psoriasis treatment; recent research bears this out, showing that berberine inhibits keratinocyte growth (psoriasis is characterized by skin cells dividing at a rate about 100 times greater than normal).[3] Other berberine-containing herbs such as barberry, goldthread, and goldenseal may be used, although goldenseal is a less appropriate choice because of the expense and extinction issues discussed earlier. Any of these can be taken up to 10 capsules per day for this purpose.

The Ayurvedic herb *coleus*, or an extract of its compound *forskolin,* has also been shown effective for its historical use in treating psoriasis and eczema. Standard dose is 50 milligrams of forskolin extract 2 to 3 times per day; up to 8 capsules of the whole herb may also be used.

Other good skin healing and tonic herbs include *nettle leaf* (for eczema, 1 ounce as tea daily), *burdock root* (for dry, scaly skin and psoriasis, 5 to 10 capsules daily), and *red clover flower* for general internal cleansing (5 capsules per day).

Yucca root is the main treatment for adult acne in Britain (its saponin compounds are believed to be steroidal and anti-inflammatory). *Oregon grape root* is also excellent for acne. Both can be taken in capsules, 2 to 10 per day. A third acne herb is *cleavers leaf* (5 to 10 capsules per day).

Calendula flower ointment and *chaparral* tea both make good soothing external skin treatments.

DETOXIFICATION

Blood

For blood detox, use the protocol listed in the previous chapter, on page 337. *Garlic* and *guggul* are especially good. *Sulfur* is also a classic blood cleanser. Sulfur is reactive, binding with materials that the body is trying to eliminate. *Sulfur, honey, and cloves* is an Ayurvedic blood cleansing formula used to treat acne and adult skin conditions.

Liver

For liver detoxification, use the *root vegetables, boldo leaf, bhumy amalaki, dandelion root*, and/or *yellow dock root* as described in the previous chapter on pages 331–337. Remember, skin conditions that are the result of accumulated waste can temporarily appear worse before they get better because you are unleashing the previously backed-up wastes into the blood, and the more aggressive you are with your liver cleansing, the more of a load you're going to unleash. Use a blood-purifying herb and be patient. Over the long haul, the toxins will be eliminated and your skin will improve.

Large Intestine

See pages 328–330 in the previous chapter for ways to ensure that waste is being properly eliminated from the large intestine.

FUNGUS ISSUES

Fungus (such as "athlete's foot") takes us back to the immune system. Use the antiyeast protocol described in Chapter 18, "Herbs for Yeast (Candida)," as typically antiyeast substances work on fungus too.

Grapefruit seed extract can be used topically, full strength.

Clove oil and *cinnamon oil* may be applied topically, but are very hot; dilute them first with alcohol or vegetable oil. Start with a 10 percent solution and work up to tolerance.

Citrus seed extract taken internally will work over time to treat fungus from the inside. *Pau d'arco* shows antifungal properties as well.

Turmeric and *neem* have antifungal properties and can be used both internally and externally, together or separately.

Chlorophyll, vinegar, garlic, and *witch hazel* are all mild topicals that can be used for fungus.

NUTRITION

Antioxidants generally benefit the skin. Wrinkling is largely due to crosslinking of proteins, which can be reduced by retarding oxidative damage and free-radical destruction. Vitamins A, C, and E, selenium, and zinc are all important. Vitamins B_5 and B_6 are adrenal nutrients. They assist adrenals in making anti-inflammatory hormones.

Once again, don't rely on supplements alone. Try to eat as many of the antioxidant fruits and vegetables as you can. As we have discussed, you'll get a much wider range of the vitamins, minerals, and phytochemicals in their whole form and in concert with other compounds that may enhance their effectiveness. For example, from cabbage you'll not only get vitamins and minerals but also sulfur-containing compounds.

Plenty of pure water is crucial for the skin as well; that's common sense.

HERBAL SKIN TONICS

Gotu kola, figwort root, and **Chinese violet leaf** are all good long-term tissue healers and tonics.

Gotu kola is the standout in this category. It is a nerve tonic and has steroidlike compounds called triterpenes, which are anti-inflammatory. Another component, asiaticoside, appears to expedite the healing of wounds, such as surgical incisions, skin ulcers, trauma, and gangrene. Gota kola improves the function and integrity of connective tissue, increases blood supply to the tissue, and increases formation of structural components of the skin as well as connective tissue. It can be used as a tea (not bad tasting) and in capsules, and has been used externally as well.

Standardized extract of gotu kola has been shown to treat scleroderma (an autoimmune condition involving extreme hardening of the skin around the hands) and keloids (thick scars resulting from overgrowth of fibrous tissue, which can require surgery) effectively, apparently by shortening the abnormally long inflammatory phase of healing associated with these scars.

While most studies have used daily doses (60 to 120 milligrams per day) of an extract standardized to 70 percent triterpenic acids, gotu kola is taken as a tea in its traditional use. The tea is extremely mild tasting and can be prepared to maximum drinkable strength, using 1 to 2 ounces of herb per day for acute conditions, or you can take up to 20 capsules per day. As a long-term tonic, 1 to 2 capsules a day is appropriate.

OTHER SKIN TOPICALS

Witch hazel is excellent for inflammatory skin diseases; studies have shown it to be effective as a topical treatment for dermatitis.

Chamomile is another soothing anti-inflammatory topical. Brigitte Mars, an herbalist and writer with twenty years of experience with botanicals, writes that "a study conducted at the Dermatological Clinic of Friedrich-Wilhelm University in Germany showed chamomile was even more helpful in speeding skin healing time than cortisone. Not only does chamomile help promote skin growth over a wound, but it also can bring pain relief. Even after dermabrasion from the removal of tattoos, chamomile exhibits wound-healing abilities."[4]

Salves or even teas made from *comfrey* and *chaparral* may be used externally for dermatitis. Other generally soothing natural skin topicals include *aloe vera gel, calendula, castor oil, chickweed, arnica,* and *almond oil.*

PREVENTION

One more time: Basic good diet and exercise as outlined initially, along with as "low-impact" a life as possible in other ways we've discussed, will help prevent toxic buildup in the first place. Some inflammatory skin diseases are believed to have a psychological or stress-related element, and exploring that angle might be helpful as well.

Part III

Dealing with Disease the Natural Way

Other Specific Conditions

Part III is an herbal remedy resource addressing common illnesses and conditions Americans face that haven't already been covered in other chapters. (For example, premenstrual syndrome was covered in Chapter 8, "Especially for Women: Natural Healing for a Woman's Lifetime," prostate conditions in Chapter 9, "Especially for Men: Natural Healing for a Man's Lifetime," and ear infections in Chapter 10, "Herbs for Babies and Children.")

Rather than try to address briefly every single health concern from A to Z, we have chosen to focus more in depth on those that (1) natural medicine excels at treating (more effectively and safely than the available conventional therapies); (2) affect large or increasing numbers of people in the United States; and (3) Karta Purkh has had extensive experience with and seen great success.

In this way, we can offer a more thoughtful analysis and detailed guidelines for the conditions most likely to concern most people. This is also more consistent with our goal of supporting major, holistic changes in thinking and living that are global throughout your life, rather than providing an exhaustive list of remedies that can be "popped" as "herbal fixes" in the absence of any real change or healthy context.

We include here cardiovascular disease and diabetes, which in most cases are preventable, but herbal treatment has a lot to offer those already afflicted. Other conditions we cover here are not necessarily life-threatening, but seriously affect quality of life for millions of people, and diagnoses continue to rise. These conditions include arthritis, allergies and asthma, and candida (yeast) syndrome.

Note: When addressing specific conditions, we offer a wide array of suggestions for each symptom or phase of healing. These are not necessarily to be used all at once. The idea is to start with one or two things, see how that works, and try something else if you aren't satisfied. It helps to have a natural health practitioner overseeing your herbal treatment program.

16

Herbs for Allergies

WHAT IS AN ALLERGY?

"Allergy" refers to any condition of the body mounting an attack on a specific substance that for most people is benign. People can experience allergic reactions to foods, chemicals, plants, animals, or a variety of airborne compounds. The substance to which you are allergic is called the allergen.

An allergy is a normal immune response gone haywire. As you have seen, the immune system's job is to identify and deal with threats to your health. When an invader of some kind enters the body, the exposure causes a reaction by the body. Usually the reaction itself is designed to rid the body of the threat. This reaction can take many forms, but one kind is an inflammatory reaction—the rushing of blood and/or mucus to the area of contact or site of invasion. This is healthy and normal. The increased blood supply to the affected area delivers healing nutrients; swelling and heat may expel the invader, and mucus may flush it out.

What is not normal is when the body mounts this type of response against something that is not in fact a threat to the body, such as grass or tomatoes or feathers. In this case, you experience ongoing inflammation from contact with something that should be perceived by your body as innocuous. This can be very distressing and uncomfortable.

A generally weakened immune system creates an environment for allergies to develop. In this state, the body considers itself vulnerable to attack, and prepares to launch a defense against any perceived invader at a moment's notice. This hair-trigger response is the body's way of preventing crisis in the long run. Pollen, cat hair, and mold are not truly invaders, and are tolerated just fine by many people.

Some natural health practitioners believe that one possible contributing factor in allergy may be our standard approach to medicating inflammation. We have been so consumed with eliminating symptoms that we rarely stop to consider whether those symptoms have a reason for being, with which we ought not to interfere. For example, when your nose runs or gets stuffed up, perhaps your body is doing you a favor, producing fluid that will flush away something offensive. Instead, you may reach for a medicine whose sole purpose is to make the mucus go away. Perhaps when you beat back the body's natural response to a foreign substance, the area later becomes a site for chronic inflammation, a rebellion against our attempt to quash its healing efforts. We may weaken that site, or make the body overdefensive in that area, or both.

WHAT HERBS CAN DO

The herbal kingdom offers many centuries-old remedies for allergy. In natural therapy, the thrust in allergy control is to nourish the body, particularly the immune system, so that the body feels confident it can control infection. The body then relaxes its intense defensive response, and the symptoms of allergy disappear. Meanwhile, on a temporary level, we use gentle natural methods to control inflammation and swelling, relieve pain, dry and soothe mucous membranes, and strengthen respiratory tissue.

So herbs can do two things for most allergies: First, they can be used short term for symptomatic relief, and second, they can be used to address and heal the underlying issues—usually immune weakness—to eliminate the allergy completely over time.

Allergies can be successfully treated without drugs. Not only can symptoms be controlled without medication, but the allergies themselves can be eliminated forever. Consistent with conventional rationale (if you can't kill it, stay away from it), it is a widely held myth that the only way to "cure" an allergy is to remove the allergen—to avoid the food or substance to which you react.

For many people, total avoidance of allergens is impractical. If you're allergic to peanuts, that's one thing, but if you're allergic to ragweed it's pretty hard to escape, and if you're allergic to the family pet it can be heartbreaking.

It's also long been thought that allergies were inherited, that we were cursed by fate and family legacy to suffer the misery of nonstop sneezing and swollen eyes. While in some cases genetic tissue weaknesses may contribute to the risk, or determine what area will be affected if you do become allergic, allergies are developed through health decisions made as we develop.

I have personal experience with allergies, and so do several of my family members. I had terrible hay fever and asthma when I was a child. Thanks to the use of herbs, I don't have even the slightest sign of either anymore. My husband once had serious asthma and airborne allergies to animals; these were permanently eliminated through a program of herbal and natural healing. The same type of healing work eliminated almost two dozen food allergies from which I suffered until my early twenties. Karta Purkh has seen literally hundreds of people manage the same kind of healing. Allergies are an unfortunate source of suffering in millions of people, but the great news is they just don't have to be.

AIRBORNE/INHALANT ALLERGIES

Headache. Nonstop sneezing. Stuffy nose. Fatigue. If you're an airborne allergy sufferer, these symptoms are your constant companions for several months (or more) every year. For those with year-round allergies, each day brings a cycle of misery, often broken only temporarily by powerful drugs—antihistamines and decongestants—often with side effects as uncomfortable as the original symptoms.

Airborne allergies usually affect the respiratory system. Some airborne allergies, like the one we call hay fever, are seasonal; others are perennially active.

Hay fever, which affects some 35 million Americans, is a colloquialism for allergic rhinitis. It involves sneezing, itching throat and eyes, sinus headaches, and sometimes coughing. It is not an allergy to hay. It can be triggered by different kinds of pollen throughout the seasons: tree pollens in spring, grass and weed pollens in summer, and ragweed pollen in the fall. Pets, molds, mildew and fungus, dust, and cigarette smoke are common household allergens that can cause symptoms similar to those of hay fever.

Airborne allergies are not only irritating (and occasionally debilitating) but are also a long-term drain to the immune system, because the body is in a constant low-grade state of attack on the allergen(s). This makes the allergic person also more susceptible to infections in general. Often a vicious cycle of respiratory allergic reaction/respiratory infection is set up, so that the person rarely has any relief from symptoms. Many a person wonders whether symptoms are "cold or allergy" at a given time.

Histamine, a necessary substance released by immune cells when the body is injured, causes allergic symptoms when the body overreacts to a sensitizing substance.

Herbal Symptom Relief

Dr. Andrew Weil notes in his newsletter *Self Healing*, "Conventional medical treatments for hay fever are unsatisfactory. Desensitization shots are invasive, expensive, time-consuming and often not effective enough to justify the trouble. Antihistamines are toxic and suppressive. Steroids are dangerous."[1]

Fortunately, natural substances can do the job well without these unpleasant side effects. We hope that more doctors will begin to learn about them and suggest them to patients.

For inhalant allergies like hay fever, herbal healing offers an array of options for symptom relief.

Cubeb berry, an aromatic relative of black pepper, comes from Jamaica, and is an excellent tonic for the tissue of the lungs and nose. It is discussed in detail on page 175 for its use as an antiviral. You could take 5 capsules per day or 1 ounce of dried herb daily as tea.

An herb long used in Native American medicine, and gaining widespread respect today in allergy treatment, is the leaf of the **stinging nettle**. This common plant offers excellent symptom relief for allergy. Of course, the stinging qualities are deactivated in the drying process.

Nettle can essentially be thought of as two different remedies, and only one is appropriate for hay-fever relief. The normal air-drying method results in a nourishing, blood-cleansing, general tonic that can be used like a vegetable (similar to spinach) or made into a tea that is good for the lungs, much like elecampane root, mullein root, or coltsfoot flower. The tea as a general pulmonary tonic can be taken in a dose of 1 to 2 ounces per day.

However, this air-drying (sometimes called shade-drying) method destroys the antihistamine compound, a bioflavonoid. Thus, to benefit hay fever, nettles must be freeze-dried or otherwise specially processed when fresh to preserve that compound. The specially-processed nettles, which are usually sold in 300-milligram capsules, should be taken at the first sign of discomfort. Take one and wait 5 minutes. If symptoms are not relieved, take another and wait 5 minutes. Do this until symptoms are resolved. In Karta Purkh's experience, most people reach that point at about 5 capsules. From there on, you will know the dose you need to suppress symptoms and can take the full dose at once at the onset of symptoms.

Nettles are totally nontoxic and do not have any of the side effects of OTC antihistamines—no dry mouth, no drowsiness. You can take as many as needed. Normally, once you've taken your dose, they last all day, but on a particularly bad "allergy day" you may need more.

Nettles taken this way are not preventive and do not build or nourish to heal the underlying allergy problem, but they are a safe and nontoxic way to live with allergies until you can eliminate them completely. The use of stinging nettles allows many people to wean off antihistamines.

Fenugreek seed is a tasty seed that's available at most grocery stores. It treats the symptoms of allergy at the time they're occurring, but because it's mild, you need to take a fair amount to get the job done. The seeds can be soaked overnight, then chewed and swallowed (or put into cereal), or a tea can be made with the seeds steeped in hot water. Fenugreek can also be ground and capsuled; 5 to 10 capsules a day for allergies is appropriate. However, due to the mildness, capsules are not the most effective form; the whole seeds used consistently in the diet to maximum tolerance are really the best way to get the effect.

Ephedra (ma huang) is a Chinese remedy discussed in more detail elsewhere in this book. Ephedra is an excellent asthma remedy, used by the Chinese for millennia. It was also the first Chinese remedy to be used in America to synthesize a drug. The compound ephedrine, which soothes spasms of the smooth muscles of the bronchia, was used to synthesize asthma drugs like Primatene. Ephedra is also an excellent nasal and sinus decongestant; pseudoephedrine, the active ingredient in OTC medications like Sudafed, was also synthesized from constituents of ephedra.

However, ephedra is not a good long-term solution for these symptoms because of its potential to cause nervous-system and adrenal overstimulation in high doses. Insomnia, nervousness, anxiety, and elevated heart rate and blood pressure may occur in some people (although most herbalists feel that from a practical point of view, these are not serious concerns when ephedra is used responsibly for the purpose of healing and not "weight loss" or as a recreational drug). We discuss these issues later in the book.

Ephedra is very effective when used concurrently with work on the underlying problems in order to eliminate the allergy completely over time. While you are taking it, it's a good idea also to take adrenal-nourishing herbs (which, in any case, will help long-term against allergies, particularly against asthma). These could include licorice root, ginseng, sarsaparilla root, prickly ash bark, cedar berry, or cubeb berry. (See pages 283–284 for more on the adrenal builders.)

Ephedra for allergies can be taken as tea (1 to 3 tablespoons crushed herb per day) or 1 to 5 capsules per day or as directed by your natural health practitioner.

Rose hip is a good source of bioflavonoids as well as exceptionally bioavailable vitamin C. It's a general respiratory soother (much like elecampane, nettle, coltsfoot, and mullein). In addition to capsules (5 per day), it can be obtained in a solid extract form, which is a good way to get enough down, considering its mildness. Solid extract is made by cooking down a tincture or other liquid preparation under mild heat to reduce the liquid. The resulting product has the consistency of shoe polish, and can be taken in doses of 1/4 teaspoon to 1/2 teaspoon, several times a day.

Kokum fruit (garcinia) is a classic Ayurvedic remedy for hives. This too-sour-to-eat citrus fruit probably owes its anti-inflammatory properties to bioflavonoids. It has culinary uses in South Asia. It can be taken in capsules, up to 10 per day.

Triphala, which has been mentioned in numerous other chapters, makes a dramatic allergy treatment. A particularly good remedy if you're one of those people who wakes up with "nasal drip" (and have to blow your nose 100 times before noon), it was taught to Karta Purkh by his teacher Yogi Bhajan. Open 6 capsules of triphala into a tumbler of water. Put the tumbler at your bedside to "soak" all night. In the morning, drink down the entire thing, including the dregs. In minutes you will experience a massive nasal purge (in Ayurveda this is considered accumulated *kapha*).

Two triphala capsules per day will also provide good long-term general immune support.

Saw palmetto berry is an excellent endocrine tonic and anti-inflammatory (5 capsules per day). (*Licorice root, black cohosh root,* or any of the other adrenal tonics listed on pages 281–288 could be substituted).

Myrrh gum is a blood detoxifier (5 capsules per day). The Ayurvedic herbs *guggul, frankincense,* and *boswellia* are all relatives and can be substituted.

Baical scullcap root, classically a liver herb in Chinese medicine, is also detoxifying and is anti-inflammatory as well, making it a good anti-allergy herb (5 capsules per day).

Pau d'arco bark is a general immune-system builder that is particularly good for allergies long term. Some herbalists don't feel the tea is as effective as other forms, but Karta Purkh has had good experience with the tea. It's a "fluffy" herb so it's hard to capsule, and since it's trendy it tends to be expensive; tea is cheaper (1 ounce dried herb per day).

Quercetin is a bioflavonoid found in citrus fruits and some other foods. It is very helpful for respiratory allergies both as a symptom treatment and as a preventive agent taken in advance of allergy season's onset. It is available in tablet or capsule form and can be taken in divided doses of 1 to 2 grams daily.

Mixed bioflavonoids may help too. Flavonoids are anti-inflammatory (inhibit histamine, leukotrienes, and prostaglandins), antioxidant, immuno-stimulating, tissue regenerative, liver protective, and capillary strengthening (reducing their permeability). Reducing leakiness of capillaries can help histamine metabolism, according to David Hoffmann in *Therapeutic Herbalism.*

A quick and convenient routine for allergy control includes the naturally antihistamine mineral *magnesium* with vitamins B_6 and C. Taken at the onset of an attack, a combination of these three nutrients will very often quell the intense sneezing and itching. Experiment to find the effective dose. Magnesium will cause loose stools, so increase the dose gradually, and use the amount that is tolerable or will control the symptoms. One or both of the vitamins B_6 and C can be added as necessary.

Bee pollen is recommended by many practitioners of natural healing to desensitize the body against local pollens. Some practitioners recommend using local pollen and starting to take it at least four months in advance of the coming hay-fever season. Karta Purkh is not sure locality is the key, since people have reported good results using pollen from all over. The locality may not be involved in the mechanism; EFAs, pantothenic acid, or other elements shared by all pollens may be involved.

Since in this case you are ingesting the allergen, you must begin very cautiously. Don't start by downing a heaping spoonful of it every day! Desensitizing means beginning with a very tiny amount and slowly reintroducing your body to the substance over a period of time to give it a chance to adjust. Start with very small amounts (less than a quarter-teaspoon) and work up to a spoonful daily. If you experience allergic symptoms, lower the dose till they disappear (stopping completely if necessary). We strongly suggest using this strategy in combination with general immune-building herbal support.

Foods to emphasize include **greens** for their superb anti-inflammatory, blood-cleansing, and cooling effects; **orange vegetables** for carotenoids; **root vegetables** for liver support; **chilies** for immune boosting, circulation, blood cleansing, and thinning of mucosal secretions; **ginger** as an anti-inflammatory and for thinning of mucosal secretions; and **onion** for quercetin, immune building, and its affinity for lung tissue.

Milk is best avoided by those with sinus problems. It suppresses the helpful thinning of mucosal secretions, and causes or aggravates symptoms in many allergic people.

FOOD ALLERGIES

In addition to inhalant allergies, natural therapeutics has a history of outstanding success with what has become a growing epidemic in the last decade—food allergies. Again, the body responds, out of hypersensitivity, to a normal food it misinterprets as an invader. By nourishing and balancing the body, enhancing digestion, cleansing the liver, and building the glandular system, food allergies can become a thing of the past.

In twenty-five years of experience in the herb field, Karta Purkh has never seen a food allergy that couldn't be reversed. In fact, he estimates that for a period of ten years, 75 percent of the people in his classes were multiple-food-allergy victims trying to learn more about how to deal with this issue. I was one of those people, and I can attest to the fact that the conditions underlying food allergies can be healed.

For five years, after being diagnosed with allergies to corn, egg, soy, peanut, chocolate, caffeine, peaches, plums, pears, apples, cherries, and a variety of beans, I avoided these foods completely. I became an expert at label reading and knew what was in everything. When I ate one of these foods, or a food containing one of these ingredients, I would get a headache and feel exhausted—which was the way I had lived daily for many years prior.

By strengthening my immune system using herbs, and then very slowly integrating the foods one by one back into my diet, I was able to train my body not to react inappropriately to them. I now consume all of those foods freely (in moderation) with absolutely no symptoms. Because of this, one of the most exciting things for me to share with people is the possibility of eliminating food allergies.

Many practitioners recommend simply removing the foods from the diet—as was initially recommended to me—which is impractical. In fact, if you merely remove the offending foods without also promoting healing and strengthening of the immune system, you wind up overconsuming the foods that remain, in the setting of a still-compromised immune system. This makes it likely that you will eventually become allergic to more of the remaining foods. It's a downward spiral that can have dismaying, even drastic, consequences.

One student in Karta Purkh's classes explained how he developed more and more allergies each time he identified and eliminated additional "allergic foods." Since his main symptoms were an almost narcoleptic fatigue and severe blackouts (for example, he would find himself walking around downtown Seattle and not know how he got there) he feared eating anything that would set him off. He cut his diet back so severely that by the time he met Karta Purkh, he was eating nothing but cabbage and white rice. Through a gradual step-by-step process that involved dedicated herbal immune-building and nutrient therapy, this young man was able to integrate more and more foods back into his diet. One year later he was eating a wide and varied diet with no return of his symptoms.

A huge percentage of Americans report daily fatigue; our tolerance for feeling bad is very large in our culture. We would suggest that many people don't know what it's really like to feel good. I certainly didn't ten years ago. Of course, often a large part of this is simply lack of good basic nutrition: not enough complex carbs, not enough (or too much) protein, too much of the damaging fats, not eating often enough. But in addition, many of the foods to which Americans have become addicted are not only displacing healthier foods, they also create allergies.

It can be hard to identify what is causing an allergy because the reaction to a particular substance or food may occur up to three days after ingestion, and the reaction may be continuous or it may be delayed. To be tested for an allergy, Karta Purkh strongly recommends muscle testing by an applied kinesiologist, if possible using the method he developed, called Kinesionics. The Association for Specialized Kinesiologists (see "Resources," page 511) can refer you to a list of practitioners in your area. Most people have told Karta Purkh that the results indicated by muscle testing more accurately matched their personal experience of food reactions, whereas skin or blood tests were less consistent with actual experience. Other available tests are the RAST, RASP, and ELISA-ACT, the latter being more sensitive and less expensive than the first two.[2] Check with your natural health practitioner for available methods.

Cravings are a classic sign of food allergy (when I received my list of food allergens I was horrified to find that many were my daily staples; this is an extremely common response, hence the term *allergic/addicted*). The first thing to do if you suspect a food allergy is to remove the food from the diet. Carefully monitor any changes after the removal of the food; keeping a diary is helpful. Try to get more in tune with your body and your life. Be attentive to common denominators when you don't feel good. This kind of elimination "challenge" can be the best and most accurate allergy test.

Once the offending foods are out of the system, the system itself must be strengthened and nourished as described below.

During the period of time when the allergens are being avoided, you will need to find substitutes for the foods. This can be especially difficult with certain foods such as wheat. For alternatives, consult the "Alternative Ingredients and Substitutes" list on page 506.

HEALING THE ALLERGY ITSELF

The underlying weakness that favors overzealous immune reaction is healed with a three-pronged approach: glandular balancing, immune building, and tissue support. We have covered elsewhere the herbs and nutrients that assist in each of these processes, so we will touch on them briefly and refer you to the full explanations earlier in the book.

Glandular tonics help the body achieve balance generally and also provide "food" for the production of anti-inflammatory hormones, particularly by the adrenals. Glandular tonics are covered in Chapter 11, "Energizing Herbs."

Immune building makes your body a more confident, less "jumpy" defender against foreign substances. Chapters 4 through 7 cover the immune system and general building; in particular look at the immune tonic herbs on pages 133–146 and the nutrients discussed on pages 146–158. (Of course, the immune-supportive dietary suggestions and a "low-impact" lifestyle should also be followed.) Bioflavonoids and coumarins are among the most anti-inflammatory of the phytochemicals found in foods.

Tissue healing supports the cells and membranes in the particular site where the allergy is manifesting. This could be lung, sinus, or skin, for example. For respiratory and pulmonary tonics, see Chapter 7. For sinus tonics, see Chapter 7. For skin, refer to Chapter 15.

These remedies really work for allergies. Kim P., a thirty-one-year-old woman who worked on her allergies after taking a class taught by Karta Purkh, used a program of immune tonics and respiratory-tissue healing herbs for almost a year to build before the allergy season hit. When it did, she kept waiting for some symptoms to show up, and since none did, finally decided it must not be a very bad year for hay fever. When she mentioned this to her doctor, he said, "What do you mean? This has been the worst pollen season ever!"

ALLERGY PREVENTION

Obviously, the basic health recommendations regarding diet, exercise, stress, herbs, and other fundamentals discussed in earlier chapters apply here. Most pathologies are different ways that individuals react to the strains and burdens of unhealthy habits and environments. At its core, just about any disease has at least a link to the function of the immune system and the potency of the healing response, with the exception of acute injury (and even then, recovery is affected by the healing response).

As we discussed in Chapter 10, "Herbs for Babies and Children," allergies can be prevented starting at birth, by not feeding solid foods too soon (under one year) and breast-feeding if at all possible, rather than using cow's milk or soy formulas. When the child does begin to eat solid food, it should be as pure and nutritious as the diet for adults. If you start on sugar-filled jars of baby food you're asking for trouble. A steady diet of candy also compromises immunity.

In both children and adults, a wide variety of fresh whole foods, free of additives and chemicals, eliminates many potential allergens.

As with most conditions, the diet, lifestyle, nutrients, and herbs that heal the problem and the ones that prevent it are virtually identical. Immune-system strength is the crux of an allergy-free body. Remove the minuses and increase the pluses. It may sound simplistic, but the body is marvelously responsive to this kind of common sense (and it's a lot more sensible than keeping all the minuses and taking drugs).

Why Allergy Shots Don't Work

A common practice when I was a child was the use of a series of injections to try to desensitize very allergic individuals. The theory with "allergy shots" is that by exposing the body to the allergen, you force the immune system to accept it, supposedly desensitizing yourself to it after a period of time.

The problem is that injecting allergens directly into the blood has many disadvantages. Injection is an unnatural route of exposure to anything, bypassing all of your body's normal defense mechanisms. Under normal circumstances, an injected allergen (or pathogen) would have to contend with the mucosal immune system and the respiratory and gastrointestinal systems before it reaches the blood. Such a blitz without warning may make the problem worse. Regularly forcing into your system something that is causing rejection doesn't solve the problem. You want to make the immune system less "jumpy" and hysterical, not bombard it more.

I have heard many stories from people who had allergy shots as children—which not only did not help at the time, but did long-term damage to the immune system. I have never actually talked to anyone, nor has Karta Purkh, who received these shots and was satisfied with the results. (Most are people who still have allergies.)

We have noticed that many people who had allergy shots as children develop asthma later in life. (In some cases we know of, asthma developed *immediately* after treatment.) This pattern makes sense. Unfortunately, many then turn to treating the asthma through more immune-suppressive drugs, which compounds the problem.

Desensitizing slowly and gently through dietary changes and herbal supplementation is the only long-term allergy cure we have ever seen. It gives your immune system the time and the nourishment to heal and balance its response.

ALLERGIES TO HERBS?

Looking at herbs to treat allergies raises a question we get asked from time to time: "Is it possible to be allergic to an herb?" The answer is that while it is technically possible, it is extremely rare. For example, Dr. Andrew Weil states that during all his decades of prescribing botanicals, he's seen perhaps one or two reactions he suspected might be allergic, and they were mild.[3] Other herbalists, including Karta Purkh, have simply never run across it.

Karta Purkh suggests numerous reasons for this. First, herbs are not overconsumed or overexposed like many of the foods people are allergic to, or like the pollens that bombard us daily year after year. Second, we don't consume the entire plant; generally there is some diluting adaptation in the form of processing, such as drying and making tea. Third, allergies tend to form more frequently to substances that penetrate the nasal membranes, lungs, or skin than to those that come through the intestine (though obviously this is not always the case, as with food allergies).

However rare, there have been a few scattered anecdotal reports of allergy to echinacea and chamomile (both in the same family as ragweed). If ingestion of an herb makes you uncomfortable, discontinue use and consult your natural health practitioner.

ASTHMA

Bronchial asthma is actually now properly called reactive airway disease, or RAD. It is usually (although not always) an allergic response, sometimes to the same allergens that cause hay fever, and is often exacerbated by stress, exercise, infection, fumes, and cold air. It's characterized by chest tightness, coughing, wheezing, and shortness of breath. These symptoms of an attack are caused by the contraction of smooth muscle around bronchial airways, and sometimes also by secretion of mucus.

From a natural healing point of view, asthma is an adrenal disease manifesting in the lungs. Long-term resolution of asthma involves treatment of the adrenal glands to support production of adrenal hormones—both stress hormones and anti-inflammatory hormones. Usually, that resolves asthma very rapidly. Note that conventional short-term treatments for asthma symptoms, like methlyxanthines, stimulate the adrenal glands or mimic adrenaline.

Long-term conventional treatment uses suppressive anti-inflammatory steroid drugs or bronchial dilators such as theophylline to mask symptoms. In natural healing, you treat the lungs with specific pulmonary herbs to tonify, soothe, and strengthen tissue. Short-term asthma symptoms can be relieved with natural remedies, but the exciting part is that even lifelong asthma can eventually be resolved permanently with the use of long-term adrenal and lung tonics.

Herbs for Asthma

Long-Term Asthma Treatment

There are some exceptional herbs for the long-term treatment of asthma. Probably the preeminent herb for this purpose is *cubeb berry*. This warming, drying peppercorn conveniently does double duty as an excellent long-term lung tissue builder, and as an adrenal builder and tonic. Take 10 capsules or 1/2 ounce as tea per day. The Chinese herb *schizandra berry* is also a good long-term lung tonic, and can be taken in capsules, 2 to 4 per day, as part of a long-term asthma reduction program.

Licorice root is another good choice as a long-term builder, since it is both a lung tonic and adrenal builder (it contains compounds that are similar to the adrenal cortical hormones). In addition, it is expectorant (clears lungs of mucus). Take 5 capsules or 1/2 ounce as tea daily.

Other good long-term pulmonary herbs you can choose from (find one you like and work it into your daily routine) are *coltsfoot flower, elecampane root, mullein leaf, nettle leaf,* and *eyebright leaf.* More information on these herbs is given on pages 188–190. The average dose for these teas is 2 to 3 ounces of the herb daily for acute symptoms, or 1 ounce for building.

Though supported by scant scientific literature, *turmeric* is widely used in Ayurvedic asthma regimes, with the same use being clinically supported by several American herbalists. Turmeric is good for so many other things that it certainly will not hurt to include it. It's anti-inflammatory (this in some way is most likely related to the mechanism for asthma), antioxidant, immune supportive, broadly antimicrobial, and so on.

Bitter herbs reduce *kapha,* the accumulation of mucus, and these include **turmeric, dandelion, yarrow, yellow dock, barberry,** and **goldenseal.** Pungent herbs also do the trick, and these include **black pepper, garlic, cinnamon, cloves, ginger, rosemary, sage,** and **thyme.**

Ginkgo biloba, one of the most widely prescribed phytopharmaceuticals in the world with over 200 published studies and abstracts, best known for its ability to increase blood flow to the head, can reduce inflammatory response. Take 2 capsules of the 50:1 extract or 4 "00" size capsules of the whole herb daily.

Coleus forskohlii is an Ayurvedic herb historically used for asthma (as well as allergies, inflammatory skin diseases, and heart problems; all of these uses have been upheld by extensive research in the last fifteen years on forskolin, a constituent of coleus). It's not a nervous-system stimulant, so it's free of the side effects associated with theophylline-based treatments. It activates an enzyme that sets off a series of biochemical reactions resulting in smooth-muscle relaxation. The dose is 50 milligrams of forskolin (the active ingredient) extract 2 to 3 times per day, or 4 to 8 capsules per day of the whole herb. (In traditional use, the whole herb is preferable, although thousands of studies using the extract of forskolin confirm the historical results.[4])

Chinese baical scullcap root has anti-inflammatory properties. According to Drs. Murray and Pizzorno in their *Encyclopedia of Natural Medicine,* the flavonoids in this herb can inhibit the formation of inflammatory compounds more than 1,000 times the strength of histamines, in a way that is similar to an asthma drug except without toxicity. They are also antioxidant and free-radical scavengers. Work up to 5 to 8 capsules per day as needed.

Nervines (central nervous system relaxants) can be useful for asthmatics. For at least some sufferers of this condition, there appears to be a stress or emotional element. (My husband has experienced two mild asthma attacks since his asthma cure seven years ago; both occurred during emotional upsets around animals.) Calming herbs such as **valerian** may help in stressful situations when the asthmatic may be more vulnerable to an attack. More of these are discussed on pages 304–309.

Finally, while supporting the lungs and adrenals, a general immune tonic should be used for steady long-term "feeding" of immune function. A mild, warming, energizing herb like **astragalus** can be a good choice; others to choose from are covered on pages 285–286.

Short-Term Asthma Relief

Short-term asthma remedies abound in the herb world as well, so that relief can be obtained naturally without the use of drugs.

The herb *khella* is available in the United States only in tincture form. This oil from the seeds of **Ammi visgana,** a member of the carrot family, has antispasmodic action on the small bronchi. This ancient Egyptian herb can be used long term with no toxicity, and the effect on the bronchi lasts about six hours, so it is particularly effective to prevent attacks. Khellin, the active principle, is rapidly absorbed through the mouth, so tincture (10 to 25 drops as needed for acute attacks) is effective.

Cranberry juice (unsweetened), *ma huang* (2 to 4 capsules or a few *sips*—not cups!—of strongly brewed tea), *white pine needle* tea, *horehound* tea, and *ginger* tea can all be very effective at the time of an attack. The caffeine in very strong coffee will work too, and black tea is traditionally used for its theophylline (the ingredient that is purified in many asthma prescription drugs).

Foods and Nutrients for Asthma

Another element of long-term asthma treatment is to include anti-inflammatory herbs and foods in the diet, since asthma involves inflammation of the bronchi and an inappropriate inflammatory reaction by the body to certain substances.

Supplementation with **essential fatty acids (EFAs)** helps by promoting synthesis of helpful prostaglandins instead of inflammatory ones that can cause mucus secretion and bronchial spasms. You can get these EFAs from flaxseed oil (1 tablespoon per day), or 1–2 capsules of evening primrose oil or the others discussed on page 142.

Onions and *garlic* are excellent anti-allergy herbs, especially for asthma. Onions contain quercetin, the bioflavonoid compound mentioned earlier, but both of these lily bulbs also inhibit an enzyme, lipoxygenase, which generates an inflammatory chemical, note Drs. Murray and Pizzorno in their *Encyclopedia of Natural Medicine*. They cite a study in which oral pretreatment of guinea pigs with an onion extract markedly reduced their asthmatic response to inhalant allergens. Onion has also been long noted in Ayurveda to have affinity for lung tissue.

Chilies are excellent food for allergies, especially asthma, both to prevent and treat an attack. In addition to being immune boosting long term, the capsaicin in chilies desensitizes airway mucosa. The effect is long lasting, so chilies can be used preventively; there is also clinical evidence that capsaicin can break an attack once it has started. Another benefit is chilies' ability to cause secretions that thin mucus.

Long-term consistent antioxidant vitamin intake, especially **vitamin C,** is important. Low dietary antioxidant intake is associated with increased asthma risk, according to a report from the Pulmonary Toxicology Branch of the U.S. Environmental Protection Agency. We have already recommended a diet high in antioxidant foods and the supplementation of certain key antioxidants for everyone, but for asthmatics vitamin C may be especially important. Vitamin C is the most prevalent antioxidant in lung secretions, and may protect against free-radical damage to lung cells. Vitamin C has also been used to prevent exercise-induced asthma, and as little as two grams has been shown to open airways and suppress histamine response in clinical situations.

Magnesium can relieve muscle spasms, including those in the smooth muscle of the bronchi. Dr. Melvin Werbach, M.D., says there is considerable evidence that asthmatics are frequently magnesium deficient[5] and a *Journal of the American Medical Association* study published in 1989, among others, showed significant improvement in subjects treated with magnesium as compared to a placebo, including a lower rate of hospital admission than for the placebo group.[6] A dose of 1,000 to 1,500 milligrams per day is usually helpful without exceeding bowel tolerance. Magnesium also reduces the histamine response (asthmatics typically show excessive histamine release, which leads to constriction of the bronchi). **Irish moss, licorice, oatstraw,** and **nettle** are magnesium-rich herbs.

Studies show that **vitamin B₆** supplementation decreases frequency and severity of asthma attacks, according to Donald J. Carrow, M.D., and Mitchell Chavez, C.N.[7]

General Lifestyle for Asthma

General good health habits are, of course, crucial if you hope to resolve asthma permanently. As with any condition, a favorable environment for healing must be created, both internally and externally. The basic healthy diet outlined on pages 107–117 should be observed generally. Any immune-weakening habits should be eliminated. If food allergies have been identified, those foods should be avoided temporarily while immune-building measures are taken.

Leukotrienes, those inflammatory substances we're already discussed, are made from the fatty acid arachidonic acid, found only in animal products. Leukotrienes are generally considered to be a thousand times more potent than histamine, a well-known cause of bronchial constriction. Meat in the diet may contribute to both allergies and asthma.

Cigarette smoking is absolute anathema to asthmatics. That means that asthmatic children, too, suffer greatly when their parents smoke. Many studies are revealing that both respiratory infection and asthma occur more frequently in children of smokers.

If you have asthma, you should feel confident that natural healing methods can support you in eliminating this disease from your life. I watched it happen myself, as my husband took on his asthma and won. Using some of the herbs described above, along with the immune-supportive strategies discussed earlier (immune-building herbs and foods, a noninflammatory vegetarian diet, healthy exercise), he eliminated his allergies and his asthmatic response to them within a year and a half. While at one time he was violently allergic to dogs, cats, and horses, we were eventually able to adopt a puppy and go to a training class two nights a week with nine other puppies—the ultimate test!—without problems.

Here's another story of someone who found a natural healing path away from asthma.

A Breath of Natural Healing: Jeff Pyatt

Jeff Pyatt, now thirty-six, was diagnosed with asthma at age five. It came and went as he got older. "I was constantly medicated," he remembers. "I took all the prescription drugs, including experimental ones, and got all the shots. I was hospitalized twice, at age eight and eleven. The second time, I was taking all kinds of medicine and was on a machine that pumped stuff into my lungs at night. Once after getting up following use of the machine, I blacked out and lost control of my bladder and bowels. It turned out the machine had overdosed me."

The asthma continued into college, when Jeff used inhalers and had frequent colds that "went to his chest" and created infections that made his asthma worse. Jeff enjoyed sports of all kinds, but found his activity curtailed due to his condition. He had to use an inhaler before exercise and took prednisone, a steroidal prescription drug, on and off, as well as theophylline-based prescription asthma drugs daily.

At twenty-three, Jeff moved to the Northwest. By now he had developed hay fever and allergies. He could not visit the home of anyone with a cat—the sneezing, wheezing, and watery eyes would drive him away immediately. A couple of years after that, his asthma took a sharp turn for the worse and he was put on prednisone again. This time, however, he did not respond. Instead, he says, "I got sicker and sicker."

Jeff was hospitalized and tests showed he had noninfectious hepatitis—liver damage. He was in the hospital for ten days and lost twenty pounds. Doctors thought he had an intestinal bacterial infection and gave him intravenous antibiotics. He still didn't get better.

"My sister is very wise," says Jeff. "She was there at my bedside and she said, 'Jeff, your body is trying to detoxify itself. The last thing you need is more drugs. Your liver is trying desperately to get rid of all the drugs you've already had.' And the doctor was on the other side of the bed saying, 'We need to put you on different antibiotics, because these aren't working.' I looked from one to the other, and I decided my sister was making more sense. That decision started a fundamental change in my life. I refused any more medication, and eventually my body healed itself, all by itself. My bilirubin is normal now; my liver is fine."

Once the crisis had passed, Jeff resolved to get more proactive about natural medicine for his asthma. He went to an acupuncturist and took classes with Karta Purkh, which fascinated him and inspired him to learn more. From what he learned, he was able to put together a program of botanicals to build up and heal his lung tissue, as well as support and strengthen his immune system.

"I haven't had a real asthma attack in over six years," says Jeff. "We've been house-hunting lately, and we went into one house and I could smell a cat and said, 'Oh, no, they have a cat!' But nothing happened! No wheezing, no watery eyes, nothing.

"I still use an inhaler about ten percent of the time. But I use coltsfoot tea regularly, and it really helps. I've learned that this is simply my weak spot, but I can control it easily now using natural means. My lungs are my barometer. I have a tendency to push too hard, do things to extremes.

Sometimes I try to do more than my body is capable of tolerating, and now I use my health as a measure of when I need to pull back. And I use herbs to keep me from getting sicker and sicker, as so many people today seem to be doing.

"I've really appreciated having access to this approach. It's helped in so many other ways. My father died of heart disease at forty-two, and a while back a test showed that my cholesterol, which has always been low, had jumped to 214, with the HDL down. The doctor said not to worry, but I had learned about the Ayurvedic herb guggul from Karta Purkh, and began to use that. When I saw my doctor again six months later, my total cholesterol was back down to one-fifty and my HDL was up. The doctor was amazed.

"And my daughter, now eight, has benefited from natural medicine. She seems to have the same weak lungs I do, and used to get such painful deep hacking coughs it would break your heart. We hated giving her cough medicine to help her go to sleep. With dietary changes, vitamins, bee pollen, and herbs, we've been able to get through whole winters without one cough, or with only a few very mild ones. I figure the less cough syrup, the better. So learning about all of these things has really impacted the whole family's life for the better.

"I believe Western medicine has its place, when extremely powerful medicine is needed quickly. But now I think, let's get beyond needing it."

17

Herbs for Arthritis

Rheumatoid arthritis (RA) and osteoarthritis (OA) are actually just two of over 100 forms of rheumatic diseases. These two are probably the most commonly known by name to the layperson, but even they are not necessarily distinct disease classifications—they may vary in cause and manifestation from individual to individual.

Still, these two well-known forms affect millions of people—and they can be dealt with effectively using natural medicine. These are conditions with which natural healing's power shines, because modern medicine has not offered much for these chronic diseases, yet herbal medicines work well without toxicity for many people.

In his newsletter *Self Healing*, Dr. Andrew Weil writes that he is disturbed by the long-term use of suppressive anti-inflammatory drugs to treat arthritis, noting that they not only don't cure the arthritis but may actually worsen the disease process by suppressing it. "Although these drugs sometimes bring relief," he says, "they can be very irritating to the stomach and can even cause fatal stomach hemorrhages. A significant number of such deaths occur each year, even among people who don't take heavy doses."[1] Many people with RA are treated with light doses of a cancer chemotherapy drug.

There are some factors that are common to both of these types of arthritis, and thus they share some common remedies. Blood cleansers (alteratives) are recommended in natural treatments for both kinds of arthritis, since accumulation of wastes and toxins can affect both. (See page 337 for a list of such herbs.) Oils are also recommended in both cases, for lubrication as well as "good" (noninflammatory) prostaglandin synthesis. Some of the same pain remedies provide relief for both kinds. And general immune support is important to the long-term resolution of any arthritis.

There are also differences that make the total treatment program for each distinct.

RHEUMATOID ARTHRITIS

From the Ayurvedic point of view, RA—also known as "inflammatory arthritis"—is a classic condition of *pitta* (fire) energy gone awry. It typically occurs in midlife, the most *pitta* phase of life. It is also more likely to occur in *pitta* constitutions—fire types. The primary motivation in RA treatment from this point of view is to control *pitta*, which is to control heat and inflammation.

RA is classified as an autoimmune disease. This means that the body is invoking an inflammatory response to its own tissue. In the case of RA, the body selectively attacks the soft tissue around the joints, especially of the hands and feet. This is very painful and results in disfiguration of the joints. They become hot, swollen, and red or purplish, as well as deformed.

No single cause of RA has been identified. There are a number of theories. Some health practitioners believe that at least in some cases, RA is one big food allergy, some people's way of expressing an overreaction to certain foods. The standard American diet definitely seems to be a factor; RA quite simply is not found in cultures that eat a plant-based diet without the fat, meat, sugar, and other refined foods found in ours.

There is also increasing evidence to support another theory, the "leaky gut syndrome," in which an abnormally permeable intestine allows large undigested food particles to be absorbed directly into the bloodstream rather than digested or eliminated. When the immune system is unexpectedly confronted with large molecules of undigested protein in the blood, it develops antibodies to their antigens (the protein "ID marks" on invaders). Those antibodies then simultaneously react to similar antigens in the tissues of and around the joints.

Suggested causes of leaky gut include weakening of the intestinal lining by penetration of candida (yeast) overgrowth, "bad" intestinal bacteria and their toxins, or—ironically—irritation from use of nonsteroidal anti-inflammatories (NSAIDs) such as ibuprofen and naproxen.

Other practitioners believe there is an emotional factor to at least some cases of RA. Dr. Weil notes, "There's a strong mind-body component to RA, and I'm discouraged with rheumatologists who act as if there isn't. The ups and downs of the disease often correlate with emotional ups and downs. I've seen the condition appear within 24 hours of an emotional trauma and disappear when people fall in love."[2]

It's important to note that all of these factors—and more—may be involved in the disease, and for some people there may be several cumulative factors that lead up to it. One person may in fact manifest RA after an emotional shock, while in another, RA may be the idiosyncratic way that individual manifests multiple food allergies.

The good news about RA is that, like many autoimmune diseases, it has in many cases been observed to go into remission in response to lifestyle—reduction in stress, changes in diet, and use of natural remedies. With consistency and dedication, it is possible to support your body into remission. Following are the most successful strategies.

The herbs used for RA are selected primarily either to cool and soothe inflammation or to cleanse the blood. The Ayurvedic herbs **boswellia** and **guggul** are related, and either is a good choice for RA as a blood cleanser and joint detoxification remedy. Guggul is the single most widely used herb for arthritis in all of Ayurveda. Six to 10 capsules per day is an appropriate dose to work up to; some people with severe cases have benefited from up to 15. Yogiraj guggul is a superior preparation of guggul.

Boswellia is marketed as a product called Boswellin, which is standardized for 150 milligrams of boswellic acids. Studies show that it improves blood supply to the joints and restores integrity to blood-vessel walls. It also appears to inhibit some leukotrienes (inflammatory messenger molecules). Boswellia can be taken in doses from 3 to 6 capsules per day.

Turmeric is another one of the most widely used herbs for arthritis in India, where it is commonly combined with ginger for OA. Turmeric is believed to have a general joint-rebuilding capability. It is used in rheumatoid arthritis and gout, both internally and as a pack on the joint.

The anti-inflammatory effects of curcumin, turmeric's extensively studied yellow compound, are well documented.[3] While typical anti-inflammatory drugs have grave side effects like ulcer formation and immune suppression, curcumin is exceedingly safe, with no known toxicity.[4]

Extremely high doses of turmeric, its alcohol extract, and pure curcumin do not produce undesired effects in any animal studied.

Curcumin has been shown to be as effective as or more effective than various steroid drugs to treat acute inflammation, without the toxicity and side effects.[5] Like capsaicin, the active ingredient in cayenne, curcumin also depletes substance P, a neurotransmitter of pain impulses, in the nerve endings. When used orally, curcumin has several direct anti-inflammatory effects: It inhibits leukotriene formation and platelet aggregation, promotes fibrinolysis (tissue regeneration), and stabilizes membranes.

As a polyphenol, curcumin is antioxidant, preventing cell and tissue destruction due to free-radical activity. It also potentiates adrenal hormone action, and supporting the adrenals is a good thing for RA because the adrenals produce anti-inflammatory hormones. (For this reason, an adrenal tonic is a good long-term herb to include in RA treatment: go back to pages 283–284 for a list of adrenal tonics.)

While curcumin has been the main focus of study on turmeric, it is unlikely that curcumin accounts for the totality of the broad-spectrum action of the herb. Subjectively, most herbalists say that they have seen better results with the whole herb than with curcumin alone for a wide variety of conditions. This has definitely been Karta Purkh's experience, and he strongly recommends using turmeric in its whole form.

Turmeric is a relatively mild herb, pound for pound. The dose for acute conditions typically would be about 1 ounce per day, or the equivalent of about 50 capsules. Since this obviously is not practical, powder is the best form. Four level teaspoons of powder is about 1 ounce. For RA, 2 tablespoons of paste should be used daily, working up to more if possible (see recipe on page 497).

Ginger can work for RA (though it is more commonly used for OA). It is a bit of a conundrum in its use for RA from the Ayurvedic point of view. Normally ginger would not be used with an inflammatory illness because ginger is pungent and warming, and increases *pitta* (fire); thus it provokes inflammation if used in large amounts for too long.

However, ginger is a well-established anti-inflammatory and can be effective if used carefully. There is much to recommend it for RA despite its warming properties. Ginger is known to block formation of inflammatory hormonal messengers—prostaglandins, leukotrienes, thromboxanes, and other "bad guys"—and to break down acids in synovial fluid (the cushioning fluid surrounding joints). Some cases of rheumatoid arthritis have reportedly gone into complete remission from eating extremely high quantities of fresh ginger in food daily, according to Jean Carper in *Food: Your Miracle Medicine.* Carper also reports that Dr. Krishna C. Srivastava of Odense University in Denmark has seen many patients cured of RA by the use of ginger.

Michael T. Murray, N.D., writes in *Health Counselor* that "in one clinical study, seven patients with rheumatoid arthritis, in whom conventional drugs had provided only temporary or partial relief, were treated with ginger. One patient took 50 grams daily of lightly cooked ginger; the remaining six took either 5 grams of fresh ginger or 0.1 to 1 gram of powdered ginger daily. All patients reported substantial improvement, including pain relief, joint mobility, and decrease in swelling and morning stiffness."[6]

Ginger also improves circulation, especially to joints, which is important for treating any joint condition because these areas of our body are not fed directly by the cardiovascular system. Without a blood supply of their own, joints must rely on surrounding tissues for nutrients and oxygen. Unfortunately, this means they heal more slowly than tissues fed directly by the blood. The more fresh blood you can bring into the area surrounding joints, the more healing benefits you'll bring to the joint. Start with 1 or 2 capsules per day and work up to 6 or 7 if results are good.

Chinese wild ginger (asarum) is also good for pain and inflammation; up to 10 capsules a day is appropriate.

Cinnamon is another herb that increases circulation to joints, but again, because of its pungency, it must be used with caution in RA. Start with 1 or 2 capsules and work up to 6 to 8 if necessary to achieve relief.

Buckbean is the leading European arthritis herb and works well for RA. It can be taken as a tea, up to 1 ounce of herb per day.

Chinese baical scullcap root is anti-inflammatory and antioxidant due to its powerful flavonoid compounds, and is liver supportive and cleansing as well. It is an especially good choice for RA because it is not warming. It can be taken in capsules, 5 to 10 per day.

Mexican wild yam has mild steroidlike properties (some steroid drugs were synthesized from its compound diosgenin). Mexican wild yam is anti-inflammatory and can be taken in capsules (3 to 4 per day).

Gotu kola is an Ayurvedic herb that enhances tissue regeneration—particularly connective tissue—and tissue healing generally. Up to 1 ounce of the dry herb daily can be brewed into tea, or 5 to 10 capsules a day may be taken.

Another Ayurvedic herb, *ashwaganda,* is primarily used in Indian culture as a men's tonic and is also used in both men and women for a long-term anti-anxiety effect. However, this herb also has anti-inflammatory and anti-arthritis properties. According to Ayurvedic doctor Virender Sodhi, M.D., ashwaganda's high steroid content produces more potent action than hydrocortisone in rats and also produces results comparable to the effects of the drugs phenylbutazone and aspirin (without the immuno-suppression and intestinal irritation). Sodhi notes that many of his patients have been able to eliminate all arthritic drugs completely ("weaning" slowly is advised, over two to three months) and are showing improvement on ashwaganda complemented by other herbs after not having taken drugs for many years.[7]

Devil's claw is a South African root that has a long history of success with joint pain and arthritis, although scientific studies have produced mixed results regarding its ability to reduce inflammation. (As usual, the whole herb is superior; the purified active constituent alone is not anti-inflammatory.) Clinically this herb does provide pain relief to many patients. The dose for capsules is 2 to 10 per day.

Sarsaparilla root from Mexico, India, China and Central America, once used to flavor root beer, is believed to stimulate adrenal anti-inflammatory hormone. The root beer taste makes it a decent tea. For arthritis relief, take up to 1 ounce of herb as tea daily.

Other herbs for RA include:

> *Black walnut leaf* for acute flare-ups (5 to 10 capsules)
> *St. John's wort leaf* for pain and long-term anti-inflammatory action (up to 10 capsules per day)
> *Chinese fang feng root* for long-term anti-inflammatory action (5 to 10 capsules per day)
> *Nettle leaf* for long-term anti-inflammatory action and blood cleansing (1 ounce as tea per day)
> *Yucca root* for joint detoxification and anti-inflammatory action (up to 10 capsules per day)

There are also nonherb supplements that are useful for many RA patients:

Bromelain, an enzyme found in pineapple, is a natural anti-inflammatory agent, with more than 200 studies documenting its effectiveness in this regard. It can be obtained in capsules or tablets, usually 500 milligrams; start with 3 per day and work up until you get relief.

Bioflavonoids are anti-inflammatory (they inhibit leukotrienes, as well as histamine, as discussed in Chapter 17, "Herbs for Allergies") and can be taken in a mixed bioflavonoid formula, as well as *hawthorn berry* or *bilberry* extracts. Eating more *berries* and *cherries* would help, too.

Vitamin E should be taken at 1,000 IU daily because it is antioxidant, anti-inflammatory, and lubricating, and may actually help stimulate repair and synthesis of tissue. *Antioxidants* are crucial to RA because most of the actual damage is the result of the action of free radicals, as well as that of inflammatory prostaglandins and leukotrienes.

Selenium should also be taken since it potentiates vitamin E, and even by itself is an excellent antioxidant. According to Drs. Murray and Pizzorno in *Encyclopedia of Natural Medicine,* it is also a cofactor for an enzyme that inhibits inflammatory prostaglandin and leukotriene production. That makes it especially significant that RA patients frequently have low levels of this mineral.

Flaxseed oil is often recommended as a good quality source of "good" fatty acids for production of anti-inflammatory hormonal messengers. Take 1 to 2 tablespoons per day, or buy light-protected refrigerated capsules and take 4 to 6 per day.

Parsley is cooling and detoxifying, and should be juiced. Drink as much as possible throughout the day.

Treating the Pain of RA

While working long term to resolve RA, many people want natural pain relief in the interim. This can be provided by the herb *meadowsweet* (1/2 ounce to 1 ounce as tea daily), *white willow bark* (same dose), or supplements of the *dl-form of phenylalanine* (also known as DLPA). The extract of the herb *feverfew,* standardized to contain .125 percent parthenolides (the active ingredient), can also work over time. Feverfew has a long folk history of use for headaches (especially migraines) as well as arthritis, and modern research is showing that it relieves pain by actually reducing inflammation, not merely as an analgesic. Studies show that feverfew can inhibit the synthesis of inflammatory compounds.

Chinese corydalis tuber and *Chinese notopterygii root* are both used for muscular aches and pains. Chinese notopterygii root is good for hot, swollen joints, so it's perfect for RA. Corydalis can be taken up to 1/2 ounce as tea per day; notopterygii is taken in capsules, 1 to 15 per day.

Tienchi root, another Chinese remedy, circulates blood to joints to relieve pain and reduces swelling; 1 to 15 capsules per day. *Chinese mimosa bark* is a mild herb for joint pain and swelling; 5 to 10 capsules per day.

Keep in mind that these herbs will not provide instant and total pain relief upon the first capsule or sip of tea, but they will help keep the pain in check over time and will last longer once they go into effect. Most of all, they are not immunosuppressive or toxic, like many of the drugs used to do the same job.

Avoid aspirin, ibuprofen, and acetaminophen. While nonsteroidal anti-inflammatory drugs (NSAIDs) are commonly used with arthritis, many natural health practitioners frown on their use because the short-term gain comes at the expense of long-term healing. One of the reasons aspirin (and the stronger steroid drugs) used long term may make RA worse is because they lower levels of PGE1, an anti-inflammatory prostaglandin that helps collagen formation and is helpful in RA and other autoimmune diseases.

Topicals for pain that many people have found effective include *cayenne oil, ginger oil, mustard oil,* and *castor oil. St. John's wort* oil or ointment is a very typical European treatment for trauma and joint pain. You should experiment with small amounts and see which works best for you; the response is very individual and idiosyncratic, but once someone finds the topical that works for him or her, it can be very effective in providing relief.

Diet for RA

The ideal diet for long-term healing of RA should be as close to vegetarian as possible. A number of studies have shown significant relief for patients following a strict vegetarian diet.

In a Norwegian study on patients with rheumatoid arthritis, the subjects who fasted, then followed a vegan, gluten-free (gluten is found in wheat) diet experienced significant improvement in pain, number of tender and swollen joints, and duration of morning stiffness. The benefits were still present after a year, even when subjects carefully reintroduced wheat and dairy products.[8]

The Arthritis Foundation's vice president for public education says this diet cannot be recommended "yet" because (what else?) "more research is needed."[9] In the meantime, we *do* recommend it. It worked not only on these twenty-seven subjects, but also in other studies that corroborate these findings. It will not harm you to eat a vegan diet—there are dozens of other benefits anyway—so withholding such valuable information until the study can be replicated some indefinite number of times does not seem prudent.

At a minimum, the following should be eliminated: meat; corn, safflower, sunflower, and cottonseed oils; all dairy products; and sugar. The following would preferably be cut, but at least minimized as much as possible: corn, wheat, oranges, eggs, coffee, peanuts, and tomatoes. Foods with artificial colors, additives, preservatives, and chemicals should also be eliminated (this rules out most processed food).

One of the problems with meat and dairy products is that they are a source of a fatty acid called arachidonic acid, which is known to convert to inflammatory prostaglandins and leukotrienes, the chemical-messenger molecules that are responsible for much of the tissue damage seen in RA. Animal proteins are also suspect in RA following the theory about leaky gut syndrome: The body reacts to animal proteins mistakenly allowed into the blood, and then finds similar antigenic sites on the tissue that surrounds joints. (Plant proteins do not have the similarity to body proteins that would allow the immune system to get confused in this way.) These are both strong reasons for the RA patient to eat a vegan diet.

Foods with *essential fatty acids, monounsaturates,* and *omega-3 fats* are good to include in the diet—olive oil, flaxseed oil, and cold-weather fish (like salmon, sardines, and herring) are excellent sources. Hundreds of studies have shown that additional supplementation with these fats provide RA relief.[10] A study in the *Annals of Internal Medicine* reported that the essential fatty acid gamma linoleic acid (GLA) from borage reduced the number of tender joints in participants by 36 percent. It not only controlled pain, but also inflammation of the joint lining.[11] Evening primrose is another GLA source that has been extensively studied with RA subjects, and black currant seed oil is yet another source that is available in capsules.

As well as the bioflavonoid fruits mentioned earlier above, **green vegetables** are cooling and anti-inflammatory, and should be emphasized daily in the diet. Juicing them (**parsley** and **cucumber** are especially good, and **celery** has the added benefit of being relaxing) is a practical way to get more of them down.

OSTEOARTHRITIS

From the Ayurvedic perspective, osteoarthritis or OA—the cold, stiff "crunchy and crackly," dry kind of arthritis, also sometimes called "degenerative arthritis" (it involves increasing cartilage destruction)—is a classic *vata* condition. *Vata* people are most vulnerable to it, and it occurs for most people in the last third of life, the *vata* stage (80 percent of people over fifty have OA). The therapeutic protocol in Ayurveda is to warm up and lubricate the joints, and to control or decrease *vata* (dry, cold) energy.

Osteoarthritis has been called "wear and tear" arthritis and has long been assumed to be an inevitable function of aging, but more recent studies show now that it's more likely due to the body's failure to rebuild and regenerate joints as it can and should. Such failure is probably due to overall depletion of nutrients, depressed general functioning, and/or a high degree of toxicity—yet another part of the "chronic subclinical everything syndrome," a phrase that Dr. Alan Gaby has coined. One recent British study suggests just that: a failure of the body's normal healing mechanism to repair joint damage.[12]

As Thomas Dorman, M.D., wrote in the *Townsend Letter for Doctors*, December 1995, "If osteoarthritis was truly a necessary part of aging, why would it affect joints so irregularly? When the shingles on your roof age they do so evenly." The collagen matrix of cartilage can be stressed by traumatic injury, obesity, and chronic lack of use as well as overuse, but the body should not necessarily lose its ability to synthesize normal collagen structures.

If OA is indeed a disease reflecting a lifestyle-induced decline in self-healing ability, that may be why natural remedies are so effective for osteoarthritis. By working on the whole body, such remedies may help restore the body's repair functions generally. Improved joint repair would be one of many possible benefits.

OA responds extremely well to several common herbs. Karta Purkh has observed many people with OA achieve enormous success with natural healing, enabling them to return to a more active and pain-free life without drugs.

Turmeric is as effective for OA as it is for RA—one of the remedies shared by the two types. With OA, it is not turmeric's anti-inflammatory properties that are needed so much as the joint-rebuilding characteristics of the herb. The dose is similar: as much of the whole powder (or paste from powder) as you can consume on a daily basis, up to 1 ounce (4 level teaspoons). For the paste recipe, see page 497.

I can personally relate a story that attests to the joint-healing power of turmeric. On a bike trip in 1995, I developed severe knee pain by the end of the very first day. Joint pain is something I'd simply never experienced (it's not generally a fire-type problem and I'm not exactly of typical OA age). But the first day of this trip was particularly challenging—seventy miles with a mountain pass smack in the middle—and I was pushing two hundred pounds (including me, bike, and gear). The second day was no better, and by the time we arrived at our destination on the third evening (after another seventy-five-miler), I was limping and seriously concerned about my ability to finish the trip.

My husband had packed for himself a full container of turmeric paste, which we kept in a small cooler. He takes this daily year round to maintain his own joints preventively (he is *vata*/air type, so this is a potential problem area for him). Indeed, although he is twelve years older than I and was carrying fifty more pounds of gear, in addition to his greater *vata* tendencies, he had not experienced so much as a twinge in any joint yet. He urged me to try some turmeric.

I'm more of a capsule or occasional tea person myself, and tend to avoid messy, bad-tasting preparations. I really did not want to eat the bright yellow paste. However, in pain and with the trip in jeopardy, I agreed to try it. Reluctantly I rolled a ball of paste about the size of a marble onto the back of my tongue and swallowed it with water. I repeated this with a second "marble." Crazy as it sounds, silently I hoped it wouldn't work—then I wouldn't have to keep eating the stuff.

My wishing did not make it so. The next morning, when I woke, the pain was gone. Not just better, but gone. One hundred percent. Despite the many wonderful results I have seen with herbs, both for myself and others, I was freshly amazed at how powerful a medicine a simple kitchen spice could be (I had not even taken a very large amount, and had expected results in several days, if at all). I grudgingly continued to use the paste throughout the trip, which was completed successfully and without any further soreness in my knees whatsoever.

For our next trip—which featured even longer daily mileage and steeper mountain passes—I started the turmeric in advance and took it throughout the trip, which was pain free and wonderful. Turmeric paste is now a "bike touring protocol" for me. And, oddly enough, it doesn't taste that bad anymore!

Ginger and **cinnamon** are excellent remedies for OA because, as mentioned above, they increase circulation to the joints and are warming. OA patients can take it in higher amounts than those with RA—up to 15 capsules per day—because the joints are cold and stiff, not hot and inflamed. **Clove** and **allspice** are acceptable substitutes in similar doses—also hot and pungent. Work up to 10 to 12 capsules per day (less if you get relief at a smaller dose).

Cayenne can also work well, both internally and externally. Start very slowly with internal use, about half a capsule, and work up to comfort and tolerance. **Chinese morinda root** is a sweet, warming tonic that warms cold, stiff joints at up to 10 to 15 capsules per day.

In conventional medicine, there is much disbelief about the possibility of repairing damaged connective tissue and reversing the course of arthritis. However, new research is showing that this *is* possible. The most promising experience yet has been with a substance called **glucosamine sulfate**, which is proving to be one of the most outstanding remedies for osteoarthritis. It has been shown to be extremely effective in both humans and animals, and is extremely desirable because it provides relief by actually helping the body to heal and rebuild joints, not just suppressing the pain.

Glucosamines are basic building blocks of connective tissue (like tendons, ligaments, and cartilage). If the body is starved for them, it cannot repair connective tissue or joint damage. Unrepaired damage means weakened, degenerated tissue, the so-called wear and tear of OA.

Supplementing with glucosamine gives the body the "food" it needs to make new connective tissue and synovial fluid. Studies have shown that anti-inflammatory drugs provide more pain relief than glucosamine supplements initially, but that after five or six weeks those patients on glucosamine begin experiencing more pain relief while those on the drugs experience a rebound effect of pain and inflammation. It's believed that glucosamine's pain relief initially takes longer because relief is due to actual decrease of inflammation, as opposed to a masking of the pain, which only returns with a vengeance when you have suppressed it.

Glucosamine sulfate comes in 500-milligram capsules and can be taken up to 3,000 milligrams per day. Response time may be 4 to 6 weeks. Once you experience relief, halve the dose for maintenance. Taper off and see at which dose symptoms reappear, then return to the next highest dose.

Pipali, an Ayurvedic herb, does four things that help OA: warms, moistens, builds, and cleanses the blood. Up to 10 capsules a day may be taken.

Other useful herbs for OA, some of them already mentioned for RA, include:

Boswellia, as discussed earlier (5 to 10 capsules per day)
Alfalfa for moistening and blood cleansing (10 to 20 capsules per day)
Horsetail for calcium balance and silicon (1/2 ounce as tea or 10 capsules per day)
Buckbean leaf, as discussed (1 ounce as tea per day)
Eucalyptus oil externally for pain relief, as needed

Flavonoids are, again, indicated here as potent antioxidants that have been shown to help preserve and enhance the integrity of cartilage. Anthocyanidins and proanthocyanidins are the flavonoids that give **berries** and **cherries** their deep blue or red colors. Eat plenty of these fruits, as often as possible. Supplements that would provide these compounds include **bilberry** and **hawthorn berry**. There are also mixed bioflavonoid supplements.

Vitamin E, at about 1,000 IU daily, can help stabilize membranes, reduce free-radical damage, and, according to some studies, actually promote cartilage synthesis and inhibit enzymes that break down cartilage, say Drs. Murray and Pizzorno in their *Encyclopedia of Natural Healing*.

Pain Relief of OA

The same pain relievers recommended earlier for RA will work for short-term relief in OA: *meadowsweet, white willow bark, dl-phenylalanine, feverfew, devil's claw,* and *Chinese corydalis tuber* in the same doses recommended earlier. The topicals mentioned previously may also be useful; cayenne ointment applied externally appears to be especially beneficial for the pain of osteoarthritis.

Again, avoid NSAIDs. In addition to their side effects, they actually hinder the healing process. Aspirin is known to block regeneration of cartilage, and some studies show that it actually accelerates cartilage destruction[13]—a classic example of how symptom suppression actually worsens the disease.

Drs. Murray and Pizzorno, in their *Encyclopedia of Natural Healing,* note an interesting study that attempted to determine the "natural course" of OA. Even though all the subjects had established, advanced OA of the hip, the researcher reported marked clinical improvement in half of them over a ten-year period. (No therapy was applied to these subjects; the express purpose was to ascertain the course without therapy.) Drs. Murray and Pizzorno point out that this outcome is far better than that produced by most medical therapy for OA and suggest that it is important to ask, "Does medical intervention in some way promote disease progression?" It appears that it can.

Diet for OA

Diet has not been specifically implicated in OA in the same way that it has in RA—that is, through food allergies, leaky gut syndrome, and so on. However, insofar as a poor diet decreases overall health and functioning, a diet filled with too many "minuses" and not enough "pluses" could certainly lead to the body's decreasing ability to repair joints (or anything else) over time. We suggest at minimum following the healthy diet recommendations on pages 107–117.

Warming, lubricating foods are good to include in the diet: these include all the warming kitchen spices. Healthy, quality oils should be used, as discussed earlier, such as olive and flaxseed oils. Quality oils considered in Ayurveda to have warming properties include sesame and almond oils. Obesity can increase genuine wear and tear on joints, so staying lean is important too.

In the early 1980s, the Arthritis Foundation published a statement that "the possible relationship between diet and arthritis has been thoroughly and scientifically studied. The simple proven fact is: No food has anything to do with causing arthritis and no food is effective in treating or 'curing' it." Today, Arthritis Foundation literature sings a different tune, acknowledging that "diet may change the way the immune system reacts in certain kinds of arthritis that involve inflammation. Researchers also are investigating the effects of food allergies and reactions; fasting, low calorie or low fat diets; and fatty acids such as fish oils on rheumatoid arthritis."[14] In addition to providing hope for a nutritionally based remission or cure for arthritis, this is a classic reminder of how science is a moving target, and that today's convictions may be overturned tomorrow.

18

Herbs for Yeast (Candida)

Mary had a vaginal infection, like clockwork, four times a year. She was thirty years old and had been having them every season for fifteen years. Each and every time she used a topical yeast drug, and the painful symptoms would disappear gradually over a few days, only to reappear in two or three months. Why, Mary wondered, could she not stop these miserable infections once and for all? No one could tell her.

Concerned about using drugs so consistently, Mary sought out an herbalist. While overnight results are rare in herbal medicine, Mary was lucky. After a thorough evaluation, the herbalist recommended a high oral dose of grapefruit seed extract. Mary's symptoms were gone by morning. Suitably impressed, Mary wondered if there were following treatments that could actually prevent her infections. Of course, this is what herbal medicine does best.

Mary immediately embarked on an herbal program to support her immune system to resist the yeast. Today, two years later, she has still not had a single day of yeast infection.

Yeast is a naturally occurring microbe to which we have accommodated over the centuries. When our immune systems are functioning well, yeast growth is kept under control. Only recent changes in lifestyle and diet have resulted in this growing problem in an increasingly immune-compromised society.

Candida occurs naturally in the mucous membranes of the gastrointestinal and genitourinary tracts, as well as on the skin. Ninety-five percent of us have yeast growing in our bodies by six months of age. Candida shares the intestines with billions of bacteria, most of which are lactobacillus types, which perform many necessary functions, including producing vitamins and lowering cholesterol. Yeast competes for space and food with these "good" bugs. If we have enough healthy intestinal flora, yeast is kept under control.

The fungus *Candida albicans*, the most common of over eighty types of yeast, is the culprit in minor conditions such as vaginitis and skin rash. In extreme cases, in people with damaged immune systems, yeast can enter the bloodstream and be fatal. There is growing awareness that a syndrome caused by the overgrowth of the common yeast, largely overlooked by the medical profession, is often the cause of a long and complicated list of symptoms in people who are chronically unwell. Candida-related complex, or polysystemic candidiasis, as this condition is known, is primarily a women's problem, but men and children are also at risk.

Systemic yeast infection represents the underlying problem of a depleted immune system. To conquer yeast syndrome, you have to support the immune system very powerfully.

In 1978, C. Orion Truss, M.D., of Birmingham, Alabama, gave the first report of a yeast-connected illness. Dr. Truss had discovered the condition ten years earlier while treating a patient for a vaginal yeast infection. When her yeast cleared up, her migraine headaches and depression disappeared. Dr. Truss's work became popular with the release in 1983 of *The Yeast Connection*, by his colleague, William G. Crook, M.D.

WHEN CANDIDA GAINS CONTROL

Candidiasis typically progresses very systematically. We can categorize these symptoms in four ways.

1. *First, imbalances begin in the digestive tract.* As the candida gains a foothold and begins to dominate the intestinal environment, people develop characteristic symptoms such as heartburn, gas, bloating, anal itching, vaginitis, fatigue, and allergy, especially to foods. As body defenses weaken, candida and other fungi can infect other body areas. People may suffer athlete's foot, jock itch, and skin and nail infections.

Once the yeast has developed in the large intestine and replaced the beneficial bacterial that should live there, it can be quite difficult to destroy, as it reproduces quickly and invades the tissue deeply. Yeast is hardier than bacteria in this way—it puts out threads that snake through cells, and the threads don't die like the fruiting body. Although yeast can't invade the tissue directly the way bacteria and viruses can, yeast, like other fungi, produces rootlike structures ("rhizoids"), which penetrate the lining of the gut.

This damage provides a site for incompletely digested dietary proteins to enter the bloodstream (sometimes called "leaky gut syndrome"). The body sees these proteins as invaders, and responds by developing an allergic reaction to the food. Candida sufferers are often plagued by multiple food sensitivities or allergies, which creates a vicious circle of immune suppression that creates further candida and allergy.

2. *Yeast cells attach themselves to mucous membrane surfaces, form a colony, and transform into a fuzzy "mycelium" (think mold on bread).* As their roots penetrate the tissues, searching for nutrients, the yeast begins to produce toxins that damage tissue and cause inflammation. Any tissue that has been colonized by yeast will be plagued with symptoms, be it vaginitis, diarrhea, heartburn, or thrush (yeast in the mouth). They may also show up in the sinuses, ears, and eyes.

As the toxic by-products circulate through the bloodstream, they can trigger symptoms in distant parts of the body. This tissue insult can result in conditions as diverse as asthma, sinusitis, lupus, PMS, and kidney stones, according to Dr. Ralph Golan in *Optimal Wellness*. Specific symptoms will depend on which organ has been damaged by the toxins. For example, damage to the brain may cause fuzzy thinking, while skin damage will cause itching and rashes.

As the immune system becomes damaged, the body becomes hypersensitive not only to foods, but also to otherwise benign levels of common chemicals, such as gas fumes, perfume, and pesticides. The yeast-damaged body becomes so overwhelmed that it can produce antibodies to its own tissues, resulting in autoimmune disease.

As the sufferer becomes more allergic and chemically sensitive, in addition to classic allergic symptoms like hives and hay fever, he or she can develop myriad reactions including, but not limited to, headache, joint pain, and nausea.

3. *The central nervous system becomes involved, and mental symptoms begin.* Dr. William Crook feels that these are the definitive candida symp-

toms. He includes headache, irritability, confusion, feeling "spaced out," and lethargy.

4. *The body develops symptoms of organ and hormone dysfunction.* The most common of these is hypothyroidism, followed by adrenal failure, but any organ can be involved. In children, the symptoms usually start with chronic ear infection and colic.

All of this translates into chronic lack of energy. After all, the body is full of an alien invader that is stealing its fuel while forcing the body to fight a protracted battle against it.

CAUSES OF YEAST INFECTIONS

Healthy people do not get yeast infections. Candida is a naturally occurring microbe to which we have accommodated over the centuries; yeast is a benign passenger in our bodies unless some balance gets upset. Only recent changes in lifestyle and diet have resulted in the current problem. All the factors known to aggravate yeast overgrowth are consequences of modern living.

Yeast overgrows for two reasons— something feeds it, or something suppresses the immune system, rendering it incapable of controlling the yeast (or both). Anything that promotes yeast growth, or suppresses lactobacillus populations, will lead to an imbalance and trigger a yeast-related disease.

Antibiotics are thought to be the single greatest contributor to candida. True, antibiotics kill unwanted bacteria, such as those that cause acne in teenagers, but they also nonselectively kill the good bacteria in the digestive tract and vagina, allowing *Candida albicans* (which is resistant to antibiotics) to flourish. It is common knowledge that women often develop vaginal yeast infections after using antibiotics.

Often people trace the first onset of candidiasis to a potent course of antibiotics, sometimes years earlier. The proper colony of beneficial bacteria is never restored without treatment. When yeast is overgrown and entrenched in the mycelial stage, the good bacteria are overwhelmed and can never re-colonize the gut.

In addition to the antibiotics we take as drugs, nearly three-fourths of the antibiotics produced in the United States are sold for agricultural use and are fed to animals. Unless labeled as chemical free, commercial meat and milk contain antibiotics. This adds to the "total load" of antibiotics consumed, and influences the balance of intestinal flora.

Yeast loves sugar. Recall that other types of yeast are used to ferment sugar in bread and beer. Simple white sugar, especially, is perfect yeast food. To make matters worse, as you have learned, white sugar also suppresses the immune response. All carbohydrates feed yeast to a certain extent, and can contribute to episodes of symptoms.

Women are more at risk for yeast syndrome, at least during their fertile years. Progesterone, produced in abundance before menstruation, favors yeast. Many women find that their yeast symptoms increase premenstrually. This hormone is also contained in oral contraceptives, which provoke yeast. When all other factors are balanced, this should not be significant, but when candida is out of control, it can be a complicating factor.

During pregnancy, women have higher blood sugar *and* higher levels of progesterone. What could be better for yeast? Some women can trace the onset of yeast symptoms to their first pregnancy. Finally, of course, women have a vagina—one more dark, moist, warm cavity for yeast to call home.

Many other circumstances favor yeast development. Incomplete digestion of carbohydrates brings food to the yeast in the large intestine. Numerous drugs, especially cortisone, encourage yeast, as does exposure to damaging amounts of environmental chemicals, such as pesticides. Allergy, glandular disorders from any source, diabetes, and trauma such as surgery contribute as well.

Yeast disorder will rarely be caused by one of these factors alone. Once yeast has gotten hold, you must address each of the building blocks that contributed to your candida problem. Fortunately, natural healing practitioners have developed powerful, effective therapies that are successful in rooting out this pest by bringing the body into balance without the use of drugs.

REGAINING CONTROL

Candida is controlled with a multidisciplinary approach aimed toward normalizing and strengthening immune function, killing yeast in the digestive tract (or other areas it has colonized), replacing beneficial flora in the intestines, and improving the nutritional status of the body as a whole.

Diet

Step one is diet. The basis of a therapeutic yeast diet is eating whole foods that nourish you, but not the yeast. You knew we were going to say it: no sugar. Yeast feeds on sugar (alcohol behaves like sugar in the body) and a high-sugar diet literally provides a large yeast overgrowth with ongoing sustenance—as it simultaneously suppresses your immune response.

The less simple carbohydrates (replaced by more complex carbohydrates) the better. Most people need to eliminate some or all fruit temporarily, and a few don't even tolerate high-starch vegetables like potatoes. The individual must "test" each of these foods to see how his or her particular case responds.

Essentially, the diet that starves yeast while supporting the immune system includes:

- Avoiding sweets and refined flours
- Adequate protein
- Large amounts of fresh vegetables
- Complex carbohydrates as appropriate to the case
- Moderate fat (monounsaturated)
- Fruit only as tolerated, generally in very small amounts
- Avoidance of all allergic foods
- Avoidance of mold-containing foods if sensitive

Food cravings can be a big problem on this diet. When full of yeast, people feel a tremendous physiological pressure to feed it with sugar. Also, as we have discussed, people with food allergies are often addicted to the food, and will have a classic withdrawal craving when it is removed. This can last up to several months, sometimes misleading the person to believe that the removal of the foods is "the wrong direction" because they initially feel worse. Patience is required as you work to rid the body of both yeast and allergies that drive you to provide them with sustenance.

Supplements for Yeast

Many natural medicines work well to control yeast. One of the most important is "friendly flora," the lactobacilli that belong in the gut.

Because the yeast has colonized the membranes of the intestines, large doses of L. *acidophilus* are necessary to overpower the candida and replace its colonies. Use high-potency powdered acidophilus from the refrigerator case. A typical regime would be 2 tablespoons per day for 2 weeks.

Capsules of live yogurt bacteria—lactobacillus, bifidobacteria, S. *thermophillus*—will also allow these "good germs" to multiply in the digestive tract, and replace and consume the yeast in the intestines.

In addition, you can use:

Caprylic acid—work up to 6,000 milligrams per day

Biotin—5 milligrams per day

Anti-Yeast Herbs

Many herbs act as antifungals. These may either kill yeast directly or control yeast over time by supporting the immune response—or both.

Herbs that contain **berberine** fall into both categories. Berberine both kills yeast and activates macrophages (immune system white cells). It also kills bacteria, and is effective in reducing microbial overgrowth of all types from the intestines, thus inhibiting the leaky gut syndrome. Berberine also enhances digestive secretions, which is always valuable in candidiasis.

Herbs that contain berberine include **barberry root (Berberis vulgaris**, from which comes the term *berberine*), **Oregon grape root (Berberis aquifolium), goldenseal root (Hydrastis canadensis),** and **Chinese amur cork tree bark (Phellodendron chinense)**. Barberry and Oregon grape are also liver herbs, while goldenseal supports mucous membranes.

Grapefruit seed extract (GSE) is a very effective yeast killer. Now widely available, it kills a wide variety of microbes, and is nontoxic. Often an initial large oral dose (3–5 teaspoons in a quart of liquid or squeezed into capsules) will kill a vaginal yeast infection overnight. (Note: take GSE with plenty of water and follow with food to avoid queasiness or burning sensation.)

This extract kills yeast and fungus quite effectively when applied topically, so it can be used as a gargle, a douche, a suppository, or topically for athlete's foot. (Some very effective natural skin sprays contain grapefruit seed extract and **tea tree oil,** another antifungal that is for external use.) As a vaginal suppository you may want to dilute GSE. Some people find the extract irritating to membranes and sensitive tissues.

Echinacea root stimulates white cell activity, and can work well in the first stages of treatment to kill the yeast. This herb is expensive, and there are serious quality considerations as discussed earlier, so it is important to shop for a powerful preparation. The recommended dose is 5 to 15 capsules per day.

Garlic is a widely recommended antiyeast herb. Several components of garlic are known antifungals, and garlic also has a long history as an immune support herb generally. Garlic doses can be quite high; the higher the better, except for extreme *pitta* types and people taking blood-thinning drugs. The quality of garlic preparations varies widely, so choose a proven form, such as aged extract or freeze-dried types.

Deodorized garlic capsules, alone or combined with berberine or a berberine herb, work well as vaginal suppositories for yeast infections. Leave the capsule in overnight—it will be dissolved in the morning.

Pau d'arco bark is a standard for yeast control through immune support. This South American herb has a broad spectrum of antimicrobial activity, and is a slow but sure way to enhance immune response over time. This herb is expensive, so tea is more suitable. Typically, the dose would be 1/2 to 1 ounce, dry herb weight, per day.

Celandine is perhaps the perfect herb for yeast problems. Classically, celandine is a well-respected liver herb, which by itself is important in candida treatment for the elimination of wastes (dead yeast along with the toxins they produce). Since celandine is not yet trendy or well known for this use, it is very reasonably priced, yet widely available. We recommend up to 10 capsules per day.

Astragalus as we have discussed, is a Chinese herb known to powerfully support the immune system over time. This herb is mild, well tolerated, and tastes good, so it is practical to use as a tea. As an immune tonic, astragalus works slowly, and should be taken for 3 months to 1 year for full effect. The dose is 1/2 to 1 ounce, dry herb weight, as tea, per day.

Ginseng kills yeast, and acts as a general stamina and immune tonic (3 to 5 capsules daily).

Eleuthero is a general tonic herb that supports the immune system long term, and is used by many herbalists to treat yeast (10 capsules daily).

Holy basil, or "tulsi," is a classic Ayurvedic antifungal (10 capsules daily).

A few other herbs deserve mention for yeast:

Oak bark kills systemic yeast (10 capsules daily), and is used as a douche for vaginal yeast.

Gum benzoin from southeast Asia kills yeast (10 capsules daily).

Myrrh gum is a classic blood cleanser and kills yeast (10 capsules daily).

Because yeast syndromes are multifaceted, getting control of yeast requires a complete approach to your total lifestyle. View the strategy as restoration of inner balance, not an attack on a microbe. The world is covered with yeast, and our bodies are covered with it—you will never be able to kill enough yeast to escape it. Since we can't hope to eradicate all yeast in our bodies, or in our environment, we must develop a strong defense that allows us to live in a dynamic synergism, or at least tolerance, with these creatures. Support your immune system powerfully and protect your "good bacteria," adjust your diet, de-stress your life, and your body can live in peaceful harmony with candida.

19

Herbs for Diabetes

D iabetes (properly called diabetes mellitus) is a chronic metabolic disorder characterized by a compromised ability to metabolize and use dietary carbohydrates, either because of insufficient amounts of insulin or inefficient use of insulin. Insulin is a hormone produced by the pancreas that is responsible for escorting glucose (sugar) out of the blood and into cells for use as energy.

In one type of diabetes, the pancreas produces little or no insulin; in the other type, the body does produce insulin (sometimes even to excess), but its ability to use the insulin is impaired. Either of these problems results in elevated blood glucose (hyperglycemia or "high blood sugar") and sugar in the urine (glycosuria).

High blood sugar is unhealthy and potentially dangerous. When insulin is not being produced sufficiently or used well, cells don't get from the blood the glucose that they need to burn for energy. Also, unnaturally high concentrations of sugar in the blood are toxic and damaging to tissues—one of the reasons diabetics are more prone to blindness, kidney disease (nephropathy) and nerve degeneration (neuropathy). Other complications include arterial plaque (atherosclerosis), heart disease (angiopathy), and foot ulcers.

It is estimated that 8 percent of people in the United States—about 12 million Americans—are diabetic. The prevalence of diabetes is increasing rapidly, at a rate of 6 percent a year. At this rate, the diabetic population will double every fifteen years. The American Diabetes Association expects the number of cases of adult-onset diabetes to double between the years 2000 and 2012.

Currently the fourth leading cause of death in the United States, diabetes is strongly associated with Western diet and lifestyle, and is rarely seen in cultures relying on a more traditional diet. As peoples around the world gradually switch from more native foods to commercial, processed diets, their rate of diabetes rises to match the proportion found in Western cultures. In the *Textbook of Natural Medicine*, Drs. Joseph Pizzorno and Michael Murray state that "the epidemiological evidence indicting the Western diet and lifestyle as the ultimate etiological factor in diabetes mellitus is overwhelming."

TYPES OF DIABETES

Diabetes is of two major types (called Type I and Type II). Type I, insulin-dependent diabetes mellitus (IDDM), is a disease that primarily begins in adolescence, and it accounts for about 10 percent of American diabetics. It involves complete destruction of the cells in the pancreas that produce the hormone insulin, the beta cells. People with IDDM require lifelong insulin injections to control blood sugar. The modern development of insulin as a drug has allowed these people to survive their illness, and natural methods offer hope for improved control of blood sugar, but there is no known cure.

The precise cause of Type I diabetes has not been discovered, but it is thought to be due to injury to the beta cells in combination with a defect in the capacity of the body to heal tissue. Possible causes of this injury may be autoimmune reactions, toxic or free-radical (oxidative) damage, or viral infection. Since the onset of IDDM is much greater during October through March, childhood diseases such as mumps, hepatitis, and measles are suspected as cofactors.

Non-insulin-dependent diabetes mellitus (NIDDM), or Type II, usually is diagnosed after age forty. Over 90 percent of diabetics in our culture are Type II. NIDDM is a disease of loss of sensitivity to insulin. Typically, insulin levels in the blood are actually increased as the pancreas tries to compensate for the high blood sugar, but the tissues have lost their ability to respond to the hormone.

Obesity, a high-fat/high-sugar diet, smoking, and lack of exercise are all significant risk factors for reduced insulin sensitivity and NIDDM. Obesity in particular is a serious contributing factor in NIDDM, with an estimated 90 percent of Type II diabetics being obese. Even in nondiabetic individuals, large body-fat gains often result in carbohydrate intolerance, higher blood insulin, and insulin insensitivity in body tissues. Progressive insulin insensitivity is now thought to be the main factor in the development of this most common type of diabetes. Many obese diabetics are able to restore normal blood sugar levels *simply by achieving ideal body-fat level.*

Diabetes Characteristics

	Type I—IDDM	Type II—NIDDM
Age of onset	Before 25	After 40
Body build	Lean	Obese
Family history	Infrequent	Very often
Insulin in the blood	Decreased	Increased
Thirst	Highly increased	Increased
Fatigue	Pronounced	Moderate
Weight loss	Pronounced	None
Blurred vision	Moderate	Pronounced
Vaginal problems	Moderate	Pronounced
Nerve damage	Moderate	Pronounced
Vascular disease	Heart damage	Arterial plaque

DIET

The United States could cut the $92 billion annual cost associated with diabetes by $26 billion if medical nutrition therapy was required protocol in the treatment of diabetes.

—The American Dietetic Association

Dietary modification is not only the key to diabetes prevention, it is absolutely essential to successful diabetes treatment. The disease is highly correlated with the "civilized" diet of refined carbohydrates, excessive fat consumption (especially animal fats), and fiber-depleted food—as well as with the overfat, depleted, and toxic bodies that result from such a diet.

Even though dietary intervention has a high success rate in diabetes, it is often overlooked in favor of insulin or drugs. Drug therapy is expensive, immunosuppressive, and doesn't heal or promote the health of the body. The consensus of natural healing practitioners around the world is that NIDDM is treatable, and even curable, without drugs.

As with many common Western diseases, the diet that is best for preventing the condition in the first place is also therapeutic, and makes an ideal foundation for other therapies. The diet that causes diabetes will also aggravate it. Not coincidentally, the ideal diabetic diet doesn't differ much from the generally disease-preventive ideal.

The diet of choice in diabetes treatment is high in complex carbohydrate and emphasizes plant fiber. The ideal diet includes cereal grains, legumes, root vegetables, and tubers (such as potato) in large amounts, and limits (or preferably excludes) simple sugars (white sugar), refined and processed grains, and saturated fat. Total fat should not exceed 20 percent of calories, with protein (lean and preferably plant based) at 15 to 25 percent and the carbohydrates described above comprising 55 to 65 percent of the diet.

This diet results in better control of blood sugar after meals and later in the day. It also increases insulin sensitivity, reduces cholesterol and triglycerides, increases HDL cholesterol ("good" cholesterol), and promotes progressive body-fat reduction, all of which reduce the need for insulin. Diabetics who adopt this type of diet reap the benefits.

Dealing with Diabetic Diet Myths

In my work with people through *BodyFueling*®, I've encountered many diabetics and noted a tremendous lack of consciousness about diet among both diabetics and their health professionals. A very outdated yet lingering version of conventional treatment severely restricts carbohydrates and encourages high protein and even fat consumption.

This rampant misinformation applies to hypoglycemia as well. I know one hypoglycemic woman whose doctor has her eating a mainly protein diet. But the human body is not meant to subsist on protein, and must perform complicated finagling to fuel itself as a result. Ironically, protein must be converted to carbohydrate, but with stressful extra work and toxic byproducts that could be avoided by just eating carbohydrate to begin with. I shudder to think of what this burden is doing to her body long term.

Knowledgeable health authorities around the world agree that both diabetics and hypoglycemics benefit from a 60 percent or so complex carbohydrate diet with 30 percent or less calories coming from fat. Despite this, the doctor mentioned above actually told this patient that a frequent-feeding, high-carbohydrate diet "would kill a diabetic or hypoglycemic."

In addition to restricting carbos mistakenly, many diabetics appear to be unaware of the dangers of high fat consumption. It is critical for the diabetic to maintain low blood levels of both triglycerides and cholesterol. This means avoiding saturated fat in meats and hydrogenated oils as much as possible (completely, if necessary), and keeping total fat low (at about 20 percent of calories). Triglyceride levels rise concurrently with dietary increases in fat and refined carbohydrates. Some researchers feel that triglyceride level is the single most accurate prediction of diabetes risk.

As a leftover from the era that supported a high-fat, high-protein diet, diabetics frequently tend to be cautious about sugar, yet oblivious to fat. In *BodyFueling*® I gave an example of a family with a diabetic child whose dinner table was laden with high-fat items. The "good" yams were the swimming-in-butter ones without brown sugar, as opposed to the "bad" ones with sugar and butter.

Jean Carper in *Food: Your Miracle Medicine* reports at least one survey whose dismal results are consistent with my observations: Only 3 percent (!) of those surveyed ate more than 50 percent of their calories from carbohydrate! Additionally, only 14 percent kept their fat intake below 34 percent of calories.

Fiber

Fiber makes up a portion of vegetables, fruits, and grains. The diet of our ancestors, until relatively recently, included 10 times as much fiber as the standard American diet. Plentiful fiber in the diet not only helps control blood sugar, but is also associated with lower rates of cancer and heart disease.

Fiber may be added to the diet in supplemental form. **Guar gum**, at a dose of 15 grams per day, can be beneficial. One study demonstrated that over one year with 14 to 26 grams of guar gum per day, diabetic patients required less insulin and had less sugar in the urine.[1] In another study,

NIDDM patients achieved a 10 percent reduction in blood cholesterol using 15 grams per day, along with better glycemic control.[2] **Pectin**, a soluble fiber from fruits, taken at 10 grams per meal, can be equally effective.

Chia seed (Salvia columbariae) is a supplement particularly rich in healthful fiber. Chia grows in the desert Southwest of the United States, and is used by the O'odham native peoples there. The seeds are 60 percent dietary fiber, with 55 percent of that fiber being insoluble. When soaked in water, the seeds' polysaccharides expand to form a wet, slimy mass. The soaked seeds can be eaten by the spoonful or mixed into cereal.

Other kinds of fiber are detailed on pages 329–330.

Specific Food Therapies for Diabetes

In addition to a well-crafted basic diet, diabetics can make therapeutic use of certain foods to help adjust blood-sugar levels. Although the biochemical mechanisms of most of these foods are not known, generally they fall into the category of botanical hypoglycemics, or plants that lower blood sugar when eaten regularly. There is no maximum "dose"; the idea is simply to incorporate as many of the foods as possible, as often as possible.

Okra is recommended by Sree Chakravarti in A Healer's Journey as an Ayurvedic remedy for high blood sugar. Many American patients who have tried this food have success with the juice of okra pods added to their diet. Okra is delicious as a steamed vegetable.

Dandelion greens have been quite successful as a botanical hypoglycemic for many diabetics. Again, the most practical form is freshly squeezed juice. For winter, the greens can be frozen and juiced daily as needed. Fresh dandelion greens can also be delicious in a salad.

Prickly pear cactus (nopal in Spanish) is used as food in Mexico. The pads are diced and prepared in a salad or as a taco.

Other foods that are generally supportive for diabetics include **cinnamon, nutmeg, turmeric, bay leaf, cashew, celery, cayenne, ginger, coriander seed, lettuce, cabbage, turnip, papaya fruit, cranberry, Jerusalem artichoke, millet, oats, barley,** and **buckwheat.** Certainly, with this many foods to choose from, one could manage to include a few each day, and still have a tasty and varied diet.

EXERCISE

Every authority on diabetes emphasizes the role of exercise in effective treatment. Exercise has a preventive effect on every symptom and complication of diabetes.

Obese diabetics are encouraged to build up the intensity of their exercise program gradually, and then to go for the maximum they can possibly do. "Thin" (usually *vata*/air) types and usually IDDM may have to be a bit more moderate, with the focus on brisk walking.

A recent study of sixty-five-to-eighty-four-year-old men demonstrated that physical activity is an independent factor in blood sugar levels, regardless of body weight and body fat; the more the exercise, the more normal the blood sugar. Several studies of strength training in older people have recently proved that they can change their insulin levels with exercise alone.

Exercise also reduces insulin resistance. The fitter the person is, the more sensitive and responsive muscles and other tissues are to insulin. As mentioned above, some health professionals believe that insulin resistance is extremely widespread in the American population, and that insulin resistance is a precursor to diabetes. This may be due in part to the sedentary tendencies of the average American.

HERB THERAPIES

General Herb Therapies for Diabetes

In addition to treating NIDDM with fundamental good nutrition, there are many herbs that diabetics can use to enhance overall health, modulate blood sugar, and prevent or treat symptoms. Combining the ideal diet with herbal therapies not only controls blood sugar, but can reduce or eliminate common complications of diabetes. Complications add to the monumental costs of this disease and cause a great deal of needless pain and suffering.

Onions and *garlic* are significant hypoglycemics. The active properties are thought to be sulfur-containing compounds (disulfides), such as allicin and diallyl disulfide. Evidence suggests that these compounds lower glucose levels by competing with insulin (also a disulfide) in the liver. The well-known cardiovascular benefits of these herbs alone (regulating blood pressure, cholesterol, and platelet aggregation) justify their use in diabetes. Even at moderate dietary levels, these herbs have potent effects. Diabetics can use these herbs liberally.

Green tea contains catechins and epicatechins, plant compounds belonging to the flavonol category. These are powerful antioxidants, and have been shown to aid in diabetes. Green tea is typically served in Asian-style restaurants, can be consumed daily as a beverage, and is available in a decaffeinated extract as a dietary supplement.

A decoction (tea) of *blueberry* (or *huckleberry*) *leaf* is considered a valuable diabetes remedy in folk medicine. The active ingredient, myrtillin, acts like insulin in the body, but is much less toxic, even at fifty times the therapeutic dose. Furthermore, its action in the body is quite prolonged, with a dose acting over several weeks. Drink 1 cup per day.

Stevia has become controversial recently in the United States because large artificial-sweetener companies are opposed to the approval of its use as a sweetener. And no wonder: Stevia is thirty times sweeter than sugar, yet has 1 calorie per 10 leaves, and is totally natural. Although not currently approved here for food use, it was recently approved as a dietary supplement. Clearly it has great promise as a sweetener for diabetics. In addition, it has a long history of use in South America in the treatment of diabetes, though scientific evidence in this area is mixed.

Bitter herbs, long a general favorite of European herbalists, are widely respected around the world, including among Asian practitioners, for use in diabetes. *Dandelion root* is a good bitter herb, and is especially synergistic with *turmeric* as a liver cleanser. Turmeric doses would be consistent with those that have been discussed at length already in several chapters; dandelion root can be taken up to 15 capsules per day. The greens can also be steamed and eaten to maximum tolerance; this is very effective.

Other good tea herbs include *eucalyptus leaf, burdock root, senna leaf* (caution: this is laxative), *string bean pod,* and *olive leaf*. Any of these can be taken in doses of 1/2 ounce to 1 ounce of herb per day as tea.

Juniper berry and *cedar berry* taken in capsules (5 each per day, good combined) are known to produce results clinically.

Desert tea stimulates respiration and cardiac response, which can be suppressed by diabetes. It reduces blood sugar and is a diuretic, causing the body to rid itself of excess glucose through the urine and reducing edema (water retention).

Ayurvedic Herbs

Diabetes, called *madhumeha* in Sanskrit, has been known in Ayurveda for thousands of years. Many successful Ayurvedic remedies have been developed for diabetes.

The bark of the *asana* tree is one of the few remedies that is thought to have an effect on Type I diabetes. In *Ayurveda, Life, Health, and Longevity*, Dr. Robert Svoboda, the only American to graduate from an Ayurvedic medical college in India, says that asana bark has been reported to actually regenerate the insulin-producing cells of the pancreas, but only if the disease is of recent origin. Drs. Pizzorno and Murray confirm this in their *Textbook of Natural Medicine*, and suggest that asana is the only substance, drug or otherwise, that is known to have this effect.

Asana is also another rich source of epicatechins, an antioxidant compound found in green tea. It can be taken in capsules, 4 to 8 per day.

Gurmar (Gymnema sylvestre) means "killer of sweet" in Sanskrit. When chewed, the leaves block sweet taste on the tongue, reducing the appeal of sugar foods. Successfully and safely used for more than 2,000 years in India, it is now being recognized by modern science as a promising remedy for both Type I and Type II diabetes. Confirmed effects include lowering blood sugar, blood fats, triglycerides, and cholesterol, and repair of liver, kidney, and muscle tissue. The leaves can be chewed, or dried leaves can be taken in capsules (1 to 10 daily).

In one recent study at the University of Madras, gurmar showed potential for pancreas repair, raising insulin output to normal levels. Another study reported that 25 percent of participants were able to discontinue all diabetes medication with the use of gurmar alone. In clinical tests in India, 3 to 4 grams of gurmar daily over a period of three to four months reduced glycosuria, or sugar in the urine.[3]

It's theorized that gurmar indirectly stimulates insulin secretion by the pancreas, since it has no apparent effect on carbohydrate metabolism. Pharmacological and clinical studies show that gurmar also acts on taste buds and the surface of the intestines, which share similar tissue structure. An organic acid in the herb, called gymnemic acid, is similar in molecular structure to glucose. Thus gurmar molecules can substitute for glucose molecules to fill sugar-detecting taste-bud receptors before they can be activated by sugar molecules. They also plug similar receptor locations in the intestine, preventing absorption of sugar molecules there. This significantly reduces the metabolic effects of sugar during digestion. Reduced absorption of sugar means reduced blood-sugar level.

Gurmar also lowers blood sugar to normal, not below normal, in most patients.[4] Of course, blood sugar should be monitored carefully to avoid a hypoglycemic effect.

Fenugreek, regarded in the United States as an exotic kitchen spice, is an effective blood-sugar-lowering herb. Since fenugreek actually tastes good, it's practical for people to use on a daily basis. One study showing its effectiveness used fenugreek seed baked into flat bread, which proved effective for reducing blood sugar in NIDDM.[5]

It is not known whether the active principle in fenugreek lies in the high soluble fiber content, or in another unknown compound. But fenugreek is effective in both types of diabetes, is cheap, well tolerated, and at 28 percent protein content is a favorable food source.

Fenugreek has one disadvantage: the dose necessary to produce results. One recent successful study used 100 grams (about 3½ ounces) per day. While Asian people, used to consuming large herb doses, may comply with this regimen, herbalists in the United States have found that the typical American diabetic may have resistance to the large amount required. Commonly, fenugreek seeds are eaten after being soaked in water overnight (you can then munch it by the spoonful or mix into cereal).

Karta Purkh spoke with one person who used to be an insulin-dependent diabetic and now treats the disease purely with fenugreek seed—4 heaping tablespoons a day. That's a lot, but it's nothing compared to injecting insulin.

Bitter melon (also known as balsam pear or bitter gourd) is widely cultivated for food in Asia, Africa, and South America. It's commonly available in Chinese restaurants and in Asian food stores. It's a longtime diabetic folk remedy, and studies have demonstrated its hypoglycemic effect.

Bitter melon looks like an ugly cucumber. It's green and covered with gourdlike bumps. It can be steamed or sautéed and eaten as a food. The fresh juice, dried herb, and water decoction (tea) are all active. Studies show improved glucose tolerance with use of the fresh juice. Two ounces per day is recommended. The juice is difficult to make palatable, so plug your nose, and take a 2-ounce shot—down the hatch!

Like some other herbs mentioned earlier, bitter melon seems to have some action on the pancreas, as well as a component with insulinlike action. Researchers have coined the term **plant insulin** to describe bitter melon. The insulinlike molecule in it is almost identical to cow insulin, widely used by diabetics. Bitter melon also contains potent detoxifiers that protect the pancreas from free-radical damage, which is widely thought to be a cause of Type I diabetes.

Jambul fruit, native to India, now grows throughout the tropics. It's also called **jamun,** rose apple, or java plum. The fruit and its seeds are considered in Ayurvedic medicine to be some of the most powerful hypoglycemic herbs. Doses of as little as 1 teaspoon of powdered dry herb per day (mix into food or put in capsules) can be effective. Jambul is thought to be particularly synergistic with okra. Sree Chakravarti explicitly recommends this combination, suggesting that you should see significant blood-sugar reductions in about 10 days.

Neem leaf is one of the most useful plants grown in Asia, and historically every part of the plant has been used—root, bark, gum, fruit, leaves, and seeds—for a variety of purposes, from immune stimulation and antimicrobial properties to ulcer treatment. The leaf is useful for diabetes because it lowers blood sugar by stimulating insulin secretion. One of the most cooling and bitter herbs, neem also improves digestion and detoxifies the liver. It can be taken in capsules (5 to 10 per day), prepared as tea (up to 1 ounce per day), or cooked into food.

Guggul gum is a sticky resin that exudes from the bark of **Commiphora mukul.** Guggul is widely regarded as the foremost cholesterol-lowering herb in the world. It's an effective herb for managing all fats in the body. In diabetes, it normalizes cholesterol, triglycerides, and body fat, thus reducing the chance of arterial deposits and hardening of the arteries (atherosclerosis). Guggul also prevents abnormal blood clotting.

This combination of actions is dynamic for reducing retinopathy (eye damage), neuropathy (nerve degeneration, usually starting in the feet), and gangrene, which are all common, very serious complications of diabetes. A famous Ayurvedic preparation, **triphala guggul,** includes guggul mixed with the three fruits of *triphala* (amla, haritaki, and bibitaki). This combination is the most respected obesity remedy in Ayurveda.

Myrrh gum is an herb that is related to guggul but is more well known in the West. It may be substituted for guggul. Either guggul or myrrh gum can be taken in capsules, 6 to 8 per day.

Kutki contains a wealth of medicines for diabetes. It stimulates digestive secretions, which in turn stimulate pancreatic insulin secretion. Kutki also enhances immune function and normalizes liver function. Kutki assists the liver in storing blood sugar in the form of glycogen, which is essential in diabetes management. It is also sometimes used to protect the liver from the toxic effects of antidiabetic drugs. One to 3 capsules a day may be taken long term.

Amla fruit by itself is a good diabetes remedy. Sometimes called Indian gooseberry, it's the world's richest known source of vitamin C and the most widely prescribed Ayurvedic medicine (it's the base of the popular tonic **chyavanprash**, an antioxidant fruit jelly, as well as one of the three components of the Ayurvedic tonic **triphala,** discussed earlier). Amla fruit jelly can be eaten from a spoon or spread on toast, 1 teaspoon or more per day.

Such a valuable herb that it is considered sacred in India, **holy basil,** or **tulsi,** increases uptake of glucose in the peripheral tissues of the body. Therefore, tulsi potentiates the action of all other diabetes medicines, whether insulin or neem leaf.

Holy basil has also demonstrated anti-stress action, which can be helpful to anyone but may be especially useful for diabetics, who may be more susceptible to stress-related conditions.

The leaves of the **stone apple** tree (also called **bilwa**) stimulate the pancreas to secrete insulin. One teaspoon of fresh leaf juice per day is the typical dose.

Black pepper is revered in Asia as a blood purifier. Black pepper is very drying in action, and can help with water retention. It also enhances circulation. For a medicinal dose it should be taken in capsules (2 to 8 per day).

Ginger root acts both by stimulating pancreatic cells and by lowering lipids (cholesterol and triglycerides) in the blood. Since ginger is particularly synergistic with onions and garlic and those are also good for diabetes, these so-called trinity roots should be eaten together as much as possible.

Shilajit is not an herb per se, but a mineral pitch from faces of rock cliffs in the Himalayas. Shilajit is believed to be fossilized remains of plants. It not only lowers blood sugar but is used for detoxification and blood purification and arthritis. It should be taken in capsules, 5 per day.

Herbs for Diabetic Complications

Diabetics often develop cardiovascular, circulatory, and nerve diseases. In addition to the tissue damage caused by high blood-sugar concentrations, Type II diabetics are especially prone to heart disease, because they tend to be overfat or obese in addition to having weakened or damaged blood vessels and poor circulation. About 65 percent of diabetics have high blood pressure.

There are many excellent herbs that can be used preventively and therapeutically to protect and heal the heart, vascular system, and nerves. We will briefly list key herbs here, but you should refer to the next chapter, "Herbs for the Heart," for detailed information. Doses can be the same as those recommended specifically in that chapter.

The bark of the *arjuna* tree from India is the cardiovascular panacea of Ayurveda. Sree Chakravarti specifically recommends this red bark as the main herb for diabetic conditions involving the heart. It's similar to hawthorn berry in its actions, much less studied, and not as widely available, but also less expensive and produces the same wide range of results.

Ginkgo increases peripheral circulation, particularly to the brain. Obviously, increasing circulation can be only beneficial to a diabetic patient, and ginkgo's mechanism—antioxidant protection of cells and vascular integrity—is particularly helpful. Protected venous membranes are more flexible and allow more oxygen-carrying red blood cells to squeeze through to the capillary-rich brain and eyes; it also makes capillaries less likely to burst. Ginkgo also protects the nervous system and may be especially useful in preventing degenerative eye diseases. A study in rats showed that ginkgo is an effective regenerator of motor nerves, so this herb may be applicable to diabetic neuropathy.

Bilberry, another antioxidant with circulatory benefits, contains compounds called anthocyanosides, which improve blood flow to the heart and extremities by protecting cell walls and capillaries from oxidative damage. This herb has a particular affinity for the eye and prevents degenerative eye disease. Studies also show that bilberry can reduce plaque deposits on artery walls, increase heartbeat strength, and thin the blood.

Hawthorn berry is another excellent cardiotonic and circulatory herb. It has demonstrated an ability actually to slow and strengthen the heartbeat, increase blood and oxygen flow to the heart by dilating coronary blood vessels, and prevent irregular heartbeats (arrythmias) by improving metabolic processes in the heart. It is especially helpful for relieving angina. It is also antioxidant and, like bilberry and ginkgo, can counter free-radical damage to cells and capillaries. It has been shown to reduce blood pressure, cholesterol levels, and atherosclerosis.

Gotu kola leaf is a superior nerve tonic with a long history of use in India, China, and the islands of Indonesia as an anti-aging tonic and wound-repair remedy. In addition to circulatory benefits, it has a regenerative effect on connective tissue and nerves, increasing blood supply to the tissues and accelerating the formation of the tissue's structural components. Studies show that gotu kola is effective in treating numbness, leg cramps, and venous conditions.

Borage leaf is good for arterial cleansing. Two to 15 capsules a day.

Motherwort leaf strengthens the heart. Two capsules a day.

Alfalfa leaf lowers blood pressure and cholesterol. Two to 15 capsules a day.

Spices that promote circulation include *cayenne, cinnamon, ginger root,* and *clove.* Cayenne also lowers cholesterol and blood pressure and increases vasodilation (widening of blood vessels). Take to comfort level.

Other Supplements

Chromium is a trace mineral that is key to glucose metabolism. It potentiates insulin function (i.e., enhances the action of existing insulin), though scientists don't yet understand exactly how. Supplementing with this mineral may reduce blood glucose by binding with GTF—glucose tolerance factor—which helps insulin bind to certain cell receptors to allow glucose to enter cells. Chromium may also improve tissue responsiveness to insulin. Scientific views on its effectiveness are mixed, but since chromium is not known to be toxic even at high levels, a daily supplement of the picolinate or nicotinate forms (designed to be more bioavailable, or easily absorbed) is a good idea.

Vanadium is a naturally occurring trace mineral, often used by body-builders because of its ability to "push" blood sugar from the blood into muscle cells, thus theoretically reducing the likelihood of it being converted to and stored as fat and also supposedly making a harder, denser muscle. From the diabetic's point of view, the fact that vanadium seems to be a potent "insulin mimicker" suggests that it can take up some of the slack. Vanadyl sulfate is the most common form and probably the safest; other forms may be toxic in high doses, so stick to the sulfate form. Dosage should not exceed 15 milligrams per day, and the mineral must always be taken with carbohydrate food.

Magnesium deficiency is common in diabetes and is also linked to heart disease, neuropathy, and retinopathy, all potential diabetic complications. The American Diabetic Association even recommends that diabetics supplement with magnesium.[6]

Antioxidant vitamins, minerals, and phytonutrients are important for everyone, as we've emphasized, but they may be especially indispensable for diabetics because many of the complications associated with the disease can be linked at least in part to oxidative damage, and such damage may even play a role in pancreatic breakdown itself. Thus daily supplementation with vitamins A, C, E, selenium, mixed bioflavonoids and mixed carotenoids is highly recommended.

SUCCESSFUL TREATMENT—A COMPLETE LIFESTYLE

As we emphasize in every case and for every condition, the whole body and the whole life must be considered. Herbs are only a piece, and although they represent an effective piece, an unsupportive lifestyle can detract from their effectiveness. Diabetics must be willing to alter their lifestyles substantially in order to achieve completely natural regulation of blood sugar, and to avoid common diabetic complications. Effective treatment requires an integration of every possible available therapy.

NIDDM is the result of a long period of chronic metabolic insult, and can require years of persistent effort to reverse. Patience is necessary. As you proceed, feel encouraged by knowing you are headed in a positive direction.

In addition, there's no need to feel that caring for yourself this way is "treatment" for "sickness." That's an unnecessarily dry, even grim, perspective. Certainly diabetes represents a system malfunction, but the natural way of addressing diabetes is not that far removed from the way we recommend *all* people eat, supplement, and generally live their lives for best health. Ironically, except for some of the diabetes-specific herbs we mention, the ideal diabetic diet and lifestyle are the same ones we would all do well to adopt—for prevention of this disease and countless others, and for general good health, fitness, and vitality.

So remember, you're in good company. Some of the healthiest, fittest people in the world are choosing to care for their bodies in exactly the way that is recommended for diabetics.

The excellent historical success of people around the world with natural treatment of diabetes gives us hope. Along with modern studies that confirm the efficacy of many of these treatments, they show that Type I diabetes can be controlled and that the vast majority of Type II diabetes sufferers may be able to reverse the condition fully. Type I diabetics probably will continue to use some insulin for life, but the dose can be reduced very substantially.

Note: *Never should a diabetic suddenly stop using diabetic drugs, especially insulin!* Under a physician's guidance, it may well be possible to gradually reduce the dose substantially and successfully, ideally to zero. Diabetes should always be monitored by a health professional, since rapid decreases and increases in blood sugar can be dangerous, and diabetics are at risk for various complicating conditions.

20

Herbs for the Heart

We do not want to give the impression that herbs alone can treat cardiovascular disease of any kind, nor that treatment after the fact is the ideal way to handle it. Clearly, prevention is the way to go when it comes to cardiovascular disease, and prevention is well within most people's reach because the causes of the disease have been well established. Heart disease and stroke are epidemic in the United States (responsible together for more than 1 million deaths annually, holding the number one and three spots for leading killers of Americans). Yet they are, in the vast majority of cases, preventable through lifestyle choices. We have covered these lifestyle issues in some detail already, and my book *BodyFueling*® covers them in even more detail.

No herb or any other medicine can take the place of a healthy diet, exercise, and stress management, nor can they compensate for unhealthy habits. But as an adjunct to lifestyle elements, botanicals can be very supportive of efforts to improve heart and cardiovascular health. People who have just begun making dietary changes or who are recovering from medical interventions for these diseases can do very well using these herbs to complement their efforts.

Guggul is the supreme cholesterol-lowering herb in the world, works the fastest, and has the most scientific evidence behind it. A typical dose of the pure gum in capsule form would be 6 capsules a day. We have known countless people who experienced significant drops in cholesterol as well as triglycerides (blood fats) using this herb.

Turmeric normalizes cholesterol. One component, dimethylbenzyl alcohol, reduces serum cholesterol (in the blood), while curcumin removes accumulation of cholesterol in the liver. Anticholesterol actions include reduction of intestinal cholesterol uptake, increased conversion of cholesterol into bile acids, and increased excretion of bile acids. Turmeric also reduces arterial plaque and inhibits platelet aggregation. It is known to reduce smooth muscle damage in the artery, the beginning step in atherosclerosis (hardening of the arteries). Turmeric would be a wise choice in fighting artery disease or in recovery from bypass surgery or angioplasty.

Turmeric can be taken up to 1 ounce a day in capsules (as noted earlier, the whole herb works much better than the standardized extract, in Karta Purkh's opinion) or as powder in various forms such as paste (see page 497 for recipes and uses). Paste makes more sense since 1 ounce equals 45 to 50 "00"-size capsules.

Arjuna, a red tree bark used extensively in Ayurveda, is in Karta Purkh's opinion the premier cardiovascular herb in the world. If ever there was a true herbal panacea, this is it for the circulatory system. Arjuna treats tachycardia (heart palpitations and increased heartbeat), arrythmia (irregular heartbeats, which can increase with age and can be precursors to heart failure), hypertension (high blood pressure), circulatory insufficiency (decreased blood flow to the heart), and angina (pain resulting from decreased oxygen flow to the heart). It strengthens the heart muscle, slows and steadies the heartbeat, lowers cholesterol, and increases oxygen to the heart.

While arjuna is prepared as a beverage tea in Asia, experience shows that Americans have difficulty with the taste, and prefer capsules. Up to 1 ounce of the dry herb may be taken per day. Between 2 to 10 capsules daily on average, but up to 20 may be taken as needed.

Hawthorn berry does all of the things that arjuna does as described above; however, it's much more well known (more trendy and thus more expensive). It's extremely popular in Europe, where governments in several countries have approved it for cardiovascular use. In Europe it is used as an extract, and some of its benefits are believed to be the result of antioxidant flavonoids.

Anti-arrythmia drugs do not have a great record of effectiveness or safety, but hawthorn berry is often combined in Europe with the toxic drug digitalis (extracted from the plant foxglove). The addition of hawthorn makes the drug safer by drastically reducing the amount of digitalis used (digitalis is so strong that the wrong dose—an overdose—can kill). Studies document reduction in angina heart pains in patients using hawthorn, allowing them to reduce or discontinue use of nitroglycerin (another very potent pharmaceutical used to treat angina) or digitalis.[1]

No overdoses of hawthorn have ever been recorded in medical literature, even after 100 years of widespread use, according to Herb Research Foundation president Rob McCaleb.[2] Five to 20 capsules daily may be taken as needed. Hawthorn is a tonic that works over time, not an immediate treatment.

Bilberry is a circulation-enhancing herb we have discussed at length in several other places, but it deserves mention here because its effects on blood flow overall are useful from a heart-health point of view. Like hawthorn berry, bilberry (the European blueberry) is antioxidant rich, and its compounds (anthocyanosides) strengthen capillaries, maintain strength and flexibility of cell walls and venous membranes, reduce oxidative damage to these tissues, and thus allow blood and red cells to squeeze through smaller spaces without bursting the vessels. Bilberry has been shown to reduce deposits on blood-vessel walls, increase circulation to the head, eyes, heart, and limbs, and act as an anticoagulant. Like hawthorn berry, no toxicity has been reported despite a long history of popular use.

Bilberry extract usually comes in 60-milligram tablets; take 2 to 4 daily.

Garlic is one of the world's most researched foods and herbs and has amassed an impressive list of medicinal properties. Thousands of research papers have been written on garlic, and among its most prodigious effects are those involving the heart and circulation. It lowers LDL cholesterol (while maintaining or even increasing HDL cholesterol) and triglycerides, thins the blood to reduce clotting, and lowers blood pressure. In addition, studies show that it prevents oxidation of fat and cholesterol, and oxidation of these fats is the first step toward atherosclerosis.

Include several cloves daily (up to a bulb, unless you are *pitta*/fire type) and/or take 2 to 10 capsules or tablets.

Ginger does for heart health what the conventional aspirin-a-day recommendation is supposed to do—only ginger does it better, without side effects. The drug aspirin can cause problems such as stomach and intestinal irritation and bleeding. Ginger inhibits thromboxanes and platelet aggregation (clotting), and thus is useful for preventing both strokes and heart failure—yet ginger is anti-inflammatory. Capsules of dried powdered ginger may be taken (2 to 10 capsules per day, working up slowly) or lightly cooked fresh ginger may be used in food to maximum tolerance (again, working up slowly).

Butcher's broom, from the Mediterranean, has been used historically for heart health to "sweep" cholesterol deposits from arteries. It can cause queasiness, so start with 1 capsule a day and work up to 5 or so. *Borage leaf* is another arterial-cleansing herb from the Mediterranean; up to 15 capsules per day is appropriate.

Tienchi root, a Chinese herb similar to ginseng, is valued in traditional natural healing for its multiple effects on the heart. It increases coronary blood flow, increases oxygen consumption by the heart, regulates the heartbeat, lowers blood pressure, reduces cholesterol, and dissolves clots. Take up to 5 capsules per day.

Two other general cardio-builders from Chinese medicine are *akebia leaf* (5 to 10 capsules a day) and *Chinese foxglove root* (*not* to be confused with digitalis, the common and toxic foxglove plant that grows all over North America), 1 to 5 capsules per day.

Black pepper is a classic Ayurvedic blood cleanser and also increases circulation (1 to 5 capsules per day). *Long pepper* ("pipali" in India) is yet another revered Ayurvedic blood cleanser (also 1 to 5 capsules). *Trikatu,* the Ayurvedic remedy that means "three pungents" (black pepper, pipali, ginger) is a superior blood cleanser (1 to 5 capsules per day).

Motherwort leaf is a good heart-strengthening tonic at about 2 capsules per day.

Alfalfa leaf is a general builder and particularly good for lowering blood pressure or cholesterol. It can be taken in tea or capsules to maximum tolerance.

Rosemary is an astringent, cleansing herb that can be helpful at 1 to 10 capsules a day or 1/4 ounce as tea.

Green tea contains polyphenol compounds (such as the flavonoid catechin) and antioxidant compounds. It is known to lower cholesterol levels and thin the blood. In addition to adding it to your daily routine as a beverage, you can try capsules of concentrated extracts standardized for 15 to 50 percent polyphenols. Follow package directions.

Ginkgo biloba is discussed at length other places in this book; it is a long-term remedy, and as a tonic can be useful to cardiovascular health because of its protective effect on small capillaries. As a daily tonic, try 3 capsules of 50:1 extract standardized to contain 24 percent ginkgoflavonocides, or 6 to 8 capsules of the whole ground leaf.

Coleus, the Ayurvedic herb discussed earlier for its use with asthma, allergies, skin disease, and depression, has also been used traditionally for cardiovascular conditions. Numerous studies bear out this use, particularly for angina, high blood pressure, and congestive heart failure. The mechanism by which forskolin (the active ingredient, whose extract has been studied much more than the whole herb) relaxes spasms of the smooth bronchial muscles also serves to relax arteries and increase the heart muscle's contraction force. Coleus also lowers blood pressure and inhibits platelet aggregation (clotting). As with other uses, 50 milligrams of extract 2 to 3 times daily or 4 to 8 capsules of the whole herb is typical.

Cayenne and *ginger* are two spices you can use liberally to tolerance (advised against only if you are *pitta*/fire type constitution or are currently dealing with *pitta* imbalance or excess). Cayenne increases circulation and lowers cholesterol and blood pressure; ginger increases circulation. With both, start small and increase slowly to tolerance in food or capsules. **Mustard seed** is another warming circulation enhancer (1 to 5 capsules per day).

Fish oil and *olive oil* are "good fats" that should comprise all or most of the fat in a heart-healthy diet. They are LDL lowering, HDL boosting, and anticoagulant. They are also not as easily oxidized (oxidation leads to artery-hardening buildup) as processed vegetable fats such as sunflower, safflower, and corn oils.

Folic acid is a B vitamin. One of folic acid's several functions in the body is to reduce the amount of homocysteine (an amino acid) in the blood. Recently, researchers have seen mounting evidence that large numbers of people have especially high levels of homocysteine in their bloodstreams, and that this substance can injure blood vessels, causing hardening of the arteries, thus contributing to heart attacks and strokes. Folic acid can apparently help reduce blood levels of homocysteine to a safe range.

Kilmer McCully, M.D., first proposed this theory in 1969, sacrificed his career to it, and was asked to leave Harvard Medical School because he hadn't proved his theory. Only recently have mainstream researchers taken an interest in his work. A recent study showed that .065 milligrams daily of folic acid reduced blood homocysteine concentrations by 41.7 percent.[3]

In the late 1960s a rare genetic disorder was discovered—homocystinuria—that would cause early atherosclerosis. Half of its sufferers would die of heart attack or stroke before the age of thirty. In this condition, homocysteine is not converted into other amino acids because of a genetic defect. The resulting high levels of homocysteine promote atherosclerosis and blood-vessel damage.

People without this genetic defect can still have high homocysteine levels, which are associated with low intake of folacin, B_6, and B_{12}. These vitamins help the normal conversion of homocysteine into amino acids the body can use, so that it does not rise to unhealthy levels.

A moderately elevated homocysteine level is now considered by many researchers to be an independent risk factor for heart disease. Research indicates that when the intake of folacin, B_6, and B_{12} is low, heart attack risk increases.

This does not mean that smoking, obesity, high cholesterol levels, high blood pressure, high-fat diet, and so on are no longer risk factors. One woman I talked to had interpreted the media blitz on this issue as saying that "400 milligrams of folic acid per day will prevent heart disease no matter what else you do." Not true. Take the 400 milligrams of folic acid, but don't throw all other caution to the wind. Get enough of these B vitamins *and* take good care of yourself in general, eat a wide variety of healthful foods, don't drink or smoke, and exercise moderately.

Magnesium deficiencies have been documented in significant percentages of heart-disease and high-blood-pressure study subjects. Magnesium is important for proper functioning of the heart and vascular system. Unfortunately, the same dietary and lifestyle habits that are disease causing in their own right—high fat, high sugar, alcohol, stress, and high-phosphate processed food and sodas—all aggravate magnesium deficiency. Magnesium is a natural smooth-muscle relaxant and "calcium channel blocker," a natural and mild version of the drugs used for cardiac arrythmia, for example. A daily supplement of 1,000 milligrams is a good idea for at-risk patients.

Vitamin C is known to relax and widen blood vessels. Take 2 to 3 grams per day.

> Note: Be cautious with your consumption of anticoagulant foods or nutrients if you are already on anticoagulant medicines or if you have a family history of hemorrhagic stroke. These include vitamin E, garlic, onion, fish oil, olive oil, chilies, and ginger. (Incidentally, some food for thought: Patients taking anticoagulant pharmaceuticals are warned by their physicians against taking vitamin E and garlic. If those substances are powerful enough to be "additive" to the drug, thereby *over*thinning the blood, might they not be powerful enough to thin the blood instead of the drug?)

21

Herbs for Headaches
and Other Aches

HEADACHES

It's estimated that 150 million lost workdays annually can be attributed to headaches, and hundreds of millions of people take drugs for them. Is there a better answer?

Generally, prevention is the best way to handle headaches. Almost always they are a sign of something else, part and parcel of a larger picture of health problems. Chronic headaches that are unresolved should be evaluated medically.

For garden-variety, occasional headaches we can make some recommendations for handling them naturally, assuming that you handle the long-term issues and remove from your life the likely causes of your headaches.

Headaches can have many different causes. Tension, injuries, infections such as the flu, high blood pressure, too much caffeine, digestive distress, sinus problems, ear problems, jaw and teeth conditions, eyesight issues, too much sun, food allergies, bad posture, muscle tension, spinal misalignment, PMS, low blood sugar, pollution or environmental toxins, liver congestion, brain tumors, and more can cause headaches. Of course, you can narrow this list considerably by paying attention to the circumstances that commonly surround your headaches.

Occasional headaches can be treated effectively using the following herbs.

You can go back to aspirin's natural roots by seeking relief from the herbs themselves. **White willow bark** was a precursor to aspirin. Salicylic acid (the chemical name for aspirin) was first purified from the plant in Italy in 1838.[1] Try 1 ounce as tea (capsules are not practical with this mild and spongy herb). **Cinchona bark** is synergistic with willow bark for pain—5 to 10 capsules usually works well.

Meadowsweet, like willow bark, contains salicylates (a class of compounds), and yielded those chemical components for the synthesis of aspirin; in fact, the root word for aspirin comes from the botanical name for meadowsweet: *spirea*. It relieves nausea and vomiting as well as pain, so it's good for headaches with accompanying digestive distress. Again, up to 1 ounce as tea is the usual dose.

These can take longer to go into effect than aspirin, but many people find that the effect also lasts longer, and most people can use them indefinitely without concern about irritation to the stomach lining.

Turmeric is analgesic. Like capsaicin, an active ingredient in **chilies**, it depletes the pain-transmitting neurotransmitter called substance P. Capsaicin increases circulation and is scientifically proven to reduce pain neurologically. Both can be used for headache—chilies in very small amounts in capsules, working up to comfort level, and turmeric in capsules or up to 1 tablespoon of powder in water or as paste (see page 497 for recipe and uses).

Chinese corydalis tuber and **Chinese notopterygii root** are both used for headache pain as well as muscular aches and pains. About 1 to 1½ ounces as tea is usually effective.

A tried-and-true "folk remedy" that I personally have found to work better than anything I might swallow is *peppermint oil* around the temples, forehead, and neck. This does a remarkable job for tension headaches. Like so many remedies, the topical use of essential oils as analgesic is now being scientifically verified after hundreds of years of traditional use. Naturopath Don Brown reviewed one study that suggests a handful of mechanisms to explain peppermint oil's effectiveness—among others, peppermint oil inhibits substance-P induced smooth muscle contraction in animals and relaxes pericranial muscles by blocking calcium channels. Brown also notes that a study comparing topical essential oil treatment with acetaminophen is currently under way in Germany.[2] Eucalyptus oil has also been noted as being effective for headaches, and a paste made by mixing ginger with either peppermint oil or eucalyptus oil also works well for some people.

MIGRAINES

Migraines are headaches that result from spasms of intracranial blood vessels, which causes dilation of extracranial blood vessels. There appear to be two kinds of migraines. One is referred to as "classic," and involves a distinct, hard-to-describe spacey sensation beforehand called an aura, sometimes with visual disturbances. The other is called "common," and has no aura. Either may involve sensitivity to light and noise; some start on one side of the head.

Migraines are usually a multifaceted situation and require investigation and step-by-step balancing to get them handled. Some natural health practitioners believe there is a food-allergy component to migraines (Dr. Joseph Pizzorno, N.D., a president of Bastyr University naturopathic college in Seattle, declares that 80 percent of migraines are due to food allergies[3]). Others relate migraines to overall toxicity, especially liver congestion or candida overgrowth. Stress also appears to be a major factor, and severe muscle tension can contribute. Certain foods are widely discouraged for migraine sufferers because of compounds in them that seem to trigger expansion of blood vessels. These include chocolate, cheese, beer, and wine.

Prescription migraine medications can be toxic, are often ineffective, and, according to Dr. Andrew Weil, can cause a rebound headache once you stop taking them, making them if anything a last resort.[4] Fortunately, natural medicine offers several standout remedies for treating migraines. Here are the most effective and substantiated ones:

In Karta Purkh's observation, *ginger* is the absolute best remedy for treating a migraine at the time when it develops, and is one of the few things that will work at the time. Stir 2 tablespoons of ginger powder into water and drink it at the onset of the "aura," preferably before the pain starts. Usually that will knock it cold. The migraine may try to restart in about four hours, in which case you have to do this again.

Freeze-dried feverfew is used as a preventive, and often can be effective after a few days. You only need to take enough to prevent the migraines, so it's important to experiment with dose. The dose you need may be higher than is indicated on packaging—up to 6 or 8 capsules per day. Feverfew extracts are sold in 125-milligram capsules or tablets standardized for 0.2% parthenolides (the active ingredient).

Feverfew was discovered in the 1940s as a cure for migraine by British gardeners, who noticed that a tea brewed from its leaves relieved painful headache symptoms.[5] Research shows that the herb reduces inflammation and fever, slows blood vessel reaction to prostaglandins that cause vessel dilation, and lessens the number and intensity of migraines. Feverfew also short-circuits the release of serotonin by hooking onto blood platelets. Unless held in check, serotonin triggers blood vessels to dilate and constrict, causing the "aura" and excruciating pain.

Studies at the London Migraine Clinic and at the University of Nottingham clearly demonstrated that feverfew effectively reduced the number and severity of migraines in participants. Follow-up studies have shown that feverfew inhibits the release of blood-vessel-dilating substances from platelets, inhibits production of inflammatory substances, and reestablishes proper blood-vessel tone.[6]

One woman I know, Jeannette R., uses feverfew as a preventive after years of debilitating migraines (she would throw up all day and be almost unable to move). After she had tried several drugs, her doctor told her there was nothing else he could do. Based on her own research, she began taking feverfew and has not had a migraine for over four years. For her, only 1 tablet per day is all it takes.

Rosemary is recommended by many natural healing practitioners for migraine prevention. Use 1/4 ounce of the herb as tea daily. This is also effective for nonmigraine headaches.

BACK PAIN

Back pain can be handled with the same pain relievers described above. Back pain can be a mechanical problem requiring the care of a chiropractor, osteopath, physical therapist, or orthopedist; chronic back pain is also highly responsive to mind-body approaches (we recommend Dr. John Sarno's *Healing Back Pain* for more on this). However, herbs can be a useful adjunct to other therapies to relieve pain and inflammation naturally without side effects.

For example, **Chinese ox knee root** is used in Chinese medicine specifically for back and knee pain, and **Chinese morinda root** is indicated specifically for low back pain. Other herbs, foods, and spices that heal muscle and other soft-tissue inflammation and injury include *turmeric* (as directed earlier), **Arnica montana** (homeopathic—8 pellets per day), **feverfew** (1 ounce as tea or capsules), **ginseng** (capsules or powder), **licorice root** (tea to tolerance or 5 capsules), **cinnamon** (10 to 20 capsules), **cinchona bark** in combination with **white willow bark** (they are synergestic; see "Headaches," this chapter), **yucca root** (10 capsules), **Chinese wild ginger** (10 capsules), and **Chinese notopterygii root** (10 capsules).

Chilies, garlic, celery juice, saffron in milk (1/2 teaspoon of herb cooked in milk, an Ayurvedic remedy for acute trauma), **raw potato juice, cherry, pineapple juice**, and **sage, parsley, rosemary,** and **basil** are also all anti-inflammatory for pain.

Herbs that promote healing include **gotu kola, turmeric, sarsaparilla root, hawthorn berry, arjuna, frankincense, myrrh, guggul** or **boswellia,** and **devil's claw**. These are also anti-inflammatory and provide some pain relief.

One seventy-five-year-old man Karta Purkh talked to had experienced chronic back pain for forty years, had tried everything, and nothing was doing the job. After discussing the problem with Karta Purkh, the man decided to try **cayenne**. He started taking a little bit, increased his tolerance, and within a week his back pain had completely disappeared for the first time in forty years. Six cayenne capsules a day controlled all pain. This may sound simple, but such a cure can be very profound in daily life.

22

Herbs for Digestion

D igestive trouble is probably as common as headache when it comes to low-grade health irritations that interfere with people's daily lives. (An anti-ulcer medication is currently among the world's best-selling prescription drugs, and the market for heartburn drugs tops $1 billion.) And there are probably as many possible causes for "stomach upset" as there are for headache, including poor diet, nutritional imbalances, stress or nervousness, infection, candida-related conditions, allergy, pharmaceutical use (especially nonsteroidal anti-inflammatories, or NSAIDs), or food poisoning, to name a few.

For a long-term and big-picture approach to dealing with digestive problems, we make the same basic recommendations as we do for headaches: Simply, a healthy person should not experience such pain or distress more than very occasionally. If you have consistent, ongoing digestive problems, you should see your health practitioner for an appropriate diagnosis to rule out any serious conditions as the cause of your discomforts. Then consult a skilled natural health practitioner if you want to pursue a holistic approach to dealing with the problem.

Speaking of holistic approaches, we must once again remind you that basics must be handled before you can expect much from treatment, regardless of the remedies you choose. Digestive problems are often caused by, or at least exacerbated by, unhealthy lifestyle choices. If you are living a high-stress life and eating a high-fat, high-meat, high-sugar diet (or eating only infrequently, and then only junk food), and/or drinking, smoking, and taking drugs, digestive distress would not be a surprising outcome. In that case, simply cleaning up those issues alone may resolve your problems. It will be difficult for any remedy to truly help heal you in an environment that is unfavorable to healing, and if the problem is not eliminated at the source(s).

Drugs that only mask your symptoms and allow you to continue the overall lifestyle abuse are inadvisable. By simply blocking an effect and not addressing the cause, you not only will fail to heal the condition permanently, but you can also cause further problems.

For example, popular OTC ulcer medications called H2 antagonists (such as Pepcid, Tagamet, and newly OTC Zantac) actually suppress the stomach's production of gastric juices (rather than just neutralizing them after they have formed, as "older" antacids do). Prolonged use can mask the normally severe pain of gastroesophageal reflux, in which stomach acids back up into the esophagus and eat away at its inner lining.[1] They also cause other digestive upsets because stomach acids are important to digestion and nutrient assimilation. Blocking a key function of digestion can cause nausea, constipation, diarrhea, and nutrient deficiencies. Liver damage, hair loss, headaches, dizziness, depression, insomnia, impotence, and other side effects are also possible from these drugs.[2] And they don't cure ulcers; continued reliance on the drugs is required for continued relief. Rebound recurrence is standard with these medications.

With that in mind, the occasional digestive upset can be soothed and healing can be supported with gentle, natural substances. These herbal remedies are divided by categories of digestive problems.

NAUSEA

The following herbs can be used to treat nausea.

Ginger—Antinausea is a use for ginger that has been well known in herbal medicine for a long time, but has just recently come to the attention of the medical profession. At least four double-blind trials show ginger's efficacy against nausea.[3] Ginger has been found to be effective for relieving motion sickness, seasickness, postoperative nausea and vomiting, and chemotherapy-associated nausea and vomiting. Ginger even beats the OTC drug Dramamine hands down in controlled studies—with just 2 capsules of ordinary ginger powder. And because ginger works locally on the digestive system and not on the central nervous system, it does not cause drowsiness. Fresh ginger powder can be capsuled by you or purchased precapsuled (which may be more convenient but possibly less potent). Powder can be used to make tea as well. Ginger tinctures are also available.

To prevent motion sickness, take two capsules 1/2 to 1 hour before the trip and then again as needed. Crystallized ginger can be chewed to prevent nausea. (Be aware that it contains sugar, however.) Studies show that giving ginger prior to surgery can reduce postoperative nausea that sometimes results from anesthesia. For morning sickness, first consult your own natural health practitioner. See pregnancy cautions on page 206.

Meadowsweet—Soothing and also good for headache pain. Take 1 to 6 capsules or 1/2 ounce as tea.

Black horehound leaf—This combines well with meadowsweet and chamomile. Take 1 to 10 capsules or 1/2 ounce as tea.

Cinnamon—Take 1 to 6 capsules, or make a tea out of 1 teaspoon of powder to a cup of water.

Spearmint, peppermint—These are soothing and cooling as well as antinausea.

CONSTIPATION

The following herbs can be used to treat constipation. Also see Chapter 14, "Herbal Renewal: Cleanse, Detox, Rebuild," for more information on herbs for constipation. Do not use if you have diarrhea or abdominal pain.

Senna leaf—This one is stronger than most of the others listed, considered to be "purgative." Originally from India, it's now a popular European remedy. One to 5 capsules or 1/8 ounce as tea.

Cascara bark—A bitter Pacific Northwest bark that's as strong as senna, it must be cured for 1 to 2 years to reduce potency. One to 5 capsules a day.

Aloe vera—The juice offers a soothing effect on membranes and a liquefying effect on intestinal contents, along with bowel stimulation. Can be taken as juice (2 tablespoons) or 6 to 8 capsules per day.

Triphala—Extremely gentle and mild for all ages; 6 to 8 capsules will stimulate a bowel movement in about 8 hours.

Buckthorn bark—Yet another purgative (slightly milder than senna or cascara); 1 to 5 capsules per day.

Rhubarb root—Also called Asian rhubarb or turkey rhubarb. This one's on the mild side. **Licorice root** and **butternut bark** are even milder options, as is *rose petal*, an Ayurvedic remedy. All may be taken at a dose of 2 to 10 capsules per day.

Slippery elm bark is a demulcent, meaning it contains mucilage, a coating, healing, gelatinous substance. So does **marshmallow root**, which may be used with slippery elm or by itself. Two to 4 heaping tablespoons of either powder, mixed with water (or into yogurt, oatmeal, applesauce, honey, or maple syrup) makes a paste that increases stool motility and nourishes and heals mucous membranes of the digestive tract.

Castor oil—A good way to moisten the stool, and purgative in its own right. Take 1 to 2 tablespoons.

Wheat bran, rice bran, psyllium seed, chia seed, flaxseed—All sources of fiber, which creates bulk so the large intestine has something to grip on and squeeze. Flaxseed also exerts its own laxative effect. Insoluble fiber (bran) additionally has a "scraping action" to clean the intestine. One-quarter teaspoon, increasing to maximum tolerance as needed.

Fruit pectins—Provide soluble fiber that absorbs toxins in the intestinal tract. Whole-food sources include apples, bananas, citrus, carrots, and oats; can also be purchased as powder or supplements.

DIARRHEA

The following herbs can be used to treat diarrhea. Diarrhea that lasts for more than a few days with no improvement, especially in children, should be checked out by a health professional.

Cinnamon—A classic Ayurvedic diarrhea remedy; 1 to 10 capsules as needed.

Cloves—Another warming and effective diarrhea remedy from India; 1 to 10 capsules as needed.

Acacia gum—This Middle Eastern herb effectively "binds" the stool; 1 to 10 capsules as needed.

Cranesbill root—This very effective North American diarrhea remedy can be used as a powder; 1 to 2 tablespoons stirred into water or bland food, or 1 to 10 capsules as needed.

Blackberry root—A European and North American remedy; 1 to 10 capsules as needed.

Haritaki—One of the three fruits that goes into the Ayurvedic remedy triphala, this bitter, astringent fruit by itself treats diarrhea in small doses (1 to 3 capsules). (Interestingly, in larger doses it is laxative.)

Kutaj—Another excellent Ayurvedic remedy; 1 to 10 capsules as needed.

Carob powder—An excellent stool tightener; take 2 heaping table-spoons mixed into yogurt, honey, or even just water, several times a day as tolerated. This is also a good long-term strategy for chronically loose stool.

Dried blueberry—This popular European remedy should be used to comfort level. Do *not* use fresh berries, which could make diarrhea worse!

Live *acidophilus* and *bifidus* culture—These are not herbs; they are cultures of the helpful and friendly bacteria that colonize and dominate the healthy intestine. A regular daily dose of **Lactobacillus acidophilus** and **Bifidobacterium bifidus** can often clear up diarrhea quickly.

From a natural-healing point of view, loose stool may be caused by lack of proper large-intestine bacteria. The use of antibiotics and other drugs, faulty diet (highly refined, low fiber), candida overgrowth, and other factors can upset the natural balance of intestinal flora, and diarrhea can be one of the outcomes. Many parents find that their babies or children develop chronic diarrhea after a course of antibiotics because the beneficial bacteria in the colon have been killed. (This can happen to adults, too.) Diarrhea resulting from this is often completely cured by large doses of potent aci-dophilus. Buy only the live, active "super" cultures in a high-potency form (usually refrigerated in powder form or capsules at the natural-foods store).

GAS

The following herbs effectively treat gas.

Asafoetida—Called *hing* in Ayurvedic medicine, this garlicky-smelling spice containing sulfur compounds can be used in capsules; 2 to 3 as needed.

All seeds from the umbellifer family (which also includes carrot)—including *fennel, dill, ajwain, cumin, caraway, anise,* or *coriander*—make exceptionally effective anti-gas remedies. Of these, fennel is probably the premier anti-gas remedy in the world. All can be used in capsules (1 to 10) as needed, or as tea, or cooked in food. Cardamom, from the same family as ginger, is also excellent for relieving gas.

Clove and *sage* are also excellent anti-gas spices, each appropriate at 1 to 10 capsules.

GENERAL DIGESTIVE TONICS

The following herbs can be used as general digestive tonics, to prevent or control garden-variety indigestion. These remedies may work by warming the digestive tract, stimulating digestive secretions, and/or soothing the membrane.

Asafoetida (hing) may be used in capsules or juice as described above. Its sulfur compounds are detoxifying.

Bittermelon contains a compound with insulin-like action—a "plant insulin" that helps regulate blood sugar. Bitter herbs also stimulate digestive secretions. You can take a 1- to 2-ounce shot of juice (remember, it's bitter!) before a meal, once a day.

Green bitter orange fruit, gentian, barberry, and *goldenseal* are all bitter "digestants"—they stimulate digestive secretions such as bile, saliva, and gastric juices. They should be taken up to 20 minutes before or with a meal (2 or 3 capsules of any one of those).

Peppermint is a good cooling, soothing heartburn preventive, either a strong cup of tea or 2 capsules per meal. *Spearmint* is a good substitute.

Dashmula (Sanskrit for "ten roots") is a warming, stimulating Ayurvedic combination that may be taken in capsules (1 to 5) or powdered in food.

Aloe vera makes a soothing general digestive tonic, as described earlier. It's cleansing and anti-inflammatory.

Mugwort leaf is a digestive stimulant; take 2 capsules with a meal.

Meadowsweet soothes and protects membranes, relieves nausea, reduces hyperacidity, and is a pain-relieving anodyne. Take 1 to 3 capsules per meal, or 1 to 2 teaspoons of the herb brewed as tea.

Papaya leaf contains papain, an enzyme that assists with protein digestion. Take 1 to 3 capsules or tablets per meal.

Wild cherry bark is a mild digestive soother and healer, good for kids because the tea is tasty. One cup of tea per meal or 2 capsules if preferred.

Slippery elm bark and *marshmallow root* are excellent general soothers as detailed earlier; use 2 to 4 heaping tablespoons of the powder daily as needed.

Cardamom, clove, and *cinnamon* all make excellent warming, soothing digestive tonics, especially as tasty teas, 1 to 2 cups per day (use 1 teaspoon of the herb to a cup of water). They may be used singly or combined, to taste.

Ginger promotes healthy digestion by warming the intestinal tract and stimulating gastric juices, gallbladder activity, and muscular activity of the stomach and intestines.

Basil and **bay leaf** are mild, warming digestive tonics that may be used as tea or in capsules, 1 to 2 per day.

ULCER

This inflammation and erosion of mucosal lining in the gastrointestinal tract causes pain and burning, and in cases that are allowed to progress, hemorrhaging. Medical understanding of this condition has a volatile history. Formerly accused villains such as spicy foods have been cleared, and formerly prescribed remedies like milk have proven harmful. Once believed the result of smoking, alcohol, and stress, ulcer is now largely attributed to a bacterium, *Helicobacter pylori*.

In fact, this is a well-documented example of a medical paradigm shift: Dr. Barry J. Marshall, the Australian scientist who gathered clinical evidence to support the theory that ulcers are often caused by a bacterium, was vilified when he first presented substantial data at a conference in 1983. In 1995, his data was validated and he won an Albert Lasker Award—almost fifteen years after he was first castigated for his "ridiculous" theory. Now *Helicobacter pylori* is the widely accepted explanation for ulcers.

Most natural healing practitioners agree that even if this bacterium is the culprit, there is a multitude of environmental factors that allow the bacteria actually to proliferate in the gut, including depletion of friendly bacteria and overproduction of stomach acids, to which stress, poor diet, and pharmaceutical drug use certainly contribute. As Dr. Michael T. Murray, N.D., succinctly puts it, "H. pylori can be compared to flies on garbage. The flies do not cause the garbage."[4] Ulcers can also be found in people with normal levels of hydrochloric acid. That's why natural healing focuses on supporting the patient's tissue-healing and -repair mechanisms (which can be depleted and weakened by poor self-care and bad habits), rather than simply suppressing stomach acids.

Suppressive prescription drugs for ulcers can cause rebound effects and mask serious problems (as described at the start of this chapter). Since the acceptance of *Helicobacter pylori* as a cause of ulcer, antibiotic therapy is sometimes now prescribed as well. However, natural health practitioners frown on this too, as antibiotic use destroys healthy intestinal flora and thus causes a host of other digestive difficulties. Ironically, the ability of H. Pylori to take hold in the first place means that friendly bacteria—which normally outnumber and control the "unfriendlies"—must be depleted to begin with. How does that happen? Antibiotics, for one.

Some very popular drugs are also known to be ulcer causing, including aspirin, cortisone, and the nonsteroidal anti-inflammatories (NSAIDs), such as ibuprofen, prescribed for a wide variety of conditions. NSAIDs can cause fatal stomach hemorrhages even among people who don't take heavy doses, with a significant number of deaths every year, according to Andrew Weil, M.D.[5]

NSAIDs cause one-third of bleeding ulcers, according to James Fries, professor of medicine at California's Stanford University. Ironically, many NSAID users chase drugs with more drugs, taking antacids to suppress the abdominal pain caused by the NSAID, masking the very symptoms that would point to a bleeding ulcer. "An excessive concern with pain relief gave us an epidemic of ten thousand to twenty thousand deaths from bleeding ulcers each year, and hospitalizations from the same condition for another one hundred thousand to two hundred thousand," Fries said at the American Medical Association's Science Reporters' Conference.[6]

Natural Ulcer Treatment and Prevention

Thus lifestyle once again represents the foundation for ulcer prevention and healing. Ulcer responds remarkably well to natural therapies without harsher medicines. And natural therapies, as always, work best when general health is supported by good diet, exercise, and stress management, elimination of clearly unhealthy habits, and avoidance of ulcer-causing drugs. All of these are cornerstones for self-healing and tissue-repair capacity.

For both prevention and healing, cigarettes and alcohol should be eliminated, and plenty of fiber should be included in the diet (low-fiber diets may contribute to ulcer, because fiber helps create a layer of protective mucin in the stomach and intestinal linings, and that can absorb excess gastric juices). It's also important to avoid yeast-producing dietary habits, such as a high processed-sugar intake, since yeast can alter the intestinal lining.

Milk should be avoided, even though in the past it has been touted as a remedy. Milk triggers the release of the hormone gastrin and actually increases stomach-acid production and inflammation. According to Dr. Murray, population studies show that the higher the milk consumption, the greater the likelihood of an ulcer.[7]

Besides, milk can cause other digestive problems. In *Food: Your Miracle Medicine*, author and nutritionist Jean Carper notes that lactose-intolerance symptoms are often misdiagnosed as much more serious bowel conditions. She quotes one internist who has seen hundreds of people spend years and thousands of dollars trying to find the cause of their bowel symptoms; when he tells them to eliminate dairy products, the immediate and radical improvement changes their lives.

The following herbs and foods can be used to treat ulcer naturally.

Cabbage—Juiced and in soup, cabbage should be taken to maximum tolerance for ulcer (minimum 2 glasses per day, up to 4 if possible). It is highly effective for actually healing the ulcer, probably the leading natural remedy for this condition. The mechanism is unclear, and some natural healing authorities believe there is more than one mechanism. Some theorize that a substance isolated from cabbage, first dubbed "vitamin U" by researcher Dr. Garnett Cheney in the 1950s,[8] may actually control the proliferation of *Helicobacter pylori*. Others point to the tissue-healing and anti-inflammatory compounds in cabbage, including sulfur compounds and the amino acid glutamine. Whatever the case, it works—and it heals, doesn't just mask symptoms.

Licorice root—Also a widely respected natural ulcer remedy, licorice root can be taken at about 6 capsules a day for best effect. You can also chew wafers, 2 to 3 before each meal. The wafers seem to be more effective; it is theorized that DGL may trigger release of salivary compounds that stimulate regeneration of stomach and intestinal cells.[9]

Be sure to use deglycyrrhizinated licorice root (DGL). This has the adrenal-stimulating compound glycyrrhizin removed, so that there is no risk of raising blood pressure regardless of dose. (We discuss the differences between whole licorice root and DGL on page 481.) The flavonoid compounds that remain in the DGL are believed to stimulate normal defense and repair mechanisms.

Licorice root, like the compounds in cabbage, doesn't mask ulcer symptoms or block the function of digestive-tract-lining cells. Instead, it actually helps the membrane lining of the GI tract repair itself. Numerous studies show that DGL licorice prevents ulcer recurrence better than prescription acid blockers.[10] For short-term relief and long-term prevention, head-to-head comparison studies have shown DGL to be more effective than Tagamet, Zantac (formerly prescription, recently approved by FDA for OTC sale), and antacids.[11] In fact, Zantac and Tagamet have the highest recurrence rate among anti-ulcer treatments.[12] And a month's supply of one of these H2 antagonists costs four times as much as the monthly dose of DGL.

Cayenne pepper—Once hot spices were implicated as a cause of or aggravating of ulcers, but recent studies show that they do not cause or worsen ulcers. A few studies actually suggest that—believe it or not—hot peppers can help. Capsaicin is theorized to stimulate nerve fibers to release a hormone that signals for more blood flow to the area.[13] Small amounts to tolerance, long term, may actually stimulate a protective response.

Ginger, a well-known anti-inflammatory, also appears to increase the production of stomach-protective substances for an anti-ulcer effect. It is also an excellent general digestive tonic, as described earlier.

Peppermint tea is cooling and soothing. Brew strong and drink as needed.

Good membrane soothers include *alfalfa leaf* and *plantain leaf* (for either, 1/2 ounce tea or 2 to 5 capsules) and parsley leaf, juiced, to maximum tolerance. *Marshmallow root* or *slippery elm bark* are mucilaginous, coating soothers and may be taken daily as described above.

As discussed elsewhere, *goldenseal* and *turmeric* are also excellent membrane healers. Goldenseal may be taken in capsules, 3 to 5 per day until the ulcer is healed. Turmeric is membrane healing and anti-inflammatory, and can be taken up to 1 tablespoon of powder per day or 5 to 10 capsules. Turmeric can be taken indefinitely to promote healing and tissue repair, and to prevent recurrence.

TURMERIC

Turmeric deserves special mention before we close this chapter. Ayurveda's leading digestive tonic and remedy, it works for almost every category of discomfort listed above. It treats typical indigestion by increasing mucin and enzyme secretions in the gastric juices. It reduces gas, and kills intestinal parasites. Hemorrhoids respond particularly well to turmeric, which, in addition to oral use, can be applied topically as a paste. Turmeric-based hemorrhoid creams are widely available in Asia. (The paste is bright yellow, however, so you can end up being yellow where you don't want to be yellow! Only temporarily, though.)

One of Karta Purkh's most dramatic stories is one he observed at the office of an Ayurvedic doctor. A patient was brought in pumping bright red blood from the rectum; they were heading for the emergency room and wanted to know if there was anything that could be done before crisis intervention. The doctor mixed 2 heaping tablespoons of turmeric and 2 heaping tablespoons of parsley powder into a bowl of yogurt and had the patient eat it as quickly as possible. Within five minutes, the bleeding completely stopped and never started again. He went to the hospital, but was not treated. With continued treatment using food and herbs at home, the individual was able to take care of the whole problem.

Part IV

Living It: Herbs in Practice

23

Living It: Herbs in Practice

his chapter will cover a range of practical issues and "how-tos" for integrating herbs into your daily life. Forms and preparations, dosages, sources and standards, storage, and related topics will be covered. We'll also discuss how to choose herbs and herbal practitioners, whom to trust (and not) in a crowded and unregulated environment, generic one-size-fits-all herbal products, and when to consult a medical doctor.

FORMS AND PREPARATIONS

There are a number of forms in which herbs can be used, and several common ways to prepare them. There is no one best way—the "ideal" form and preparation varies from herb to herb, as well as from person to person.

Some herbs are almost equally effective and beneficial in a variety of forms; others have one definite best preparation and other ways of preparing them that are adequate but not nearly as effective. Still others may have one and only one way they can be effectively used.

"Best" is usually defined as the way to get the most active ingredient out of the herb. However, in other cases the "best" preparation or form may be the only way to use the herb safely. For example, stinging nettles are only used dried, so that they no longer sting. And only special processing such as freeze-drying, preserves their antihistamine compound. Cascara bark must be dried and aged so that its effects (laxative) are mellowed; when fresh these effects are more harsh than anyone would wish to experience. Thus some herbs must be processed in some way, while others are more effective with less processing.

Some active ingredients are more soluble in alcohol than in water, and these herbs are best taken as a tincture. Some herbs are more soluble in water, milk, or oil. Some are not soluble in liquid at all and must be dried and powdered.

"Best" may also be defined as how the individual is practically able to consume it. If the "best" way to obtain the active ingredients of a particular herb is dried and powdered in a capsule but your child cannot swallow a capsule, then this is not the best way for her to take the herb. For her, a tincture would be better—because taking it is better than not taking it at all, and the difference in effectiveness between capsules and tincture may be marginal.

Another consideration in determining the "best" form is whether the herb is weak and mild, or very strong and potent. Mild herbs are best brewed as tea, not only because their mildness makes them inherently drinkable, but also because you'd have to capsule so much of a mild herb to get an adequate dose that you would be faced with a possibly prohibitive number of pills to swallow. With such herbs, it may be easier to drink a lot of liquid, and you can brew it strong to reduce the amount of liquid consumed.

By the same token, very strong herbs may be too bitter, too astringent, or just plain too awful tasting to consume as tea. And if an herb is so strong that only a few capsules will do the trick, why go to the trouble of making tea?

Fresh versus Broken Down

Most herbs are processed in some way before we consume them; it's rare (though of course not unheard of) that we walk out to our gardens, snips a leaf off of a medicinal herb, and chomp it down. Most often, that leaf (or the root, rhizome, flower, or berry) is dried, brewed into a tea, ground and put in capsules, or soaked in alcohol or glycerine.

People often ask, "But doesn't processing reduce an herb's potency?" They want to know if it's worth using at all if it's processed. The answer is yes. The ideal in most (though not all) cases would be to use the herb fresh and whole. If you ingest a fresh herb whole, you are assured of getting 100 percent of the active ingredients at their fullest strength. However, for many reasons that ideal can be unattainable. It often simply isn't practical or possible to consume an herb totally unprocessed.

First, processing provides convenience. Most of us don't have time to wildcraft or go out and gather our own herbs. Second, fresh herbs don't last—usually some kind of processing is necessary to preserve an herb if you plan to keep it for more than a few days. Third, if you relied only on fresh harvests, there would be times during the year when the herbs you needed were not growing.

Fourth, some herbs are not as safe or effective when fresh (though these are a small minority), such as stinging nettles and cascara bark, as mentioned above. Raw garlic also upsets some people's stomachs; if so, cooked or even dried garlic is going to be better than none at all. (If anything makes you feel really bad or uncomfortable, you should discontinue using it.)

Fifth, processing sometimes allows for more acceptable taste. If drying, powdering, and capsuling a valuable herb makes it consumable, whereas its acrid odor might preclude its use any other way, then there is value in that processing—because the herb gets used.

In most cases it's true that some active ingredient or nutrient value is lost, to some degree, each time an herb or food is processed or cooked. Powdering and drying may cause some active constituents to be lost, or to lose some potency. Simmering a decoction lets some volatile principles evaporate away. Brewing a tea doesn't necessarily release all of the constituents of the herb into the water. Making a tincture doesn't assure that all of the compounds are released into the alcohol or other base.

But even though all of that is true, herbs produce results even in an imperfect world. What we are able to get out of them clearly yields value. We know that most herbs are consumed in these ways, and most herbs used in successful experiments were processed in one of these ways. So whatever sacrifices in quality or potency we accept do not seem ultimately to compromise effectiveness. For example, when I boil into a broth astragalus that has already been dried, I have gone about two steps down the processing line (drying the herb; cooking the herb), but the broth has definitely worked wonders for me as a cold and flu preventive.

Going for perfection, and then achieving nothing because that goal made life impossible and you gave up, is the most ineffective way to use herbs. If we dismiss processing because it might reduce effectiveness by some unmeasurable but probably marginal degree, we would eliminate the use of many herbs.

Tea

Teas are the most popular way to take herbs in most other cultures of the world. In the traditional cultures that were the origins of holistic natural medicine, teas (and broths and soups) are a cradle-to-grave part of everyone's lifestyle.

Even in our own culture today, tea is the best form of choice if the herbs are mild; it is also usually the least expensive. Some advantages of tea use: The entire herb is usually used; no binders, additives, or alcohol are involved; it's usually inexpensive, easily swallowed, and convenient for high doses. Disadvantages: It can be time consuming, inconvenient to prepare, bad tasting, and require high-volume intake. Tea also spoils more quickly than capsules or tincture and doesn't travel well.

Making Tea

There are many ways to make an herbal tea or broth. The two most common are *infusions* and *decoctions*. For an infusion you steep the herb in water that has already boiled; for a decoction you simmer or boil the herb itself.

Infusions are best for delicate flowers, soft leaves, berries, and herbs with strong odors or volatile oils. Examples would be nettle leaves, passionflower, chamomile, or coltsfoot. To make an infusion, pour boiled water over herbs in a container and seal the container tightly (this will prevent volatile oils from escaping). A French coffee press is ideal for this. Keep the tea in a warm place and steep for a minimum of 30 to 60 minutes (or for a maximum of 12 hours). The active ingredient in most herbs comes out in the first hour of steeping.

Decoctions are best for sturdy, coarse, tough herbs that need to be broken down—roots, barks, tougher leaves and stems, as well as peppercorns. Examples include astragalus, dong quai, or willow bark. Herbs with volatile oils are usually not decocted because the volatile oils are dissipated by evaporation. To make a decoction, place the herbs directly in a pot of water and bring to a boil. Reduce heat to simmer, and simmer covered for 30 to 60 minutes. Expect liquid to decrease by half. Strain. If possible, squeeze the used herb to "wring out" the last of the "juice" after straining.

For either an infusion or a decoction, a standard rule of thumb for quantity is 1 ounce of herb to every pint (2 cups) of water. For convenience, you can make either infusions or decoctions in large "batches" and store them for up to a week in the fridge. They can be consumed cold straight out of the fridge (for speed and convenience, this is my strategy), although for certain illnesses a warm (reheated, if necessary) tea is beneficial, such as to reduce chills or induce sweating. Keep the tea in a tightly sealed container, preferably glass.

For some herbs, cold water, milk, or other substances are actually more effective in drawing out the active ingredient than hot water. With some teas, the active ingredient is not soluble in water. It takes more sophistication to understand these nuances as you get farther and farther into herbal medicine. An experienced herbalist can educate you about the more intricate distinctions involved in preparing the herbs you use. However, if you are not aware of these subtleties you will still get value out of the herbs you take; this simply goes back to the issue of ideals versus realities. For example, when it was suggested that my husband use the herb gotu kola to make a tea in milk to maximize its active ingredients, he simply never used it. When Karta Purkh assured him that the tea in water was better than no tea at all, he began to use the tea daily. This was a classic case of the compromise being more effective, in practice, than the ideal.

Regardless of the type of tea, whenever possible you should use filtered, purified, or spring water—rather than tap water—to make tea. (Hopefully you are drinking purified water on a regular basis anyway.) Also, try to avoid metallic containers. (Metals from the container can interact with tea ingredients.) Prepare teas using glass, enamel, or earthenware pots. If you must use a metallic container, use stainless steel.

Two excellent tools for making tea are the plunger-style French press normally used for coffee (large ones can be purchased for as little as $20), and an Asian herb cooker (also called a tea cooker), which can be purchased at most large Asian groceries for $60 to $80. The French press is good for infusions (pouring boiled water over the herbs and steeping, then pressing). The herb cooker keeps the herb at the right temperature for the right amount of time.

Teas brewed mildly (beverage strength) can be taken in doses as high as 4 to 8 cups a day for adults, depending on the condition. (Teas that should not be taken in such high doses are ephedra [ma huang], rosemary, and green tea.)

For a strong decoction, use 1 ounce herb to 1 pint (2 cups) water. When squeezed out, this should yield about 1½ cups of strong medicine tea, a typical daily dose. This can be taken by sips or by the tablespoon (2 to 4 per half-hour or hour). This is especially useful for children.

Dried/Capsuled Herbs

In almost all cases there will be some loss of nutrient or active constituents due to drying and cutting or powdering, but there is still obviously a great deal of value remaining in dried capsuled herbs or they would not be such a popular way to take herbs.

Capsules have many advantages: Drying and grinding preserves fresh herbs that otherwise would die; the process also reduces volume and concentrates the herb. The properties of some herbs are actually enhanced by drying. Other benefits include the use of the entire herb, convenience, absence of taste, long shelf life, and easy dosing.

On the downside, capsules are also more expensive, slower acting, and sometimes hard to swallow and/or digest.

Pills are an American medicine phenomenon. Other cultures do not use pills and capsules the way we do. Herbal medicines are typically taken as powders in Ayurveda, teas and soups in China, or tinctures in Europe.

In my family, I'm actually the most "Western" herb consumer. I prefer capsules for most of my herbs. My husband brews teas by the quart and swallows spoonfuls of cayenne pepper and turmeric daily. I drink astragalus broth because it's relatively mild and the benefits are so great, and I can also cook it into grains. And I'll drink the occasional willow bark tea or nettle tea. But almost everything else I take is capsuled. Some could be taken other ways, but then I might not take them at all.

We believe in doing what works and getting you started, not in being elitist about ideals. Some books say that capsules are bad because they promote or condone Western thinking: the expectations involved in taking a pill, the accompanying anticipation of unrealistic results. But we have to face that this thinking is exactly where most people are starting from when they begin experimenting with herbs. Capsules are a way for many people to get their foot in the door.

Start where you are and work up slowly. Taking an herbal pill instead of a pharmaceutical drug may be the first step in going natural; other steps may follow as you get into it and see results. Using herbal medicine is a slow process of experience and education; it didn't happen overnight for me or anyone I know. You'll do best if you start the process expecting that.

It's true that when you take "herbal pills" you have to realize you don't usually, for the most part, take one or two and instantly get better. *Quantity is different* and can be a problem if that is not understood. Still, herbal medicine does work in capsule form; the "pill-popping" *attitude* simply has to shift in its time. Just as I don't believe people should abandon all efforts at healthy eating if they can't eat "perfectly," I believe that if compromises for convenience keep you using herbs, then by all means make them.

Syrup

Syrups are mainly used by children. They are especially good for coughs and sore throats, since they are soothing and bring the herb in contact with the affected area. As discussed in Chapter 10, "Herbs for Babies and Children," there are a few commercially made herbal syrups, but not nearly as many as there were at the turn of the century when natural healing was closer to the forefront of medicine. Syrups can be made at home by adding honey or glycerine to a tea. Michael Tierra, in *The Way of Herbs*, suggests boiling a quart of water with 2 ounces of herb down to a pint of liquid, then adding 1 or 2 ounces of honey or glycerine.

Tinctures

Tinctures are liquid herbal preparations that have a much longer shelf life than teas. In a tincture, there is a base liquid used specifically for its abilities to preserve the herb and its components, retard spoilage, and draw out the active ingredients.

Tinctures are less expensive than capsules, yet still travel well. They are fast acting, easily swallowed and digested, and never lose potency. However, they may taste bad, often contain alcohol, all of the active ingredients may not be extracted, and the whole herb is not used. The necessary dose may also be more than you want to swallow.

The majority of commercial tinctures are made with alcohol as the carrier substance. Alcohol is a good preservative and in the case of most herbs is excellent at extracting active components. The herb is soaked in a solution of alcohol and water for a period of time. This can be done at home as well: Soak the herb in alcohol for 2 or 3 weeks and shake the solution several times a day. Vodka, whiskey, and other clear alcoholic liquors may be used. *Never use rubbing alcohol (isopropyl alcohol) for use internally!*

Other carrier solutions may be used at home and are available commercially as well, although they are harder to find. In some cases, alcohol is not the best medium for the herb's active constituents. It may destroy some nutrients and it breaks apart volatile oils.[1] Also, although the actual total amount of alcohol consumed when using an herbal tincture is extremely small, some people still prefer to avoid it completely; in the case of children especially. Vinegar and oil have been used from time to time, but both have very limited uses. In a few cases, water may be used.

After alcohol, the next most common and valuable base solution for tinctures is glycerine. This clear liquid with a syrup-like consistency is extremely useful for children, and that is its most common application as a tincture medium. It has excellent preservative properties—rivaling those of alcohol—and also does a good job of extracting many herbs' natural ingredients, although many herbalists feel this is not true in all cases and that alcohol remains superior overall. It has an advantage over alcohol for extracting volatile oils, but is less effective for gums and resins.

Glycerine is also naturally sweet, and this is another feature that makes it excellent for children's tinctures, since it can help to conceal the taste of bitter herbs. It is completely nontoxic, emollient (it is produced from fats and is an ingredient in many moisturizing lotions), and may have detoxifying properties of its own. Also, since it is a natural by-product of fat breakdown, and not a sugar, it does not raise blood sugar despite its sweetness.[2]

Steven Horne, A.H.G., suggests making herbal glycerites (glycerine-based tinctures) by simmering the herb in a mixture of 40 percent water and 60 percent glycerine.[3] (Glycerine can be purchased at any drugstore.) Strain, bottle, and store in a cool, dark place (the tincture does not need to be refrigerated).

Tincture Dosages

Karta Purkh feels that, unfortunately, tinctures are one of the most widely misunderstood forms of natural medicine. The primary misconception involves dosages. There is a very widespread impression (fostered largely by the dosages printed on the bottles) that you can put 3 drops of a tincture in some orange juice and get all better. These dosages are absurd, as are the 1-ounce dropper bottles in which these tinctures are most often sold.

Tinctures are *not* some superstrong medicine—they are no better or stronger than any other herbal medicines. "Maximum 1 to 10 drops" is rarely the dose that's effective; it's just the manufacturer's way of being cautious and conservative. It also reflects the company's anticipation of your expectations; it may be assumed that you simply won't take any more than a few drops.

This doesn't serve anyone, because it may render ineffective what could be a helpful product. Like herbs in any form, the dose needs to be adequate to be therapeutic. When inadequate doses predictably don't work, it reinforces the myth that herbs are "weak" or ineffectual medicine. Someone takes 5 drops of echinacea tincture and the cold doesn't disappear, so they write off herbs as medicine forever and tell all their friends.

A more realistic dosage for most tinctures is half an ounce per day *for adults*. Of course, in that case, one of those uneconomical little 1-ounce bottles represents a 2-day supply, usually for about $10. In Europe, where tinctures remain the most common form of herbal medicine, tinctures come in more sensible pints and quarts, so that appropriate dosages by the teaspoon or tablespoon are economical. Tinctures could be one-quarter to one-fifth of their current United States price if they were sold in such larger sizes.

At any rate, buy tinctures in the largest size you can find them and forget the eyedropper—use a spoon.

Tea Bags with Names

Your health-food store and even grocery store shelves are filled with boxes of name-brand tea bags, some of which claim to be medicinal. Unfortunately, they're not, although many of these may make very pleasant beverages.

These teas are the company's way to introduce you to the herb world in a palatable way. But they are beverages, not medicines. They are probably about nine-tenths flavoring and one-tenth active ingredient. Each tea bag generally contains about one-fifteenth of an ounce of herb, whereas medicinal teas generally require one-half to one full ounce of tea to a cup of water. And you pay for the tea bag itself. Obviously they are not an economical way to get your herbs.

It's fine and wonderful to drink a beverage with a bit of herb in it. But don't expect therapeutic results or you will be disappointed in "herbs" without ever knowing what they can really do when taken in proper medicinal doses.

GENERAL DOSAGE ISSUES

Adequate Dose Is Essential

As you have just seen with regard to tinctures and tea bags, dosages can be a problem with herbal medicine—but not in the way many people think. While in rare cases people have taken too much of an herb that should only be taken in small quantities, and it *is* crucial to distinguish those few herbs, the prevailing problem in herbal medicine is people not taking enough. This greatly undermines the effectiveness of herbal treatment.

There is a handful of herbs that are so strong that just a small dose has significant effects—but that's true of every drug. Yes, drugs are standardized and have standard dosages. But they need this, precisely because they are so strong. Most herbs aren't, and in fact are so mild and dilute that for a therapeutic effect you need to take a lot, much more than the standard dose of pharmaceuticals.

Most of us have been drilled to think in terms of pharmaceutical doses—and in terms of instant results. This thinking does not apply to herbs. You cannot take one herb capsule and expect the same kind of results as you might get from one drug capsule.

In most cases throughout the book, we have listed appropriate doses for recommended herbs in specific situations. **Doses where listed are** *per day,* **for one 150-pound person.** These doses represent *average* effective and safe doses based on any one or a combination of the following:

- The experience and observation of traditional healers in their cultures
- The experience and observation of American herbalists, other natural health practitioners, and educators, including Karta Purkh
- Effects suggested by scientific studies

It is always prudent to start with smaller doses and work up *as needed.*
When we specify capsules, we always mean "00" size gelatin capsules. Size "0" holds about half as much herb material. Size "0" may be appropriate for children. For adults, the "00" size is more practical. These can be purchased as "empties" and filled with bulk herb purchased from an herb pharmacy. When you buy bottles of precapsuled herb, it is often not possible to control whether you get "00"- or "0"-size capsules (not to mention the quality and freshness of the herb).

Throughout the book we also alert you to those uncommon herbs whose normal doses should be limited because of their natural potency. These cautions should be taken seriously.

Take with Food

Herbs, especially capsules, are best taken with food. Taking herbs with food vastly reduces the risk of nausea or other digestive discomfort, especially when increasing dosages. Also, I have found that capsuled herbs filled with light material have a tendency to "float" (the sensation that they have not traveled all the way to the stomach, but are rising back up the esophagus). "Chasing" the capsules with some food as well as plenty of water is helpful in this case. Warmer liquids are generally better than cold ones for swallowing capsules.

Divide Your Doses

You greatly reduce the risk of discomfort by dividing your herb doses throughout the day. You may want to take herbs with two or three different meals. In addition to being more comfortable, this ensures a more steady and even supply of the active ingredient throughout the day.

Increase Gradually

With any herbal medicine it's prudent to start with a lower dosage and increase the dosage as necessary to achieve the desired result. When you reach the desired effect, continue and sustain that dosage for as long as necessary. If you reach a point of discomfort (most commonly in the form of nausea, gas, or other digestive distress), reduce the dose and sustain it when you reach a comfortable level.

Give It Time

The time frame for improvement with herbal medicine depends a great deal on the condition being treated, the herbs being used, and the relative health of the individual. Clearly, a person with a cold can expect different results than a person with chronic fatigue syndrome. A simple vaginal yeast infection will clear up more quickly than systemic candida. A skin fungus may disappear faster than a hormonal imbalance.

In addition, a person who eats a healthy diet, exercises, and abstains from harmful substances will metabolize herbs more quickly and efficiently, and generally be better equipped to put the "tools" to good use, than one who eats poorly and abuses drugs, alcohol, and cigarettes. The more layers of imbalance or toxicity you have, the longer herbs take to work.

An example: A decade ago when my menstrual cycle was way off and I was generally unhealthy and imbalanced, it took several months of using several herbs and foods to achieve hormonal balance and stimulate the onset of menstruation. Today, if my period is one day late, I can take a single small capsule of the Chinese herb dong quai and guarantee my period will start within 12 hours. A single capsule of this herb would not have stimulated menses in me ten years ago and probably wouldn't in most women right now.

Because these factors are so variable, it is very difficult to define an adequate time trial for herbal treatment. We can, however, offer a few general guides.

For an acute condition, you should see improvements within one week and resolution within two weeks. For chronic illness and disease patterns, especially long-established ones, it can take three to six months to see improvements and one to two years to reverse damage. One rule of thumb, according to herbalist Linda Rector-Page, N.D., Ph.D., is one month of healing for every year you have had a condition, illness, or other health problem.[4]

Fortunately, in such cases, symptoms can usually be relieved long before the actual source of the disease is healed. Symptoms can generally be dealt with almost immediately (within days) while the underlying causes of the symptoms may take months, or in tough cases even years, to respond fully. Thus, the irritating symptoms of sinus allergies might be in check by tomorrow, but the allergies themselves might not be eliminated until next year.

You can generally be more aggressive with herbal treatment in an acute situation, since treatment will be short term and the condition should be self-limiting. For longer-standing conditions requiring long-term treatment, truly aggressive treatment is difficult to maintain (though for very serious illness this is sometimes necessary). Sometimes milder, gentler herbal protocols that are "livable" on a long-term basis are required—along with a liberal dose of patience—for indefinitely sustained treatments.

STORING HERBS

Exposure to heat, light, and air minimizes the quality of any herb.

Like fruit juice or milk, prepared herb teas are perishable. They must be used within three to seven days, and that's when they're refrigerated. Signs that a tea has "gone bad" include it being sour, bubbly, fermented or, of course, fuzzy.

Room temperature is fine for dried herbs, and a plastic bag with a twistie tie is recommended to keep it airtight. You may want to put the plastic bag inside a paper bag to avoid light exposure. Glass jars with rubber sealed lids are excellent for storing bulk herbs. Dark (amber) jars are better. You'll note that most tinctures come in amber or brown bottles. Well-prepared and properly stored tinctures generally last forever.

BUYING HERBS

Where you buy your herbs definitely matters. All herb sources are not equal; quality and reliability can vary greatly. Because the herb marketplace is still relatively unregulated and without uniform standards, it is very important to find suppliers you can trust and whose quality is consistent and dependable. The majority of sellers are well intentioned, but virtually every field of business has its shady characters whose interests are in profits alone, and the herb market is no exception. Excellent suppliers and sources are out there—you just have to know what you're looking for.

When and how herbs are harvested, how long they spend in transit, how well preserved they are, and how regular a store's turnover is all have a bearing on how effective your herbs are once you get them. A responsible, knowledgeable, and stable supplier can be counted on to buy and carry properly handled, high-grade products.

Fresh Bulk Herbs

Dried, cut, powdered, pressed—bulk herbs become the teas you drink and, if you make them yourself, the capsules you take. The best place to buy most bulk herbs is an herb pharmacy.

Herb pharmacies are like the apothecaries that were everywhere at the turn of the century. They were the pharmacies of that time, and dispensed an enormous range of herbal medicines in every possible form. As drug pharmacies became the standard, the herb pharmacy disappeared. Now, herb pharmacies are making a bit of a comeback, although they are still, unfortunately, quite rare. Our hometown of Seattle is extremely progressive, with two.

Herb pharmacies make a much higher grade of herb available to the consumer. Herbs are graded after harvesting, and the top 15 percent goes to professional herbalists. The bottom 85 percent goes to the health-food store market, and the quality is much more mediocre. This doesn't mean that health-food-store herbs will hurt you; they just may not help you as much or as quickly because the potency may not be as high. This may mean taking more to get the same effect, which is more costly in the long run.

In the short run, herbs from an herb pharmacy will cost you a little more. But for a 20 to 30 percent higher price, you may get up to ten times the active ingredient in an herb by buying it from an herb pharmacy.

Another advantage of herb pharmacies is that they are generally run, owned, and staffed by professional herbalists. They are better able to educate you and answer your questions. (While we do not recommend you get the bulk of your education from anyone who is trying to sell you products, it can be useful to have someone skilled and conversant to talk to when you need assistance.)

These shops generally sell only herbs, so you know they are specialists and that all of their attention is focused on the herbs. In a health-food store, herbs are usually a very tiny portion of the products and revenue, and they get lost in the shuffle. Very rarely is someone at a health-food store truly knowledgeable about the bulk herbs they're selling.

If there is no herb pharmacy in your city or town, some herb pharmacies will ship herbs anywhere in the country. Our local herb pharmacy in Seattle is one of these. See "Resources," page 511.

Supplement Capsules and Pills

Packaged herbal supplements can be purchased at an herb pharmacy as well. Sometimes herb pharmacies capsule and package their own "house brand" of many popular herbs. These are usually of better quality than mass-marketed commercial brands.

However, if you do buy herbs at a health-food store, you can do okay buying packaged supplements—better than buying bulk herbs there. Sometimes health-food stores will carry the same popular brands as the herb pharmacy. Seek well-known, reputable brands. We recommend Zand Herbal, Eclectic Institute, Yogic Herbs, Herb Pharm, Gaia, Crystal Star, and NF Factors.

One way to ensure herb-pharmacy quality in your capsuled herbs is to make the capsules yourself. I have chosen to do this, and rarely buy prepackaged capsules, because I like to know for a fact what's in the capsules. I want to know that it's fresh, well handled, and potent, premium quality. I can ensure this by buying ground, powdered herbs from the same

herb pharmacy where we get herbs for teas, then purchasing empty capsules and filling them using a capsule maker.

The capsule maker is a plastic contraption that can be purchased at any
herb pharmacy and some health-food stores. It costs about $10 and makes
capsule-filling go very quickly. I have made my own echinacea, isatidis,
dong quai, licorice root, guggul, ginger root, and eleuthero capsules, among
others. I highly recommend this method of obtaining herb capsules—
although, again, if you're not up to making this effort, capsules manufactured by quality companies are certainly better than no herbs at all.

Tinctures

Tinctures are another herb preparation you can make on your own (as
described earlier in this chapter). You can also purchase prepackaged tinctures in herb pharmacies and health-food stores. Again, herb pharmacies
may sell their own "house brand," which is made at the store with fresh,
high-quality herbs. They may also sell popular brands, as will health-food
stores and some co-ops and grocery stores that emphasize natural foods.
As of this writing, Herb Pharm makes the only full line of tinctures in larger, economical bottles (although Wise Woman Herbals makes large size
glycerites for children).

Homegrown and Homemade

Your own herb garden can be a delight, and learning how to grow,
wildcraft, and harvest herbs can be a fun hobby with great health benefits
as a bonus. In this manner, you can have the ultimate quality control,
knowing your source and the handling intimately. You can dry your own
herbs and use them for tea, or cut or grind them to make capsules.

However, it's important to educate yourself well and know what you're
doing, so that you use the right portions of plants, don't confuse safe plants
with the few but potent dangerous ones (foxglove or lobelia, for example),
and handle them properly once they are harvested to ensure maximum
benefit. There are books about how to plan and grow an herb garden, and
many cities offer classes or field trips to teach about growing herbs or rec-
ognizing and harvesting them in the wild. Take advantage of these before
attempting to become your own herb supplier.

Beware the Wannabe Herbalist

When you go to an herb pharmacy or health-food store, the job of the counter-people there is to sell you something and get your money. Your job is to get what you are there for and get out of there. The clerks generally should not be expected to give you truly educated information about a remedy for what ails you. We apologize to those who actually can—they do exist—but our general experience has been that when a health-food-store clerk latches on to what ails you or what you are looking for, he or she will take you on a tour of the store and find you many products to meet your "needs" other than (or in addition to) the ones you came in for.

This is less of a problem at herb pharmacies than health-food stores, but even there, the professional herbalist(s) who own and manage the store may not staff the cash register. You should not be obtaining health advice from a cashier. Herb pharmacists can help educate you, but there is a fine line between customer education and "prescribing." And no one, even if they are very knowledgeable and qualified when it comes to herbs, can make an appropriate diagnosis after two minutes of talking to you.

It is never a good idea to go into a health-food store or even an herb pharmacy and say, "What do you have for [xyz condition]?" You should determine what herbs are best for you with the help of a qualified herbalist or other natural health practitioner, or through your own thorough and intensive study. Know what you are looking for and don't be swayed by the recommendations of clerks, unless you know them well and trust their judgment.

Costs

Herb costs can vary as widely as quality. Unfortunately, cost is not necessarily a harbinger of quality, either. It's crucial, again, to know and trust your sources to ensure that you not only get what you pay for, but that you pay a fair and decent price.

As we discussed above, herb pharmacies are generally 20 to 30 percent more expensive for bulk herbs and other items as health-food stores, but in exchange, the quality increase can be many times that. Still, herb pharmacies are not necessarily the most cost-effective sources for absolutely everything. Herbs that have become very popular to the point of being trendy will be extremely expensive even at an herb pharmacy.

We wish that we could offer you a simple, foolproof strategy for cost-ing out your herbs that would work across the board for all products and all suppliers. But we can't, because herb costs and price-to-quality ratios vary so much locally, and even in a single locale from store to store and product to product. What is necessary for every herb consumer to do is, through research and some trial and error, develop a personal strategy for obtaining herbs at the best possible prices.

For me, if there is an herb that I want to try that I don't already have experience in obtaining, this means sitting down for an hour with a phone and my list of trustworthy herb pharmacies, mail-order companies, herbalists, and healers, and calling around to price herbs. The prices can vary widely. As I mentioned in an earlier chapter, Chinese herbs can be radically cheaper at Chinese markets than at an herb pharmacy—the most dramatic example being the astragalus I purchase from a Chinese grocery at $8 a pound, where the same stuff at the herb pharmacy costs $80 (eighty!) per pound.

A qualified local herbalist can be a huge help in this process, directing you to the best sources for the best herbs both for price and quality. Herbalists know the ins and outs of the herb trade, are usually familiar with the products and prices of most local retailers, and may have inside information about your local market.

Note: An herbalist should guide you to the most economical and appropriate sources for each recommended herb, not only try to sell you his or her own brands. People who always want to sell you only one prod-uct or brand should be avoided.

I get my herbs from a diverse, eclectic range of sources: a local herb pharmacy, a doctor of Chinese medicine, a Chinese market, a Colorado herbalist, an Indiana mail-order company, a local health-food store, and even my local supermarket.

So to find reasonably priced quality herbs: Shop around, compare prices, ask experienced friends about their sources, and consult with an herbalist.

GENERIC, ONE-SIZE-FITS-ALL SUPPLEMENT FORMULAS

There is a huge distinction between the kind of herbal healing we are writing about and that qualified herbalists practice, and the one-size-fits-all, often multilevel-marketed herbal "blends" that are unfortunately the only way much of the public sees herbs. Let's look at some of the problems with these types of supplements (which are often mistaken for representing "herbal medicine") and the approaches to marketing and using them.

By generic we don't mean "no-name" brands. On the contrary, the kind of supplements we are referring to may have very fancy names, often used to suggest high-tech-ness in general or specific benefits. By "generic" we mean not specifically targeted at a particular need, type of person, or condition.

Lack of Specificity and Personalization

For example, we would rather see you look at the myriad specific issues (preferably with the help of an experienced and qualified practitioner) that may be factors in a health condition, and target those factors with the appropriate herbs, than take a one-size-fits-all "Herbal Cleanse and Detox" formula or "Herbal Yeast Syndrome" remedy. Better to know what (or if!) you need to cleanse and why, what mitigating or secondary factors may exist, and what herbs that meet those needs are also best for your body type and lifestyle.

When you choose single herbs for specific conditions, you can control not only which herbs you take but how much of each, in what form and what concentrations, and in what ratios (if you take more than one). You can also control the source and the quality to a much greater degree.

One-size-fits-all formulas may contain herbs you don't need, and exclude the ones you do. You can buy a formula with eight or ten herbs in it that are not related to anything you are necessarily trying to accomplish. At worst, you can waste a lot of money and get discouraged. This is especially true if you are trying to address a specific health issue rather than simply seeking to optimize health.

There's nothing wrong with formulas per se. Formulas, in fact, are how the majority of herbs are used in traditional medicine of other cultures. But the formulas used in these cultures are either classical formulas that have a long history of use for specific purposes, or they were developed just for the individual by the herbal practitioner. Most formulas sold in the

United States are simply the ten or twelve trendiest herbs with which American consumers are familiar, stuffed into one capsule. One product with the word "herb" in the name contains no herbs at all!

You should choose a formula based on a specific issue or desired outcome, not for some general, undefined "health benefits." Our bodies' organs and systems work together, and disease issues are often interrelated, so it is certainly useful in many cases to use a combination of herbs that work synergistically, and/or on different levels or aspects of the problem. But in that case you're still working on something specific; all of the herbs in the formula have a purpose. And you're better off choosing each of those herbs yourself, or with the guidance of a practitioner who knows how to tailor a program to your needs.

Wasteful Usage

Another problem with the mass-marketed or multilevel-marketed (MLM)–type herb formulas is their use of popular and overharvested herbs because they are trendy rather than because they are the most effective herb for a formula. This is truly a waste for herbs like goldenseal and echinacea, which are so popular that every company feels it must have its own combo formula with them in it. If we use these herbs for everything whether we need them or not—especially if companies throw them into everything just to sell more product—there is a very real danger that we won't have them when they really would be most appropriate.

Lack of Information

Mass-marketed, generic supplements are typically not presented by people who are deeply knowledgeable about herbs in general. In some cases they are relatively clueless even about the specific product they sell. The herbs are being marketed solely as a way to capitalize on consumer interest in herbs, with little or no regard for how effective the herb is, let alone how educated the consumer is.

The MLM (multilevel marketing) rep is rarely a great resource for learning impartial information about herbal medicine as a whole. He or she may even have limited information about the formulas being sold. (I remember one rep for a diet product trying desperately to explain to me the supposed difference between losing "fat" and losing "body fat.") Often the materials, if there are any, don't say anything substantive; they may go on endlessly in marketing-speak that never really amounts to much.

All kinds of companies are trying to take advantage of the blossoming interest in herbs by manufacturing and marketing their brands of newly popular supplements. For example, one catalog sells a supplement for the eyes that it says contains "Ginkgo **balboa**"! (The herb is called *Ginkgo biloba*.) Elsewhere in the catalog, a different product manufactured by a different company claims to contain "Ginkgo **bilboa**"!

Bad Reputation

Another strike against generic-use, mass-marketed, and multilevel-marketed herbal formulas is that they make too easy a target for anyone interested in discrediting herbal medicine. Poorly made formulas hyped for dubious purposes such as "getting thin," "maxing muscle," or "spiking energy" are an embarrassment to the responsible herb industry. They provide naysayers an opportunity to criticize herbal medicine when in fact they are criticizing something that has nothing to do with taking feverfew for migraines or guggul to lower blood fats.

And if you cannot tell the difference between XYZ Company's "Super! Duper! En-R-G Formula" and responsible, medicinal use of whole herbs for health and healing, doctors and regulators may use that as a handle to "prove" the supposed folly of giving you access to substances that allow self-treatment. Thus it is in your interest to be able to distinguish quality, professional sources and products.

Cost

The unfocused, generic formulas usually cost a lot more than single herbs that you might target to specific conditions. With these types of commercial products you can spend a lot of money and get very little in return.

Tips for Avoiding the "Generic" Traps

- Seek specialists. Get herbs from a qualified herb pharmacy or trusted mail-order company that specializes only in herbs. See "Resources," page 511.
- Stay away from herb formulas sold by network-marketed (multilevel-marketing) companies and distributorships.
- Stick to single-herb products as much as possible.
- Avoid herbs with cheesy ads. This may sound subjective, but usually the more tacky the packaging and promo, the less trustworthy the product. Liberal use of "all caps" and exclamation points can be used to communicate something that isn't really there, often in lieu of facts and information. Do you trust products that scream, in big block type, **"WOW!!!!! YOHIMBE INCREASES SUPER SEXUAL PERFORMANCE!!!!!!!!"** (I don't.)
- Don't buy herbs from anyone who promises instant results. These are the herbal world's "quick-weight-loss" counterparts. In individual cases, obesity treatment may warrant the use of herbs or sensibly prepared herbal formulas in conjunction with other interventions, including dietary and lifestyle changes. But in the vast majority of cases, that is not the context in which consumers purchase these supplements. Most often they are expected to work *in lieu of* any lifestyle or habit changes—and they are promoted that way.
- Don't buy the cheapest herb on the market. This is not to say that you can't find economical herbs and supplements, but use common sense. If 400 capsules of a relatively trendy and popular herb costs $3.99 when it costs $25 everywhere else, you're probably not getting a quality product.
- Know what you are trying to accomplish. Learn about herbs overall and the best herbs for your goals or condition. Know the basics of the energetics and tastes of herbs as defined by Eastern herbal medicine, and what results they generally produce, as outlined in Chapter 2, "History of Ayurveda: Ancient Healing Wisdom." Chances are great that once you do this, few if any generically marketed herb formulas will appear to be a better choice for you

than fresh single herbs or single-herb preparations ("simples") from a reputable herb pharmacy.

- Seek professional support. Sometimes the best way to get results from herbs is to have them tailor-matched to your body type and condition by someone who is experienced with one of the traditional Asian healing systems, and uses kinesiology, acupressure, or pulse reading along with medical tests where appropriate to assess which herbs are right for you at the time.

REGULATION

Currently, the regulation of herbs in the United States is in flux. Under the Dietary Supplement and Health Education Act of 1994 (DSHEA), the FDA issued a set of proposed regulations that created a separate category under which herbs would be regulated: as dietary supplements, which also includes vitamins, minerals, enzymes, amino acids, phytopharmaceuticals, and the like.

Dietary supplement products may make what are called "structure or function claims." That is, it may indicate that the product benefits a structure or function of the body, but it cannot claim to cure or mitigate any disease. (If it did, it would be classified as a drug and have to undergo the normal FDA drug-testing and approval process. This is unfortunate because, as we have discussed, herbs clearly can mitigate disease and yet this does not make them "drugs." Many herbs that can mitigate disease have been historically used that way for hundreds of thousands of years. And there just isn't financial incentive to put unpatentable natural products through the quarter-of-a-billion-dollar FDA testing and approval process.)

Labeling issues were also addressed by this act: Dietary supplements must list all ingredients and their amounts, and botanical products must indicate the part of the plant from which the ingredient is derived. Manufacturers must be prepared to substantiate claims and must include the disclaimer: "This statement has not been evaluated by the Food and Drug Administration. This product is not intended to diagnose, treat, cure, or prevent any disease."

The FDA has a committee working to establish quality controls, as directed by the act, and at the time of this writing these recommendations are not final.

Many herbalists and other experts in the field respect Germany's system and suggest it would make a good model for us. The German system has encouraged a great deal of research and understanding in herbal medicine. Pharmacognosist Varro Tyler, Ph.D., in *Herbs of Choice*, suggests that regulatory reform should "permit claims, as for any other drug, based on a doctrine of 'reasonable certainty,' utilizing information gathered from all sources, including reference works, practicing physicians, patients' anecdotal testimony, folkloric sources, etc." He notes that this prevails now in Germany and Canada.

The Herb Research Foundation and American Botanical Council have proposed that a special category called "traditional medicines" be created to allow claims for botanicals that have a long historical use for particular health conditions. We strongly support this common-sense idea.

CHOOSING AN HERBALIST
OR NATURAL HEALTH PRACTITIONER

Throughout this book, we have presented many reasons for this field's undeserved status as a target of skepticism and persecution, and offered many reasons why these attitudes are unwarranted and you should let down your guard. Now we must suggest something that seems to run counter to that bid: You must be cautious about choosing an herbalist. This can be difficult, because currently there is no such thing as an "herbalist credential." There are naturopaths, medical doctors, osteopaths, and chiropractors who are herbalists, and those who are not. Then there are simply people who are herbalists, who have apprenticed with a master in the field, and who have more knowledge of these healing methods than many people with "credentials."

Indeed, some of the most proficient people in the field may have no credentials whatsoever, and that makes it all the more confusing. People from other cultures, or who have apprenticed with masters of other cultures, have sophisticated instincts born of contact with people for whom herbal medicine is truly second nature.

Karta Purkh notes, "In other cultures, the spectrum of folk knowledge goes from the layperson right up to the highest medical professional. In other cultures, laypeople might have a long, animated conversation about whether turmeric is warm or cool; they talk about such things the way we talk about sports scores."

Unfortunately, Karta Purkh estimates that a large percentage of people who call themselves herbalists are independent product reps who have taken a one-day workshop on their company's one-size-fits-all herbal blend product(s).

Also, herbalists who are not licensed health professionals technically are not allowed to diagnose health problems. That means that if you want to see an herbalist for a problem, you may need to see a medical doctor first for a diagnosis, then consult the herbalist. This can be difficult because medical doctors often do not want merely to diagnose you and then have you run off to someone else.

Another strategy is to find a naturopathic physician or other licensed natural health professional who also happens to specialize in herbal medicine. There is often confusion about the difference between a naturopath and an herbalist. They are not synonymous. An herbalist is not a licensed physician; a naturopath is. A naturopath may or may not be an herbalist. Naturopathic medicine is a wide field, and there are many different philosophies that may comprise a naturopath's specialty.

In such an ambiguous and complicated environment, choosing a qualified herbalist to work with requires care and deliberation. Unlike naturopaths or homeopaths, herbalists are not licensed by states. There are various colleges, programs, and certification courses for the study of botanical medicine and herbalism, but standards vary, certifications are not consistent, and there is no central governing body for all herbalists. Anyone can hang out a shingle as an herbalist—even without certification or experience of any kind—so it's important to know what you're looking for.

Here are some tips for finding a qualified herbalist in the current environment:

- While there is currently no accreditation for herbal healing, the American Herbalists Guild is an association in which any herbalist you consult should be a professional member. Professional members are admitted by peer review and must pass an exam and meet a minimum of clinical experience.
- Get recommendations from friends and family whose opinions on these kinds of matters you trust. Interview several practitioners to see who is the best fit for you.

- Go to classes given by herbalists to get a sense of whether their approach and special areas of knowledge suit your needs.
- Avoid "herbalists" who pitch one specific brand of product. A good herbalist will have a broad base of knowledge about many different kinds of herbs, and will be interested in teaching you how to find the best herbs in the best form or preparation at the best price, for your purposes.

Here are good questions to ask herbalists—or, for that matter, any other health practitioners—when interviewing them. Remember that you are the consumer and you may choose the person you work with. The field of natural medicine and those practicing in it are no more uniformly perfect than in any other profession. You are not obligated to work with anyone you do not trust, like, understand, or feel comfortable with. Your health professionals should be knowledgeable and experienced, but in addition, you may want them to be open-minded, friendly, compassionate, and optimistic (i.e., believe healing is possible).

1. What is your philosophy?
2. Where were you trained?
3. How long have you been practicing?
4. What are your professional affiliations?
5. What is your experience with the types of problems I seem to have?
6. What other healing arts do you embrace or recommend?
7. What is your attitude toward or philosophy about orthodox or allopathic medicine?
8. What is your experience with chronic (long-term) or serious conditions?
9. What is your diagnostic or evaluation system?
10. With what natural healing system do you most strongly identify yourself?
11. If I don't find relief or consider myself healed following your suggestions, what will you recommend as "next steps"?
12. How do you feel about the role of the patient in the healing process?

A qualified herbal practitioner or educator can help you learn to identify strengths and weaknesses using the body-typing systems of natural healing, and to determine the best herbs for your health or conditions, based on your lifestyle, health history, special sensitivities, and other considerations.

That doesn't mean that you can't take herbs without a practitioner's advice. Because of the mild and dilute nature of most herbs, you absolutely can do this safely and effectively. In some instances, however—if you want very specific or progressive results with particular issues—it is often helpful to have some education and assistance to refine and streamline your use of herbs further. A professional herbalist (American Herbalists Guild professional member) or other practitioner, such as a naturopath or a holistic medical doctor, may be able to support you further.

WHEN TO CONSULT A MEDICAL DOCTOR

Throughout this book we have encouraged the use of herbal medicine and the natural healing approaches as a first resort for many minor and chronic illnesses. We suggest that turning first to natural, "lower-tech," noninvasive, and nontoxic remedies can be more effective in the short run, healthier in the long run, safer, and more economical for you personally as well as for the health-care system.

Dr. Andrew Weil gives an example in *Spontaneous Healing* from his own experience: When a freak accident dislocated his jaw, he went to see osteopath Dr. Robert Fulford, one of his mentors in natural healing. Dr. Fulford gently manipulated his jaw back into place. Ten minutes later, driving home with all pain gone, he thought to himself, "What would you have done if you didn't know about him? Probably, I would have visited an emergency room, undergone X rays, and been sent home with painkillers, muscle relaxants, and the expectation of a large bill. Possibly I would have remained unhealed for weeks or months."

However, there absolutely are situations where you should consult a medical doctor. See a doctor when:

- You have been seriously injured and are experiencing shock, severe bleeding, head trauma, or another life-threatening condition.
- An infection is not responding at all to natural alternatives.
- You have lumps, masses, sores, or lesions anywhere on your body that remain after a few weeks.

- Any condition you have been trying to treat with other methods shows no improvement after several days or weeks.
- You feel, for any reason, that you require medical attention.

Being Your Own Healer

Each patient carries his own doctor inside of him.
We are at our best when we give the doctor who resides within each patient
a chance to go to work.

—Albert Schweitzer, noted German physician

The more you learn, the better you will be able to care for yourself; the more specifically and purposefully you will be able to target your own specific health needs, strengths, and weaknesses; and the more powerful a consumer you will become. You will be able to weed through the endless plethora of health headlines, rhetoric, and contradictions, selecting the useful and discarding the worthless. We have included an extensive recommended reading list in the back of this book, and we enthusiastically encourage you to select more books in the areas that interest you and keep learning.

The idea of taking charge of your own wellness is one that is just beginning to find the public, and we hope it will soon burgeon into the norm for our culture—not to replace the trained physician, but certainly to take the unnecessary and inappropriate burden off of him or her. I think I am a good example of how informed, responsible, intuitive, and sensible a consumer can be, with superb results.

SHOULD YOU USE STANDARDIZED EXTRACTS?

One somewhat disturbing aspect of the drive in research to find out why something works is that there is always an underlying presumption that we will want to isolate it and put it in a concentrated pill. When we do this with herbs, we end up with what is called a "standardized extract," a product that contains what is *currently believed* to be the active ingredient guaranteed to be present at a specific level. Thus every unit (pill, capsule, 10 drops of tincture) contains an identical amount of active ingredient at the identical concentration. In this way, it becomes a "natural drug."

Herbalist Michael Moore, an instructor at the Southwest School of Botanical Medicine and author of several herb books, calls standardized products and phytopharmaceuticals "Little Drugs." He suggests that they not blend into the marketplace as "herbs" because they are not herbs, as they lack the diluting, buffering effects as well as the synergies of whole plants.

These extracts are an attempt to exert pharmaceutical quality control over botanical products. In an attempt to create consistency and, proponents claim, eliminate side effects, manufacturers will spend millions to make these extracts using pharmaceutical equipment and procedures. (The "eliminate side effects" argument is particularly weak, because most herbs cause few to no side effects when they are whole—and ironically, isolating constituents is *more* likely to cause side effects because of the absence of many of the balancing components.)

Standardized extracts are usually used in scientific studies since they allow researchers to produce quantifiable, repeatable results. In fact, standardized herbal extracts originated in Europe, where most of the research on botanicals has used the extracts. These are the studies on which European doctors base their recommendations of herbs to patients. This has created a market in Europe for the extracts, and now they are becoming popular in the United States.

The whole-herb versus standardized-extract argument is becoming a central theme in the philosophical tensions between holistic healing and conventional science and medicine. As we have seen, the assumption that isolation and standardization automatically make for more effective medicine is straight out of reductionist Cartesian thought, which gave rise to conventional medicine as described in Chapter 1, "Herbs: The Original Medicine." In that model, parts are of more interest than wholes and are assumed to be more relevant. There is a disregard for the larger picture, for the concept of interaction between parts, for the whole being more than the sum of parts.

What you lose when you take apart herbs is the very essence of herbal medicine. Few if any plants can be reduced to the pharmacology of specific constituents. A whole herb acts across a wide spectrum, thanks to a range of compounds that provide synergies, safeguards, and enhancements to one another. This is considered by herbalists to be a key strength of herbal medicine.

Most plant substances have thousands of identifiable chemical components, and dozens or hundreds of them may be active in many different ways. You could research for a century and possibly never figure it all out. And do we really need to maintain magic-bullet medicine if we're not trying to make an herb into a convenient pill with a good shelf life? If the whole plant works, it works. It is not necessary to identify the active components in order to make it effective.

What scientists call "inert" because it has no direct activity of its own may actually potentiate or moderate the activity of other ingredients in powerful ways. "Inert" ingredients may well have a reason for existence— to help dilute, protect, accelerate, stabilize, transport, or enhance absorption of the "active" ingredient(s). Often the isolated "active" ingredient alone doesn't work without the presence of the whole plant.

Also, many active components in whole herbs were at one time believed to be inert, even after research had been conducted. For example, components of echinacea once believed to be inert are now considered key active constituents. And there are herbs whose active ingredients still have not been identified.

A natural extract—a "Little Drug"—is still likely to be a better choice than a "Big Drug," a synthetic pharmaceutical. It is likely to be less toxic. But even if herbal extracts are less toxic than a synthetic drug, you still lose the synergy of a bounty of other compounds. That's re-creating what we did a hundred years ago when we got away from natural whole medicines in the first place. You get a fixed, consistent substance—but you don't get herbal medicine.

For all of these reasons, many herbalists are opposed to the idea of extracting an herb's active ingredient (or several) and engineering them into a supplement. The case for whole plants is very strong, and the case for "active ingredient herbalism" (as *New Holistic Herbal* author David Hoffman calls it) is dubious. If the bottom line is efficacy, most herbalists agree that herbs consistently show more activity when the whole herb is used than when isolated ingredients are applied.

Probably the strongest influence driving "active ingredient herbalism" is not efficacy, but rather the sheer momentum of reductionist scientific thinking. "Isolate and concentrate" is simply what's always been done, and it is assumed to be superior.

Full Herbal Extracts versus Standardized Extracts

It is important to make a distinction between standardized extracts and full herbal extracts. A full herbal extract (also called a "simple extract" or "crude extract") contains all or most of the whole herb's chemical components, balanced to the proportions in which those components would appear in the whole herb. It is a way to get everything the whole herb has to offer, only in a more concentrated and convenient form. The standardized extract, on the other hand, contains only one or a few of *what is presumed to be* the herb's "active" ingredients, with supposedly "inert" ingredients removed.

Ed Smith, founder and president of Herb Pharm in Williams, Oregon, points out that making a simple extract is an environmentally friendly process using biodegradable grain or fruit alcohol, water, or plant glycerine. Making a standardized extract requires the use of harsh synthetic chemicals to extract the "inert" ingredients. Such chemicals include acetone, benzene, methyl alcohol, butyl alcohol, or carbon tetrachloride. Not only are these environmentally unfriendly, but, says Smith, they are not always completely removed from the finished extract.[5] This doesn't exactly represent "natural" medicine.

Some herbalists even question full extracts, however, suggesting that simply placing an herb in a different medium can change its effect.

We are not totally negative about using extracts. Some herbs may benefit from being standardized. With expensive herbs that tempt manufacturers to adulterate with filler, a standardized extract may be able to guarantee a certain amount of active compound. And for a few herbs, standardization may provide the most practical way to get a therapeutic dose of the herb—feverfew, hawthorn berry, or saw palmetto, for example. (Even in those cases, though, whole preparations are still options.)

But because standardization may benefit a few products does not mean that most or all herbs should be standardized. If that were true, no one would have gotten any results from herbs up until the point that standardization became popular, and of course that's not the case. For example, Ayurveda and Traditional Chinese Medicine have been using herbs effectively for millennia without the "benefit" of standardization. Ironically, it is often the historical effectiveness of whole herbs in traditional uses that inspires study—and sometimes, subsequently, standardization.

CONTRAINDICATIONS
AND OTHER CONCERNS

In general, contraindications (inadvisability of combination with other herbs, foods, drugs, or other substances) for herbs are rare because herbs themselves are so gentle, dilute, and, for the most part, slow working. Because they are whole plants, made of compounds our bodies have seen since the time of our ancestors, our bodies perceive them as something akin to food. In most cases the idea of contraindicating the use of certain herbs together is analogous to the idea of contraindication for eating rice and beans together.

No herbalist wishes to produce side effects, nor does he or she expect to. For the most part, herbs should be free of side effects, and most often they are—when used by knowledgeable consumers, or by trained herbalists who typically consider the whole person and his or her body type, current levels of functioning, and various other individual co-factors.

A knowledgeable person chooses herbs that will balance or enhance his or her basic constitution and work well with his or her lifestyle. Just as certain foods do not agree with certain individuals, some herbs are potentially more aggravating to some types than others. (The Ayurvedic and Chinese systems of body typing include such considerations, both for herbs and foods, and provide exactly this kind of guidance.) Hypothetically, of ten herbs that have potentially helpful actions for a condition, perhaps two to five might be ideal for a particular individual with that condition.

In the conventional model of drug toxicology, active substances are thought always to produce a single effect in all people. Trying to understand herbs and potential reactions from within this paradigm leads one to believe that a reaction on the part of one person means the herb itself is dangerous. But in most cases you cannot predict a consistent "drug reaction" from an herb. Herbal medicines simply do not work exactly like drugs. Reactions can be predictable, but not so much due to an innate quality of the herb as from a poor match between the energetics of a particular herb and the constitutional characteristics or quirks of the whole person.

This is one of the reasons natural medicine must, and does, deal with a holistic range of considerations about a person's body, history, and current lifestyle as well as symptoms and conditions. Some herbs can aggravate one person, yet soothe another. Thus, an herb's potential side effects have more to do with the person taking it than with the herb itself. This makes knowledge, experience, and education critical to the appropriate use of herbs. And it makes simple intuition and attentiveness to one's own body perhaps even more important.

In the vast majority of cases, common sense is a person's best friend when using herbs. Indeed, serious reactions to herbs virtually always occur in situations of such obvious abuse, with such plain warning signals that potential for trouble should have been clear to the victim and anyone else observing. Among the scattered handful of possible (as yet unproven) herb-related deaths over the past several decades, unmistakably extreme uses precipitated every one. Herbalist Michael Moore writes, "We have a generation or two of people that *expect* a warning label on everything, and that have come to doubt common sense."[6]

Moore notes, "Most herb reactions occur when an herb *stimulates* metabolic processes that are already overstimulated."[7] Most possible problems with herbs, he says, will occur only rarely when a variety of factors come together to create a "potentiated state." When they do occur, they are likely to be so subtle that people who believe in herbs will ignore them, while skeptics will magnify them totally out of proportion. "There is little intrinsic danger in using herbs, since few have the potential for drug side effects," Moore explains. "The side effects are usually idiosyncratic or idiopathic, and not predictable by drug standards."[8] In other words, they occur based on the idiosyncrasies of the individual, not as a predictable reaction that can be expected from that herb on a regular basis.

In nearly twenty-five years of working with and talking to people who are taking herbs, as well as many practitioners who are working with herbs, Karta Purkh has not seen or even heard about a single instance where herbs and drugs together presented a problem. He suggests, "Don't take No-Doz with ephedra. Don't take Ex-Lax with cascara bark. Work your way in slowly and follow traditional use. Observe these rules of common sense, as well as the occasional specific caution we have given in this book." (That means if we say "This herb is very strong—do not take more than one capsule a day," do not take twelve and assume that you'll get better results.)

Many herb books provide lists of herbs that are contraindicated during pregnancy. Some natural medicine experts include only a handful of herbs on that list; others' list are very long. Our suggestion is simple: **If you wish to take *any* herbs during pregnancy, do so only under the advice, guidance, and observation of a health practitioner experienced with the use of herbs.**

24

Urban Myths and Sidewalk Talk

"Illnesses associated with herbal use are relatively uncommon, and deaths rare."

—*Health,* "The Naturals," May/June 1995

B ecause so much knowledge about herbs was originally anecdotal—even though modern research is verifying vast amounts of what was once considered "folk wisdom"—there is a capacity for all sorts of hearsay about what works and what doesn't, what's safe and what isn't. There is so much that is credible and worthwhile about herbs that it is important not to let the ever-churning myth factory divert attention from, or distort, the greater body of good. That means knowing how to separate "sidewalk talk" from valid facts.

In addition, it's important to be well informed as herbal medicine surges to the forefront of health news—predictably, in the usual mix of truth and fiction. As herbal medicine progresses back to a position of popularity, there is an increasing inclination on the part of the media to do "herbal exposés" that are deceptive, sensationalist, and sometimes irrational. It's in your interest to be able to distinguish these hype pieces from informative journalism.

Unfortunately, the myth-busting data usually only reaches professionals; the consumer just gets the mainstream media-driven hearsay that alternately hypes, trivializes, or "awfulizes" herbs. That's why we've included this chapter. We selected from a base of pervasive fallacies gathered from popular magazines, newspapers, and television shows; recurring questions from Karta Purkh's classes; and comments overheard at health-food stores, at parties, on buses, in libraries, and so on. Our clarifications will hopefully assist you in being as discriminating and analytical with similar items in the future.

Double Standards for Medicines

By far, the most common germ of concern and skepticism about herbs is a double standard for safety and effectiveness. The government, modern medicine, and the public tend to give leeway for drugs that they don't give for herbs. We have heard the claim that it's the other way around, that people will take herbs too freely and openly without questioning them merely because they are herbs. This has not been our experience, and we believe this itself is a groundless myth.

Scientific medicine has effectively instilled within the public a fear of nature. People who have been taking so many prescription drugs that they are experiencing numerous side effects will fix a wary eye and question herbal recommendations, asking, "Will these hurt me?" Most people don't talk about or worry about "side effects" when consuming the large amounts of refined sugar, fat, processed food, and artificial substances that most Americans do every day. Most don't even worry about it with drugs, despite their huge propensity for side effects.

In addition, science may use standards to measure and judge herb safety and effectiveness that are more stringent than those that are applied to conventional therapies. Science can also structure experiments in such a way as to ensure predictable results. If you feed just about anything to pregnant laboratory rats or infant mice at 100 times the normal dosage, you will no doubt find a problem. The kinds of questions you ask and how you ask them certainly steer the kind of answers you get.

It's common to use noncontrolled anecdotal information to insinuate negatives about herbal medicine, when this format is frequently dismissed by modern science as a way to confirm positive results. Mere observations from clinicians that positively reflect on herbs are almost always labeled unscientific. If hearsay is considered scientifically unacceptable to support herbs, why should it be acceptable to discredit them?

An example: *Consumer Reports* noted in "Herbal Diet Supplements"

(November 1995) that an editorial (not a study) in the *Journal of the American Medical Association* "speculated that liver damage of unknown origin might stem from herbs more often than doctors realize." The editorial also urged doctors to question patients carefully about their use of supplements.

Speculated, editorial, and *might* are the operative words here. Again, such speculation is rarely considered adequate proof for the efficacy of herbs. We could also speculate all sorts of things about drugs, too. Why not suggest that doctors also question their patients more carefully about the use of OTC drugs and the prescriptions that they themselves may have given? In fact, that's an excellent idea.

Ironically, *Consumer Reports* later published a scathing review of OTC cold and flu drugs in "Finding the Right Cold Medicine" (January 1996). After touting the "safety and effectiveness" of OTC drugs in the November 1995 herb article, CR reversed itself in the January 1996 piece to raise points such as these:

- Some combination-formula ingredients accomplish nothing "except trigger adverse side effects."

- Antihistamine is often used in cold medicines, yet it does nothing for most people's cold symptoms. It does, however, make you drowsy and possibly unable to drive or operate heavy machinery.

- Phenylpropanolamine, a decongestant, can raise your blood pressure.

- Combination cold formulas lock you into taking fixed amounts of everything that's in them even when your symptoms change. For example, if your headache goes away but the rest of your symptoms prompt you to keep taking the formula, you will be continuing to consume the maximum recommended dosage of acetaminophen or other pain reliever every six hours when it's absolutely unnecessary.

- Some formulas make no sense whatsoever. CR names one cough medicine that has one ingredient to make phlegm easier to cough up, and another to suppress coughing.

GENERAL MYTHS ABOUT HERBS

"If an herb has the power to heal, then it can harm." Technically, this is probably true. Almost every natural healing system has an adage akin to "The dose makes the poison."

But it's important to recognize that this is true of all drugs and all foods as well as herbs. It is not *especially* true of herbs. To the contrary, herbs are much more difficult to misuse than drugs because of herbs' wide spectrum of potential active ingredients, all in very small quantities, diluted by other plant material, and working through different biochemical pathways.

Doctors and scientists often assume that any active substance must have side effects, because their experience is with drugs, and drugs by their very nature will have side effects. Indeed, any rational decision regarding whether to use a drug begins with the acknowledgment that there will be side effects, and weighs that unavoidable cost against the potential benefits of the drug. But the activity of a whole plant, with all its compounds intact, simply is not comparable to the action of a single concentrated compound.

As herbalist Michael Moore puts it, "A physician's biochemical tools are drugs. By extension, docs may rightly presume that any agent capable of promoting change probably has similar potential for side effects. . . . If you are used to viewing biologically active agents as analogs to drugs, you need to suspend those standards when dealing with most herb preparations."[1]

Ironically, the expectation of side effects for drugs is such a given that side effects can come to be seen as a necessary sign of value, a warped sort of status symbol. Thus a corollary myth is: "If an herb doesn't have the power to harm, then it can't heal." Observes herbalist Moore, "Carried to an irrational extreme, some medical folks feel that anything *without* potential side effects is quackery. This, of course, leaves any alternative approach in a Catch-22 bind."[2]

Another aspect of the harm-or-heal issue is that critics cannot seem to make up their minds about whether herbs are perilously powerful or so feeble in their action as to be trivial. They seem to alternate between saying that people should not take herbs because they might easily harm themselves and saying that people should not take them because they are so useless and ineffective that they are a waste of money. Which is it? Are they weak and trifling, or are they monstrously potent? Of course, they are neither.

Keep in mind that you can easily drink too much coffee, cola, or alcohol, or eat too much fat or sugar. Those things don't even have healing abilities to balance out their capacity for harm, yet there's no move to make them illegal or restrict them. Certainly, you should not be willy-nilly about using herbs indiscriminately without knowledge and guidance, but there is inherent safety by comparison.

"Just as with a drug, the liver cannot handle large amounts of an herb; it will become overwhelmed and be unable to detoxify it." Here is another hair-splitting technicality. Practically speaking, just about any herb is far less likely than any common drug to overwhelm the liver, especially in the kinds of doses people usually use with herbs. And plant compounds are not viewed by the body as toxins, the way synthetic chemicals are. Our bodies have pathways for metabolizing plant compounds, the likes of which we have not evolved for metabolizing synthetic chemicals.

Even in extremely high doses, there is a world of difference between drugs and herbs. There are few herbs that would make you very sick in extremely high doses, let alone kill you (though several do exist). Virtually every drug on the market would make you sick or kill you in extremely high doses.

"Drugs are better because they are purified and standardized. Modern medicine has no use for medicines that cannot be purified and standardized." Purifying and standardizing drugs does not make them healthier or better (see pages 466–469 for a complete discussion of herb standardization). In fact, in most cases it makes them far more "heavy-handed" in their action, more unfamiliar to the body, and thus more toxic to the liver. What purifying and standardizing drugs *does* do is offer opportunities for patents and commercial monopolies. The leading factor in the move to drugs most likely was the limited opportunity for financial gain in natural, unpatentable products. (See Chapter 1, "Herbs: The Original Medicine.")

The article in *Health* magazine stated, "When you take a 325-milligram aspirin tablet, you get 325 milligrams—no more, no less."[3] True, and what you get is no more and no less than 325 milligrams of aspirin—a drug that can cause stomach pain, nausea, bleeding, and ulcers because of the way it works (blocking hormonelike messenger molecules called prostaglandins, including those that protect the stomach lining).

This article also quoted a liver specialist as saying that if you took sixteen 500-milligram acetaminophen tablets (Tylenol is an example of this type of pain reliever) at once, you could develop acute liver failure within four days.[4] But you could take sixteen capsules of just about any herb (exceptions are noted throughout this book) and not damage yourself in any way whatsoever. In fact, sixteen capsules is a reasonable dose for very mild herbs. You simply cannot compare whole astragalus to purified acetaminophen.

"Drugs offer exact dosages. It's too hard to dose herbs." How much to take is simply not as much of an issue with herbs, particularly if you talk to an herbalist, have a reputable herb source, and work up gradually until you get the results you want. Science is simply focused on the issue of dosage, because it is so much more relevant with drugs, and drugs are what science knows about.

The fact is that even with drugs, the dose should vary tremendously from person to person (should a 220-pound male take the same amount as a 120-pound female?), but drugs must be standardized for compliance with regulations, so those variations are unaccounted for in pharmaceutical prescriptions.

Varro Tyler, Ph.D., a noted pharmacognosist whose approach to evaluating herbs is strictly scientific, says in *Herbs of Choice*, "The therapeutic potency and potential toxicity of the active principles in many herbs is very modest, and this, when coupled with the great dilution in which they occur in the plant material, usually renders precise dosage unnecessary."

(See pages 448–451 for more information on dosing herbs.)

"Herb use is dangerous and untrustworthy because the supplement market is a confusing, hazardous minefield." There are several important distinctions to make when "the supplement market" is being discussed. One, herbal medicine is not synonymous with "the supplement market." Many people, including science and medical practitioners, assume that to give herbal medicine a try is to go to the health-food store and buy some supplements. Herbal medicine is a field, not a pill-making industry. The field is not limited to a few companies making ginseng capsules.

Herbal medicine involves practitioners trained in the ways of administering natural medicine, both in this culture and other cultures. There are professionals—herbalists, naturopaths, homeopaths, acupuncturists, Traditional Chinese Medicine doctors, and some MDs, to name just a few—trained to help you determine which ones would be most supportive for your body, your conditions, and your lifestyle, as well as in what form, where to get them, and so on.

Secondly, do not assume that all herbal medicine is "pills." All medicinal substances do not have to be in pill form. This assumption comes from a drug paradigm. In actual fact, herbal medicine encompasses a wide range of forms and preparations of botanical substances. Herbs can be consumed whole, chewed, ground up and put in capsules, brewed as tea or beverage, cooked into soups and broths, used as culinary spices, sucked, sniffed, and so on. Herbal "medicine" can be very foodlike—parsley in salad or beet juice, for example.

Third, the supplement marketplace is definitely a buyer-beware situation, but no more so than for any other food or other things we buy or consume on a regular basis. There are small obstacles, but the field as a whole is made of sound soil. The hype that does exist makes it important to be highly informed, and to know how to find and evaluate good-quality suppliers. In Europe, where there's a much more sophisticated and educated population of herb consumers (as well as a much more supportive and sensible labeling system), such issues are far less of a concern.

It is only fair to take into consideration that in our culture, most fields—despite a generally trustworthy core—are surrounded by hype. In fact, there is a tremendous amount of hype around pharmaceutical drugs. There is hype around everything from movies to milk to Mother's Day. Almost everything in America is hyped in some way, so there is no reason to single out herbal medicine.

"There is no way to know what will happen if you take an herb." There are over 100,000 studies available on the effects of over 1,000 common herbs, in terms of both effectiveness and safety. They exist; they have been discussed, written about, compiled by independent nonprofit organizations, and published in respected journals all over the world.

In addition to the voluminous amount of research data, there is also the issue of clinical, historical, and anecdotal evidence. While many conventional scientists refuse to acknowledge such standards of proof—as we discussed earlier, in Chapter 3, "Perspectives on Research"—others consider hundreds or thousands of years of consistent observation to be relevant, and you may agree. Says pharmacognosist Varro Tyler, Ph.D., in *Herbs of Choice*, "It might be surmised that herbs consumed by humans for generations, centuries, and even millennia must be reasonably safe." We would say the same holds true for efficacy.

"Any result from an herb must be the placebo effect. In most cases the person would have gotten better anyway, since most ailments are self-limiting." If this is true, then even with a pharmaceutical that has been studied, there is no way to tell what would have happened without the treatment. In fact, there is no way ever to really, truly tell what really caused healing. The assumptions that must be made, the logic that must be used, even the degree of faith that must be applied in the case of any natural remedy, is true of any synthetic one as well.

And there are dozens if not hundreds of examples of chronic ailments that most certainly are not self-limiting—asthma, arthritis, amenorrhea, to name just a few. These rarely respond without intervention.

"If you asked fifty different health-food-store clerks for a remedy to boost immunity, you'd get twenty-five different answers. There's no way so many different herbs can all do the same thing." Why is it assumed to be implausible that there are *numerous* substances in nature that offer the same benefit or perform the same function—for example, an immune-enhancing effect? (In fact, that is exactly the case.) Why would there be just one, and why would fifty different people all name the same one when there might actually be thirty well-known ones?

Also, if you ask an experienced natural health practitioner about your immune system, he or she will take a history, learn about your past and present health and illnesses, ascertain your body type, and recommend herbs based on all of those specific things. That's a lot different from asking a store clerk an extremely general question—something we recommend you never do. We agree that asking health-food-store clerks for advice is inadvisable. See our commentary and recommendations on this on page 455.

"A single herb cannot accomplish all of the different things that many claim to do." If you understand the tonic concept, it doesn't seem strange at all that a substance from nature has many different uses, effects, and purposes. Many foods have many different uses, applications, and effects. Herbs are foodlike. Most plants have thousands of compounds and constituents, and anywhere from dozens to hundreds may be active in the human body. Why would all of those compounds be capable of only one effect?

Plus, herbs that boost functioning—for example, immune function—are going to work for a lot of things. If you boost immune function, your own body can better overcome scores of different conditions. If you can improve liver function, all kinds of seemingly unrelated conditions may clear up. This is the kind of healing the Chinese excel at, and herbs that help your body heal in many ways are the kinds of herbs they prize most.

Skepticism of wide-ranging action comes from the drug paradigm. Botanicals are not designed in a lab to target one thing specifically and narrowly. Drugs are purposely made that way; nature doesn't create plants that way.

"You shouldn't take herbs because they may be adulterated with real drugs, fillers, or the wrong plants." Theoretically, this happens. Practically speaking, in twenty-five years as an herbalist and educator, Karta Purkh heard about this happening no more than a couple of times—and he never came across it himself personally because he selected his sources knowledgeably and carefully. Again, reputable sources are the key (and this is true for any product). Such incidents are certainly the exception, not the norm, in the herb industry.

Keep in mind, also, that poisoning, tampering, or improper handling situations have occurred with all kinds of products, both food and drugs—Tylenol, Jack in the Box hamburgers, and baby food, to name a few.

"All herbs are good for just about everything." Most herbs have more than one healing property, but that doesn't mean they heal everything. Most have a primary use that's out in front of all the others. A small, wonderful handful are excellent choices for dozens of things (some examples are ginger, turmeric, licorice, nettle, clove, ginseng). A fair number of others are equally good for two or three things (such as saw palmetto berry for benign prostatic hyperplasia and for general thyroid building, or cubeb berry for lungs and adrenals and as an antiviral).

But each herb is an individual plant, with distinct qualities and complexities. Some herbs are really primarily best for one thing. They usually do have other effects—a single whole plant has so many naturally occurring compounds that it's bound to do a few different things. But if your primary goal is to achieve a particular effect, it makes sense to choose an herb that "specializes" in that result. Chinese morinda root may relieve depression, but that's not its main claim to fame, so for depression you would be better off taking an herb like St. John's wort, whose best and most well known capability is against depression. To get the best result for your dollar and for your effort, choose the herb whose primary, not secondary, function is the one you need.

All herbs are not tonics; to the contrary, tonics are relatively rare in the wide world of botanicals. A common mistake is long-term use of herbs that are best suited to short-term use for acute conditions. An equally common mistake is using herbs that really are tonics or long-term builders when attempting to remedy an acute situation. Since tonics are "jacks of all trades, masters of none," you won't get the best results for your time and money this way. For a full explanation of tonic and adaptogenic herbs, see pages 129–133.

MYTHS ABOUT SPECIFIC HERBS

"Licorice root causes high blood pressure." This may be true for a small number of people with existing high blood pressure if they take very large amounts of the herb. To state this as a general caution is out of context, however; it is not a practical concern for the majority of people.

Like many herbs, licorice has many different properties and active ingredients. Primarily, it's a glandular tonic that increases endocrine output, and it is a soothing digestive healer. The active ingredient that causes the glandular effect, glycyrrhizin, is the one that could raise blood pressure in some individuals.

For digestive purposes, the effectiveness of licorice is now well documented for ulcers. The licorice used for this purpose is de-glycyrrhizinated (DGL) licorice. There is no chance that this type of licorice will raise blood pressure. (But since the adrenal-building ingredient has been removed, this type cannot be used for adrenal-building purposes.)

The real value in this example is understanding how a caution like this would come out of the Western models of research and medicine, but not in Chinese medicine. Chinese practitioners simply don't see this sort of side effect. A conventional scientist might say, "Well, that's because the Chinese don't take blood pressure." It's true that Chinese practitioners do not regularly belt someone's arm and measure blood pressure with a monitor, but they do have ways of determining if that is a concern for someone.

Of course, Chinese medicine's ways of testing energy in body systems are not recognized by most conventional scientists. But the fact is that in their own ways, the Chinese do test for and deduce the energetics and body types of patients, and simply wouldn't recommend licorice root for someone who would tend to have those reactions—someone hot with a fast metabolism who tends toward inflammation, for example. The Chinese will not recommend certain things to certain people because of incompatibilities they recognize in advance.

If you randomly give 5,000 people a large dose of licorice daily over a long period, without sensitivity to the kinds of things the Chinese look for, you are bound to get reactions from a few people whom a Chinese practitioner never would have treated with licorice. This is all difficult to quantify from a conventional point of view, but the Chinese practitioner is not seeking to "prove" any of this because their standards of proof have already been met. They will say that their great-grandfather taught their grandfather who taught their father, and now they do the same—so what's the problem?

"Echinacea is not effective after two weeks; it wanes and loses its power." A mistranslation of a 1989 German study turned this fallacy into folkloric gospel that has penetrated every mainstream magazine; even doctors and herbalists otherwise well versed in natural medicine are spouting it. This is simply one of those goofy things that didn't ever actually get confirmed by anyone, but someone said it so now it's "true," to an alarmingly persistent degree. You will see widely recommended a protocol of four days on/four days off, or one week on/one week off.

The fact is, effectiveness waned at a point in the study after the subjects stopped taking it! (In fact, the invader-engulfing activity of white blood cells was sustained for five days after the echinacea was stopped, indicating a positive lasting effect.) The original article was in German, and the duration of the dose apparently was not translated or was mistranslated.[5]

In fact, echinacea was used by Native Americans as a long-term tonic for centuries, and Daniel Mowrey, Ph.D., author of *Tonic Herbs*, lists echinacea as an immune-system tonic (for long-term use).[6] And one study showed greater immune reactivity after ten weeks of continuous echinacea use than after two weeks of use, just as the immune response was greater after two weeks than before echinacea was used.[7] This implies progressively increased immune responsiveness with continued use, which is consistent with the clinical experience of practitioners we respect as well as personal experience.

The Ephedra Chronicles

Ephedra is the oldest known Chinese herbal remedy. Also called ma huang, it contains the natural stimulant compounds ephedrine and pseudoephedrine, from which the active ingredients in OTC asthma drugs and in decongestants were synthesized. The Chinese use it for a variety of purposes, and it is an excellent natural sinus decongestant and asthma remedy.

Ephedra has been used safely as a medicine for thousands of years. More recently (much to the chagrin of many herbalists and other natural health practitioners), ephedra has been promoted for "weight control" and in irresponsible "herbal high" street-drug knockoffs (more on this later in this chapter), sometimes in combination with other stimulants, which can augment potential side effects such as high blood pressure and heart palpitations.

Ephedra has made the news recently because investigators linked it to several deaths. The links have not been proven, and other possible cofactors have yet to be explored, but regulatory authorities are reacting. Local and state governments are proposing, and sometimes passing, bans or limits on ephedra-containing products. In August of 1995, a coalition of state drug regulators wrote to the FDA asking the agency to restrict ma huang to prescription use only.

The Texas Department of Health proposed (though later withdrew) a potentially precedent-setting attempt at regulation that's a textbook example of the double standard described earlier: It would have banned the sale of ephedra (ma huang) and ephedrine-containing dietary supplements, while preserving the sale of pharmaceutical products containing the same extracts, including Primatene, Breathe-Aid, Bronkaid, ephedrine-based nose drops, and "generic equivalents."

But if the FDA considers ephedrine-containing products to be safe, then they are equally safe whether sold by a drug company or a natural products company, and all should be available. Why take only the natural versions of a substance off the market? Where is the logic in making pharmaceutical medicines out of ephedra's compounds, then banning the natural, original source while keeping the chemically based copies?

In a paper clearly stating the inconsistencies and biases of the Texas proposal[8] (and, by extension, of similar proposals that have followed from other states since then), Herb Research Foundation president Rob McCaleb pointed out that tea and coffee have an ancient history of use as stimulant beverages. Ephedra too is a long-used stimulant beverage. Except for ephedra, we legally classify these stimulant beverages as foods.

Why is this? If it's because the ephedra is concentrated in supplements, McCaleb makes another argument: When we concentrate a food, is it still a food? Instant coffee, for example, is a concentrated form of coffee, with over three times as much caffeine by weight as regular coffee. Same with instant tea. Ma huang extract is made by the same process as instant coffee, and is similarly concentrated, with about three times as much alkaloid as the whole herb.

There are other examples of food substances that are highly concentrated, yet which are nevertheless not being targeted. McCaleb rattles off a list of concentrated food extracts that could be toxic in high enough doses: wintergreen extract, cinnamon oil, almond extract, and horseradish. All of these concentrated foods can be, and are, used safely every day by millions of people. To single out ephedra is odd, unless one wishes to acknowledge that the only reason to regulate it out of existence while letting the others stand is because ephedra is used as a natural health supplement.

Other dietary supplements, such as vitamins and minerals, are concentrated forms as well. These are regulated in the United States as foods, under laws passed by the United States Congress. McCaleb emphasizes that the fact that such nutritional supplements are concentrated is the whole point, the very nature of dietary supplements: "They are concentrated ways to supplement the diet with something in a convenient form." Thus, some herbal supplements are concentrated as well.

The TDH proposal exempted the over-the-counter (OTC) drugs Vivarin and No-Doz, which contain pure caffeine. No one would call them food. Primatene is an OTC drug that contains ephedrine, the major active chemical purified from ma huang. Millions of Americans use this drug every day to treat asthma. Sudafed contains another stimulant alkaloid from ma huang, pseudoephedrine. It too is used by millions of Americans. Pseudoephedrine has a less potent action on the heart than ephedrine but is still contraindicated in those with high blood pressure, heart disease, diabetes, thyroid disease, or prostate enlargement. Some supermarkets are taking ma huang off their shelves, yet those supermarkets still sell coffee, Primatene, and Sudafed.

Interestingly, the TDH proposal made a specific point of forbidding the sale of supplements that combine ephedrine and caffeine, implying that ephedrine and caffeine are dangerous together. Yet despite such a ban, ephedrine and caffeine would continue to be consumed together by asthmatics who use Primatene and drink coffee, or people taking Sudafed and drinking cola. Obviously, there were no plans to regulate this—no warnings on OTC bronchodilator, decongestant, and stimulant drugs to warn people against drinking coffee, and no caution on caffeine-containing foods to warn people not to take those medications.

McCaleb points out that the quantity consumed is often the only real issue with regard to safety. "The best we can say about the safety of any food or drug is that it is safe 'when used in reasonable amounts by normal consumers' . . . nearly anything can be abused: coffee, Primatene, butter, ma huang . . . [and] there are people who may be especially sensitive to certain things. For example, many people can't drink milk, eat peanuts, or use caffeinated beverages. Some cannot safely use Primatene, as the label warning states."[9] I must also ask how substances like tobacco and alcohol can escape bans while an herbal product such as ephedra is marked. The outrage is disproportionate to a highly questionable degree.

Note: While the specific Texas proposal analyzed above was withdrawn, another very much like it has actually become reality in Nebraska. In July 1996, the Nebraska State Legislature passed a law prohibiting the over-the-counter sale of any ephedra- or ephedrine-containing supplement product. These products are now controlled substances that can only be dispensed by written prescription. As described above, FDA-approved OTC drug products are exempted. Only *dietary supplements* containing ephedra or ephedrine are restricted. Meanwhile, the state of Ohio has amended its total ban on the sale of all mahuang products.

Herbal supplements should be regulated in a way that is consistent with the way foods, OTC drugs, and most vitamin products are labeled and sold. That means determining at what levels the substance is safe for "average" consumers, making recommendations for dosages, and requiring cautionary labels warning those with certain health conditions to avoid the products or seek medical advice before using. Scientific experts have testified to the FDA that ephedra should not be banned, but rather sold with label warnings and dose limits.

Consumers share the responsibility with the herb industry and health professions to act sensibly with regard to herb use. It may be that dieters ruined ma huang for the rest of us—taking too much for the wrong reasons, in the wrong context. Herbal "high" products are another misguided use (see later in this chapter for more on this). Good things can always be used for bad purposes. To blame the results of this kind of usage on the herb itself is illogical.

When I belonged to a health club a few years ago, I overheard more about ephedra from people trying to lose "weight" than I ever heard about it anywhere else. When ephedra is plucked out of context of its use in Chinese medicine, that phenomenon is not ephedra's problem. It's people, their thinking, and what they are trying to do to their bodies that creates trouble. These problems come from our culture.

In addition, to use the dieter as an example of the average medicinal herb consumer is extremely misleading. It is predictable, and should be taken into account, that people in our "weight"-obsessed, dieting-happy culture will overinterpret the potential benefit of an herbal stimulant. They will assume that "more is better" if it is suggested that a substance will make them thin. Historically, dieting consumers are more likely to take any strategy (whether diet or pill) to extremes. And the lack of overall good health among many dieters makes them poor subjects for determining how an herb or any other substance might affect people in general.

It is also unfortunately predictable that companies will package herbal stimulants accordingly to appeal to this huge market segment. I don't agree with this because I think "weight" loss in general is misguided, and I think the idea that any one pill of any kind can "handle" a lifestyle issue that has many different factors needs to be put to rest.

Herbal medicine is also not about "herbal stimulants." I personally had great results with ma huang for energy and warming early in my herbal treatment—but I was using it medicinally, I discussed it with an herbalist, and I discontinued its use when I didn't need it anymore. I also used the whole herb as a tea, not pills. Many of the herb users I have interviewed used ma huang short term with absolutely no problems.

Finally, if ephedra were so dangerous, the Chinese would not have prized it so highly for more than 5,000 years. It's certainly an insult to Chinese medicine to suggest that Chinese practitioners wouldn't know if one of their most valued botanicals was picking people off left and right.

The whole ephedra "scene" is a perfect example of why the problem is lack of education and cultural thinking patterns, not the substance itself. This is why we have worked so hard to evoke a larger, integrative context to surround your use of herbal medicine. Information on specific remedies and their uses, alone, is too easily misused in a void.

The Herb Research Foundation publishes an "Herbal Stimulant Factsheet," which compares the caffeine and ephedrine content of various foods and drugs. It also discusses the relative safety of such products, and provides contraindication information about people who should avoid either substance. See page 512 for more on the Herb Research Foundation.

The Comfrey Chronicles

Pyrrolizidine alkaloids, or PAs, are the class of compounds in question with comfrey and some other herbs. In substantial doses under certain conditions, they apparently can cause the destruction of liver tissue by creating a condition known as hepatic veno-occlusive disease, in which the cells lining the veins in the liver proliferate and choke off the veins. The presumed basis for this condition is that a portion of ingested PAs are converted by liver enzymes to a toxic substance that destroys liver tissue. It is the liver's attempt to alter the compound, to make it excretable, that turns it into this reactive toxic substance.[10]

According to the *Journal of the Canadian Association of Herbal Practitioners*, there have only been four cases in the world literature of comfrey toxicity since 1980. Before that, no human toxicity was ever recorded. The four cases each involved very high consumption levels along with significant other complicating factors, including other illness and other potential sources of toxicity.

Again, the rare problems with herbs invariably happen in this way: Someone whose health is already compromised, who is using many other substances, totally unsupervised, and without proper information, abuses the herb. For example, the twenty-three-year-old man who died of hepatic veno-occlusive disease (HVOD) after eating enormous amounts of steamed comfrey on a regular basis also had a history of following fad diets.

According to *FDA Consumer*, the forty-seven-year-old woman who developed liver disease was consuming up to ten cups of comfrey tea a day and taking comfrey pills by the handful for more than a year in an attempt to cure her stomach pains, fatigue, and allergies.[11] (No herbalist we know recommends taking any single herb in such exorbitant amounts, even short term, let alone for a year. You work up slowly, and ten cups of something plus handfuls is clearly excessive. Also, if a problem doesn't go away in due time, you don't keep taking it for a year and not address it.) It is also not clear what disease she originally presented with, but she definitely was ill before beginning to take comfrey.

In another case, a thirteen-year-old boy with colitis had been taking prednisone and sulphasalazine for years, but when he stopped the drugs and took comfrey, his later development of liver disease was subjectively attributed to comfrey, not the drugs.

A press release by the National Institute of Medical Herbalists, which contests laboratory research on comfrey's safety, speaks of "two insupportable assumptions. First, that the naturally occurring complex in the plant . . . can be regarded as a mere physical dilution of alkaloids; and secondly that the human metabolism is identical with that of the rat which is susceptible to these alkaloids, and not with the sheep which is resistant to them." In other words, the isolated alkaloid used in experiments should not be considered to reflect the action of the whole herb, and what happens to rats should not be assumed to be what happens to people.

Critics of the most quoted paper on the subject have pointed to the young age of the rats and the extremely high dosage, which was twenty-eight times the body weight—obviously a larger dosage than a human could possibly consume, even over nine weeks (it would mean eating

5,000 leaves!)[12] The infant rats were also injected with isolated extracts, not orally consuming the whole herb as humans would.[13]

Herbalist Margaret Whitelegg, B.A., director of research of the National Institute of Medical Herbalists, writing in *The Herbalist* in August 1994, points out, "Tea, almonds, apples, pears, mustard, radishes and hops, to list only a few items, all contain substances which, if extracted, can be shown to be poisonous when tested under conditions similar to those used in the comfrey experiments. Must we then ignore our experience of the usefulness and wholesomeness of these foods because controlled trials and scientific evidence have not been published to establish their safety?"

Despite the shaky premise for comfrey's dismissal, many herbalists do now advise against internal consumption of comfrey, since many people would rather not take the risk. While we think the possibility of a comfrey user meeting the same fate as these four isolated cases is close to zero, there are certainly other herbs that can be used for any purpose that comfrey might. We have not suggested comfrey as a remedy anywhere in this book. We cover it here to clarify the facts surrounding an issue you may read or hear about, and as another illustration of how safety concerns can be disproportionate to the facts or based on distorted, illogical, or incomplete information.

Comfrey as an external remedy is soothing and healing to the skin and there are no reports of safety concerns for its external use.

The Chaparral Chronicles

Chaparral, like comfrey, is an herb that's drawn negative publicity to itself and to herbs in general after an apparently idiosyncratic reaction by a small handful of people. Some publications cite the case of one woman who needed a liver transplant after taking the herb chaparral for ten months; six other cases of acute nonviral hepatitis (rapidly developing liver damage) have also been attributed to this herb by some accounts.

Now for the facts: Like other cases discussed above, only anecdotal evidence existed to suggest that the chaparral caused the problem. There is no evidence to suggest that chaparral is inherently hepatotoxic, and all cases involved medical histories compatible with prior liver disease.

Pharmacognosist Varro Tyler, Ph.D., notes in the PBS documentary *The Medicine Garden* that many thousands of people took this herb over many decades with no problems whatsoever, and he believes it is quite possible that the problems arose from the herb being adulterated. (Still, the herb industry voluntarily took it off the market anyway, in December 1992, until further investigation was conducted.)

Most importantly, the FDA, in cooperation with the American Herb Products Association (AHPA), appointed a nonpartisan, independent scientific committee (medical experts specializing in gastroenterology and hepatitis research) to review and investigate these cases, and this panel concluded that chaparral be allowed back on market because it found no causal evidence of any harm. The AHPA has since rescinded its voluntary ban, with the recommendation that all consumer labeling now contain standard informational language about liver disease and symptoms, and a phone number to report unusual conditions.

Again, note that anecdotal evidence is rarely considered scientific enough to vouch for an herb's effectiveness, but it was accepted as enough to "prove" its "dangers." If six people took chaparral and experienced wonderful results with no side effects, scientists would say that's not a big enough sample and it was coincidental. But when six people took it and anecdotally had a negative result, that "counted."

In addition, almost a year after the FDA-appointed investigation concluded chaparral was not hepatotoxic, the *Journal of the American Medical Association* described one of these cases as chaparral-induced liver toxicity. This is an example of conventional medicine's need for more awareness of matters in the sphere of natural healing, and a reminder that no authority can be considered unquestionable.

Finally, it's interesting that the media fusses so about six negative herb reactions and not about the 600,000 negative drug reactions that result in hospitalization every year. By no means is even one injury or death from any product acceptable, but even if chaparral had caused six cases of liver failure, six cases among all the liver failure in this country is an unbelievably minute drop in the bucket.

"ECSTASY" IS NOT MEDICINE

The death of a Long Island college student in March 1996 after using an "herbal recreational drug" is creating a flurry of misdirected concern over herbal medicine. The media is having a field day with this "story," and fanning myths in the process as it collapses the issue of substance abuse in with the entirely separate field of medicinal herbalism.

In May 1995 a local Northwest talk show ran an exposé of herbal "drugs" (Herbal Ecstacy [sic], Cloud Nine, and Ultimate Xphoria) used by kids to get high.[14] Like similar programming and reporting all over the country, in an entire hour it failed to make the crucial distinction that Herbal Ecstacy is not herbal medicine. Herbal medicine is not about highs. Herbal formulations commercially sold to produce a "high" have absolutely nothing to do with medicinal whole herbs and teas used in traditional preparations for health.

Instead, the show lumped herbal medicine, herbal "drugs" for feel-good stimulation, and vitamins and mineral and nutritional supplements all into one basket—and it was presented, at best, as a questionable basket. This lack of distinction has been broadly perpetuated by most media as the furor has spread, including the *New York Times*, *Newsweek*, *Prime Time Live*, and CNN. (Mark Blumenthal, executive director of the American Botanical Council and editor of *HerbalGram*, sent a letter to the *New York Times* correcting numerous misleading and false statements, but his letter was not published. It is printed in full in *HerbalGram* 37, page 23.)

It's up to you to think critically when you're presented with hype that "fuzzes" the issues. For example, when it was suggested on the Northwest TV show *Town Meeting*,[15] that herbs are foodlike, the host asked, "Can you give Herbal Ecstacy to an infant?" When the response was no, he snapped, "Then it's not a food." But since when is the definition of "food" something that can be given to an infant? You wouldn't give an infant steak, Coca-Cola, french fries, or a Snickers bar, but most Americans would in fact classify those items as food. You also wouldn't give an infant rice and beans, but those are clearly foods. Everything we consume does not have to be consumable by infants. And if a drug has to be mild enough for an infant to be okay for adults, that rules out most of the pharmaceuticals approved for use in the United States, as well as cigarettes and alcohol.

It can be troublesome if an already nervous, hyped-up, anxious person with a rapid heartbeat and high blood pressure takes large amounts of a stimulating herb such as ephedra (ma huang) or yohimbe. But when a person who is already unhealthy misuses a product, neither the person's poor health nor the misuse is the fault of the product.

For example, it can be troublesome when an obese person whose arteries are so blocked that he or she may be minutes away from a heart attack sits down to a breakfast of eggs fried in butter with sausage, bacon, danish, and buttered toast. It is a problem that teenage girls will buy Dexatrim or other OTC diet pills and take five times the recommended dose assuming that "more is thinner." A person with chronic headaches can take so many aspirin that the stomach begins to bleed. Tobacco, or alcohol, and dietary fat are known to be deadly and have killed millions of people, and have no redeeming qualities. We don't ban sausage, Dexatrim, aspirin, or even cigarettes and alcohol. Nor do we see "exposés" about them. Herbs benefit and heal people, and rarely harm—yet they are the subjects of "exposés." You might ask yourself why this is.

"Herbal" substitutes for illicit drugs, hiding under the umbrella of "dietary supplements," are not condoned by the herb industry at large. In fact, the herb industry, as much as anyone, would like to see these products disappear and their manufacturers dealt with appropriately for misleading marketing. The failure of media, regulators, and health professionals to distinguish such products from medicinal herbs with long histories of safe use creates an unfortunate and undeserved image problem for legitimate herbal medicine.

MYTH: "The FDA no longer has the power to regulate supplements." A new myth has come out of the "herbal high" drug situation, since the death of one young man after using one of these products: that the new supplement law (DSHEA, described on page 457) "tied the hands" of the FDA to regulate harmful supplements. This may make paper-selling headlines and help the FDA raise consumer outrage if it wants support to topple DSHEA. However, it's totally false.

The FDA absolutely has the authority to remove these herbal street drugs, or any others, from the market, if it believes they pose an imminent threat to public health. Congress has not taken away from the FDA's power to regulate toxic products. In fact, the DSHEA gave new authority to the secretary of Health and Human Services to remove products from the market that pose "an imminent threat to public health or safety."[16]

What changed is that the FDA must now bear the burden of proof that its actions are justified. Before, excessive and arbitrary exercising of its authority kept safe substances from public access despite any reports of harm or adverse reactions. Consumers and the industry were concerned over this practice. (In one case, regarding the FDA's whimsical banning of black currant seed oil on the unfounded pretext that it was an "unsafe food additive," the FDA lost in a U.S. district court; on appeal, the U.S. Circuit Court called the FDA's arguments an "Alice-in-Wonderland" approach.[17])

The new supplement law was intended to help preserve the rights of consumers to have access to authentic herbal medicines, not shield irresponsible products from regulation. The American Herbal Products Association has acted quickly and vigorously when there is a question about a supplement, as you've seen in earlier examples. APHA developed a policy of label warnings and dose limits for ma huang products in 1994 and restricts their sale to those under eighteen. The FDA's own expert advisory panel recommended against banning the herb, instead recommending that the FDA institute a policy much like the one AHPA already instituted, but the FDA has not done it—not because it can't, but by *choice*.

WHAT ABOUT DRUG SAFETY?

Safety questions about herbs are ironic given about a dozen serious herb reactions over a period of decades, compared to drug reactions at 10 million annually. Yet the drug business continues briskly despite this, unimpeded by the kind of "exposés" to which herbs are subjected.

From a very long list we have compiled, here are a few tidbits that might help put the question of herb safety in perspective.

- More than half (102 of 198) of the prescription drugs approved by the FDA between 1976 and 1985 caused serious reactions that later caused the drugs to be relabeled or removed from the market.[18]
- 200,000 cases of gastrointestinal bleeding, with 10,000 to 20,000 deaths, occur each year due to the 68 million prescriptions of nonsteroidal anti-inflammatory drugs, or NSAIDs, used for arthritis.[19]

- In 1990, the *New England Journal of Medicine* reported that 36 percent of U.S. patients are suffering from iatrogenic disease— disease resulting from medical intervention (drugs, surgery, etc.).
- 1 in 1,000 of patients admitted to hospitals for medical rather than surgical reasons will be killed by the medicine.[20]
- Estrogen replacement therapy was encouraged for menopausal women for about fifteen years before the accompanying fivefold increase in uterine cancer risk was acknowledged. The response: Progesterone was added to the mix to make it "safer." (Now called hormone replacement therapy, Premarin is the best-selling pharmaceutical in the country.)[21]
- *Time* magazine reported in 1995 that the FDA plans to deregulate more than a dozen currently prescription drugs and approve them for OTC sale over the next few years. Pharmaceutical firms have been pressing officials at the FDA to do this for medications that the companies say are safe enough to be sold directly to the public. The eagerness to go OTC comes from the fact that law provides a three-year monopoly to a drug manufacturer when it goes OTC, before competitors may produce generic versions. That gives companies time to establish name recognition and brand loyalty. The *Time* article points out that this move will **"spur competition and prolong the financial health of pharmaceutical companies. . . . The consumer's health and well-being are not, of course, the only factors at stake in these decisions."**
- Researchers at the University of Manitoba in Winnipeg, Canada, suspect that part of the upsurge in cancers may be fueled by some of the medicines we take. Of five antihistamines tested on mice at human-equivalent doses, three increased growth in melanoma and fibrosarcoma tumors: Claritin (loratadine), Hismanal (astemizole), and Atarax (hydroxine). The drugs are not causing cancer, but they are making cancer that's already present grow faster. An earlier study found a similar effect with Prozac and Elavil, two leading antidepressants.[22]
- Research confirms that drinking alcohol while taking acetaminophen causes increases in liver toxicity.[23] In the trial of a former White House official who experienced liver failure from this combination, Tylenol's manufacturer, McNeil Consumer Products, disclosed

that they had known for years that alcohol drinkers could suffer liver damage from ordinary doses of Tylenol, yet did not make this information available to the public.

Acetaminophen has also been shown to damage kidneys—even two pills a day for a year, according to a study published in *JAMA*, increases the risk to the kidneys. Some 4,000 to 5,000 people a year suffer kidney failure from acetaminophen use. A study released in the *New England Journal of Medicine* suggests that a person who uses more than one NSAID or acetaminophen tablet per day has twice the likelihood of developing kidney failure compared to a person who doesn't use them.[24]

25

Healing Recipes

This section offers a few delicious healing recipes using both common and uncommon foods whose healing properties we have discussed throughout the book.

❧ *Yogi Tea* ❧
(© Yogi Bhajan)

This tea, a staple in Ayurveda, is immune boosting generally and healing and rejuvenating for many parts of the body. Black pepper is a blood purifier, cardamom soothes the intestines, cloves are rejuvenating to nerves as well as the digestive system, and cinnamon is for joints, bones, and digestion. All are warming. The milk is traditionally believed to aid in assimilation of the spices. You can also use soy, rice, or almond milk.

The original recipe calls for black tea, but new research shows that green tea has healing benefits of its own, including anticancer properties, thanks to its catechins—compounds that are destroyed in the fermentation process that makes green tea leaves into black tea.

DIRECTIONS

For each 8-ounce cup, start with 10 ounces of water. For convenience, make at least 4 cups at one time and store in refrigerator for reheating.

For *each* cup of boiling water add:
3 whole cloves
4 whole green cardamom pods
6 whole black peppercorns
1/2 stick cinnamon

Optional: Slices of fresh ginger root may be included for their delicious taste and because ginger is helpful when you are suffering from a cold, recovering from the flu, have digestive or arthritis symptoms, or want extra energy.

Boil for 20 to 30 minutes, then add 1/4 teaspoon of tea.
Let sit for 1 to 2 minutes, then add 1/2 cup skim or low-fat milk per cup of tea desired.
Reheat. Strain and serve with honey to taste.

♾

♾ *Turmeric Paste/Golden Milk* ♾

Turmeric is an incredible herbal remedy. It is an extremely effective treatment for stiff, sore, arthritic, or inflamed joints—probably the foremost joint remedy in all medicine, herbal or otherwise. It is also a general anti-inflammatory, liver cleanser and restorative, digestive tonic, antiseptic, antioxidant, antiparasitic, astringent, pain reliever, blood purifier, wound healer, kidney-stone dissolver, eczema treatment, and more.

DIRECTIONS

Prepare a turmeric paste. Use 1/4 cup of turmeric powder to 1/2 cup of pure water and bring to a boil in a saucepan until a thick paste is formed. This paste should be stored in the refrigerator in a sealed container. (Caution: wash all utensils and any spills immediately. Turmeric stains yellow anything it comes in contact with and is a difficult stain to remove.)

USES

The paste can be consumed in the following ways:

- By the spoonful. Roll cold paste into large, pill-like balls. Spoon to back of throat. Swallow with a large mouthful of water and follow quickly with more water.
- Stir into water, milk, soy milk, juice, or tea. Swallow quickly. (This can be done with the powder too.)
- Golden milk: The following are all variations on an original recipe from Yogi Bhajan. For each cup of golden milk, blend together 1 cup of milk, 1 teaspoon almond oil (almonds are also good for joints and are anti-inflammatory in general), 1/2 teaspoon or more of turmeric paste, and honey to taste. While stirring, on low heat, bring the milk just to the boiling point. The mixture may then be blended in an electric blender to make a foamy drink. Fruit may be added before blending, as can as much cinnamon as you can tolerate (cinnamon is also a great joint soother and restorative, especially for osteoarthritis).
- Mix turmeric paste (or just the powder) into honey or maple syrup to make a sweet paste. Swallow from spoon and "chase" with plenty of water.
- Sandwich: Mix with thick, strong-tasting food such as almond butter (almonds are also good for joints) or sesame butter. Spread this paste 1/4-inch thick on 2 slices of bread. Add condiments, lettuce, parsley, etc. Include cucumber slices.

ॳ

ॳ *Jalapeño Pancakes* ॳ

(Original recipe by Yogi Bhajan © 1982)

These extremely spicy pancakes make a tasty and extra-healthy breakfast. They contain antiviral foods (they are an exceptionally good way to ingest substantial amounts of ajwain seed) and make a protective daily meal during times of increased susceptibility or exposure to virus.

INGREDIENTS

1–2 tablespoons finely chopped ginger (or to maximum tolerance)
2–3 tablespoons finely chopped cauliflower
1 finely chopped jalapeño pepper per pancake
1–2 tablespoons ajwain seeds per pancake
Crushed red chilies to taste (maximum tolerance)
Black pepper to taste (maximum tolerance)
Bragg's Liquid Aminos (a liquid condiment similar to soy sauce),
    1/2 tsp. per pancake or to taste
Equal parts bran and organic whole-wheat flour,
    approximately 1/2 cup each per pancake

DIRECTIONS

Mix all ingredients. Drop batter onto nonstick griddle sprayed with vegetable spray or coated with lecithin (anything else and the batter will stick like glue). Cook on low heat for about 1/2 hour (15 minutes per side).

Eat 2 large pancakes per day.

ᢒ

ᢒ Luscious Immune-Boosting Broth ᢒ

INGREDIENTS

3 cups water or vegetable broth (more for milder preparation)
1 ounce (about 5 "sticks" dried herb) astragalus
1 bulb (5 to 10 cloves) fresh garlic, sliced or whole
Salt and pepper to taste

DIRECTIONS

Place water in pot and sticks and garlic under water. Bring to boil, then simmer on medium-low for several hours, until garlic is soft.

Drink hot. Eat the garlic in the broth, or remove the garlic to spread on toast or hot fresh bread. (Fire types can use less or no garlic.)

Drink the entire pot of broth at once if you feel as though a cold, flu, or other viral infection may be coming on. Drink or eat a cup or two of this broth daily, as frequently as possible—2 to 5 times weekly—to help prevent any such infection.

VARIATIONS

Try adding noodles or rice, slivered almonds, and/or carrots (cook till soft) to make a meal. Cook grains in leftover broth to add a healthier touch to a future meal. Add fresh sliced or ground ginger and diced onion as well as the garlic before cooking to increase exponentially the immune-strengthening and antibacterial properties of the soup. Shredded ginger, soft miso, green onion, and a dash of low-sodium shoyu (soy sauce) will turn this into a miso broth.

℘

℘ *Ghee* ℘
(Clarified butter)

In America, we don't normally think of butter as being healthy. And, mostly, we're right—because butter fat is saturated, it really isn't good for most of us, and is best used in very minute quantities if at all. However, Ayurvedic medicine uses a special preparation of butter medicinally, especially to cool the fire of *pitta* or lubricate *vata*. This preparation is called ghee, also known as clarified butter.

There are different ways of making ghee. Regardless of the method, the object of making ghee is to remove the solids, leaving only the liquid behind.

METHOD 1

Put butter in pan and heat on stove over medium heat. As waste comes to the top, skim off. (This should be done slowly to avoid burning.) When all waste is removed and liquid is clear, strain and store. (A gravy separator is helpful.)

METHOD 2

Put butter in pan and put into the oven at a low temperature (200° to 250°) overnight. Waste should form a crust on top and bottom. Remove top crust and strain clear liquid into storage jar.

If all the waste does not go to the top but rather sinks to the bottom, just strain the liquid, making sure that none of the waste goes into the jar.

Use 1 to 2 tablespoons a day or as necessary.

❧

❧ *Subzee* ❧
(Original recipe by Yogi Bhajan © 1980)

This Ayurvedic soup (the name refers to "vegetable stew") is a wonderful digestive and intestinal tonic and nerve soother. It's pungent and fragrant and, in addition to being therapeutic, it makes a hearty meal. The spices are all excellent tonics for inflammation, nerves, indigestion, nausea, or gas, and other ingredients are immune-boosting and nutritious as well.

DIRECTIONS

In a heavy-bottomed pot, heat the following in about 3 tablespoons almond oil and 1 tablespoon water:
1/2 tablespoon ground black pepper
1/2 tablespoon turmeric
1 teaspoon ground cardamom
1/2 tablespoon ground cinnamon
1/2 tablespoon ground ginger

When this is thoroughly blended, sauté:
1 bulb garlic, sliced
2 large yellow onions, sliced

When garlic and onions are soft and lightly browned, add a little purified water at a time as you bring to a boil, until the vegetables are covered.

To boiling water add:
2 cups of assorted vegetables (carrots, broccoli, zucchini, etc.)
1/4 cup slivered raw almonds
Salt to taste

Add enough water to cover added vegetables. Cook until vegetables are very tender.

USES

When vegetables are done, serve the soup with warm whole-grain bread or toast, or spoon over cooked rice.

✥

✥ *Preparation B (Fluorescent Soup)* ✥
by Robyn Landis

Hemorrhoids, from which half of all adult Americans suffer, are usually treated in conventional medicine by medicating the symptom, but the problem goes deeper. Its root is liver stress—stagnant blood in the liver causes an accumulation of blood in rectal veins. Speaking of roots, the root vegetables are potent liver cleansers and rejuvenators, and help to heal hemorrhoids by eliminating the source of the problem instead of attacking the symptom topically. Beets alone are a classic hemorrhoid remedy (that's why I call this soup Preparation B), but this recipe utilizes the cleansing and healing properties of several root vegetables—and as a bonus, makes a delicious meal at the same time! I nicknamed this "Fluorescent Soup" because the beets, radish, red cabbage, and carrots give the soup a glowing pink, red, purple, and orange color.

INGREDIENTS

1 large onion, diced
1 bulb garlic, sliced
2 tablespoons coriander
1 teaspoon dried basil and/or fresh to taste
5 large carrots, sliced
1 28-ounce can organic stewed tomatoes (diced, crushed, or whole)
15 to 20 radishes, sliced thin
1/2 large head red cabbage, chopped
10 large organic beets, steamed, trimmed, and sliced or cubed
    (or two cans organic diced beets, with juice)
Black pepper to taste

DIRECTIONS

Sauté onion and garlic in coriander, dried basil, and olive oil over medium heat in the bottom of 8-quart soup pot until soft.

Add carrots and cook for another 5 minutes.

Add canned tomatoes and radish, cabbage, and beets. Stir till mixed.

Fill the pot with water (or astragalus broth) and bring to a boil.

Add black pepper and turn down to simmer until all vegetables are cooked, up to an hour.

Add fresh basil before serving.

SERVING SUGGESTIONS

Serve soup with bread on the side or mix in cooked rice or other grains. Grated parmesan cheese can be lightly sprinkled over the top.

❧

❧ Antioxidant Vegetable Stew ❧
by Robyn Landis

This chunky, hearty soup is a pleasant way to get your servings of healthful antioxidant vegetables along with other healing foods. It's a tasty meal anytime, but I like it especially when I'm feeling drained or depleted, or want extra insurance against infection. This soup is loaded with carotenoids, indoles, sulforafanes, and the antioxidant vitamins A and C, among other phytochemicals known for their healing, antimicrobial, and cancer-preventive properties.

INGREDIENTS

1 large onion, chopped
1 bulb garlic, sliced
6 to 8 carrots, sliced
5 celery stalks, chopped
1/4 to 1/2 red cabbage, chopped
1/4 to 1/2 green cabbage, chopped
1 red pepper, diced
15 shiitake mushrooms, sliced (remove stems)
8 to 10 small red or white new potatoes, cut in small chunks
1 28-ounce can organic stewed tomatoes (diced, crushed or whole)
Black pepper to taste

Version 1: Italian style—2 parmesan rinds; white beans; basil, rosemary, thyme and oregano to taste
Version 2: Eastern style—Black beans; coriander, nutmeg, allspice, and clove to taste
Version 3: Mexican style—Chili beans; cumin, cayenne, chili powder to taste; top with fresh cilantro

DIRECTIONS

Sauté onion and garlic in spices of choice with olive oil over medium heat in the bottom of 8-quart soup pot until soft.

Add vegetables one group at a time and cook until slightly soft.

Add canned tomatoes and cooked or canned beans or parmesan rinds. Heat through.

Add water (or astragalus broth) to almost fill the pot. Bring to a boil.

Turn down to simmer until all vegetables are cooked, about an hour and a half.

Add black pepper and more spices to taste.

SERVING SUGGESTIONS

Serve soup with bread and cheese or cooked rice, couscous, or orzo. Grated cheese can be lightly sprinkled over the top. If you eat meat, cooked cubed meat or poultry can be added instead of the beans for protein.

♫

ALTERNATIVE INGREDIENTS AND SUBSTITUTES

If you are trying to avoid certain refined or otherwise unhealthy ingredients in foods or in your diet—and especially if you have food allergies—finding alternatives can sometimes be challenging. This list is designed to help you identify the best substitutes to standard ingredients for cooking and baking, as well as substitutes for other common foods.

In general, natural food stores, co-ops, and more upscale groceries tend to do a better job of making more of these substitute items available. Some of the larger, older supermarket chains still have a very limited selection of natural food alternatives. You might try talking to the manager of your local grocery if you are having trouble locating the items you need, and see if the store can begin stocking the items or if they can be special-ordered.

We recommend that you try to buy organically grown food whenever possible.

BAKING OR BAKED PRODUCTS

All-Purpose Flour (White)	Whole-wheat flour, whole-wheat pastry flour, barley, oat, spelt, kamut, amaranth, or rye
Cake Flour	Sift whole-wheat pastry flour. Requires more liquid.
Chocolate or Cocoa	Carob powder
Shortenings	1/3 cup canola oil and 1/2 cup unsalted butter for each cup of shortening; or one cup mashed banana for each 1/2 cup butter; or one cup puréed prunes or plums for each cup butter
Refined Oils	Unrefined oils
White Sugar, Corn Syrup	Fruitsource, date sugar, fruit-juice concentrate, honey, maple syrup, molasses, rice syrup, barley, malt syrup or powder, Sucanat (unevaporated cane juice)

OTHER FOOD

Polished White Rice	Brown rice, whole grains
Salt	Fresh herbs, fresh lemon and garlic, citrus, kelp, sesame seed, low-sodium tamari or soy sauce
Margarine	Olive oil, sesame oil, almond oil, butter (small amounts)
Coffee	Herbal or grain coffee substitute (e.g., Teecino); herbal teas
Breakfast Cereals	Whole-grain, unsweetened cereals or those lightly sweetened with sweeteners listed above
Soda Pop	Pure water, naturally carbonated waters, fruit juice
Milk	Soy milk, rice beverage, almond beverage, Amazake
Jam, Jelly	All-fruit spreads, no sugar added
Peanut Butter	Nonhydrogenated nut-butter spreads (almond or sesame butter) and soy-based spreads

Substitutes for White Sugar

For 1 cup white sugar in recipe, use		And reduce liquids
Honey	*(3/4 cup)*	*1/8–1/4 cup*
Barley Malt	*(1½ cups)*	*Not necessary*
Rice Syrup	*(1/2 cup)*	*1/4 cup*
Date Sugar	*(1 cup)*	*Not necessary*
Maple Syrup	*(3/4 cup)*	*1/8–1/4 cup*
Maple Sugar	*(1 cup)*	*Not necessary*
Molasses	*(1/2 cup)*	*Not necessary*
Fruit Juice Concentrate	*(1½ cups)*	*1/8–1/4 cup*

All whole-grain flours have different weights and consistencies. Additional liquid is usually required when replacing white flour. Begin by adding 1/4 cup liquid to your recipe.

Resources
and
Appendices

Resources

The following is a list of resources that we feel may be of interest to you, should you desire more information about any of the topics presented in *Herbal Defense*. It is grouped into five sections:

- Herbs: Information
- Herbs: Products
- Holistic Practitioners: Organizations and Information
- Insurance Companies
- Specific Support Groups and Materials

This information was compiled solely for informational purposes. We do not necessarily support or endorse all of these organizations. Also, these lists are *not* exhaustive.

HERBS: INFORMATION

3HO Foundation, International Headquarters, P. O. Box 351149, Los Angeles, CA 90035. (310) 552-3416.

American Botanical Council, P. O. Box 201660, Austin, TX 78720. (512) 331-8868. Publishes *HerbalGram*, one of the most respected botanical research and information journals in the United States, jointly with the Herb Research Foundation (see below). Its board of trustees includes the most eminent botanical experts and authorities in the country, including James A. Duke, Ph.D.; Norman Farnsworth, Ph.D.; Varro E. Tyler, Ph.D.; and Andrew Weil, M.D. ABC is planning to translate and publish the German Commission E's reports (or "monographs") on medicinal herbs, which that country uses as the basis for regulating herbs.

Blazing Star Herb School, P. O. Box 6, Shelburne Falls, MA 01370. (413) 625-6875.

The Herb Quarterly, Long Mountain Press, P. O. Box 689, San Anselmo, CA 94960. (415) 455-9540.

Herb Research Foundation, 1007 Pearl St., Ste. 200, Boulder, CO 80302. (303) 449-2265. Will supply information packets on specific herbs for $7 each. Write or call for a free brochure.

The Herb Research Foundation (HRF) is a nonprofit research and educational organization. Founded in 1983, the HRF supports, conducts, collects, and encourages research on herb safety, benefits, production, and conservation. The organization does not sell herbs, nor is it a government agency, so it is unbiased and uncensored. The World Health Organization has cited HRF as one of the most reliable sources of botanical information in the world.

HRF's mission is to improve world health and welfare through herbs, to increase the rational and informed use of herbs through scientific research and historical documentation, and to return natural remedies to prominence in modern health care in the United States and around the world, so that nature can meet more of our health-care needs for better health and longevity at a lower cost—and a better, protected environment to boot.

HRF keeps a scientific library of over 100,000 articles and references on more than 1,000 herbs and continues to gather scientific, historical, and cultural information on herbs from the ancient past to the latest research from all over the world.

Sage: Home Study Herbology Course, Rosemary Gladstar, P. O. Box 420, East Barre, VT 05649.

HERBS: PRODUCTS

Ancient Healing Ways, Rt 3, Box 259, Espanola, NM 87532. (800) 359-2940. Hard-to-find Ayurvedic products, quality herbs for herbalists and the public, books by Yogi Bhajan, Yogi tea, etc. Call for free catalog.

Auromere, (800) 735-4691, imports Ayurvedic products from India.

Eclectic Institute, 4385 Southeast Lusted Rd., Sandy, OR 97055. (800) 332-4372.

Essiac International, (800) 668-4559.

The Herbalist (herb pharmacy), (206) 523-2600, (800) 694-3727.

Herbs for Kids, P. O. Box 837, Bozeman, MT 59717. (406) 587-0180, or 1-800-735-0299 (9 to 5 Mountain Time). Glycerites for children.

Indiana Botanical Gardens, P. O. Box 5, Hammond, IN 46325. (800) 644-8327.

Nature Care, (800) 923-9338, sells hard-to-find Ayurvedic products such as chyavanprash (amla fruit jelly).

Penn Herb Company (herb pharmacy), (215) 925-3336 or (215) 632-6336.

Smile Herb Shop (herb pharmacy), 4908 Berwyn Rd., College Park, MD 20740. (301) 474-8791.

Tenzing Momo (herb pharmacy), (206) 623-9837.

Transitions for Health, 621 Southwest Alder, Ste. 900, Portland, OR 97205. (800) 888-6814. Offers a free mail-order catalog of natural health-care products for menopausal women.

Western Herb, P. O. Box 115, Index, WA 98256. (360) 793-7037.

Wise Woman Herbals, P. O. Box 279, Creswell, OR 97426. (541) 895-5152. Excellent glycerite tinctures.

HOLISTIC PRACTITIONERS: ORGANIZATIONS AND INFORMATION

American Academy of Medical Acupuncture, 5820 Wilshire Blvd., Ste. 500, Los Angeles, CA 90036. (213) 937-5514.

American Association of Naturopathic Physicians, 2366 Eastlake Ave. East, Ste. 322, Seattle, WA 98102. (206) 323-7610 referral line only; (206) 328-8510 direct line. Offers a list of licensed naturopaths around the country. Send $5, check or money order.

American Herbalists Guild, P. O. Box 746555, Arvada, CO 80006. (303) 423-8800.

American Holistic Centers, 990 West Fullerton Ave., Ste. 300, Chicago, Illinois 60614. (312) 296-6700.

American Holistic Medical Association, 4101 Lake Boone Trail, Suite 201, Raleigh, NC 27607. (919) 787-5181. Offers a list of the members of AHMA who are currently accepting new patients. Send an $8 check or money order to the association.

Arizona Center for Health and Medicine, 5055 N. 32nd Street, Suite 200, Phoenix, Arizona 85018. (602) 406-9050.

Association of Specialized Kinesiologists, P. O. Box 16169, Greece Station, Rochester, NY 14616. (814) 944-2290.

California Society for Oriental Medicine, 12926 Riverside Dr., Suite B, Sherman Oaks, CA 91423. (818) 789-2468, fax: (818) 981-2766.

Cranial Academy, 8606 Allisonville Road, Suite 130, Indianapolis, IN, 46250. (317) 594-0411.

National Center for Homeopathy, 801 North Fairfax St., Ste. 306, Alexandria, VA 22314. (703) 548-7790. Provides a nationwide directory of practitioners and homeopathy study groups. Send $6, check or money order.

Wellspring for Women, (303) 443-0321. Offers phone consultations with licensed nurse practitioners who can answer questions about herbal remedies and natural hormones, and put you in touch with doctors who can prescribe them; they can also discuss conventional hormone therapy. (A 45-minute consultation costs $120.)

INSURANCE COMPANIES

The following is a list of innovative insurance companies willing to explore coverage of natural healing and complementary medicine.

Alliance for Alternatives in Healthcare, Inc., P. O. Box 6279, Thousand Oaks, CA 91359-6279. (800) 966-8467, fax: (805) 494-8528. This company offers "The Alternative Health Plan," including coverage for acupuncture, alternative birthing centers (including midwives), Ayurvedic medicine, biofeedback, massage therapy, chelation therapy, chiropractic, herbal medicine, homeopathy, nutritional counseling, and Oriental and naturopathic medicine. The plan is available nationally and includes comprehensive coverage for conventional medical care.

The **Alternative Health Group,** (800) 966-8467. An umbrella organization of four different organizations that develop benefit packages for alternative or complementary health care.

American Western Life Insurance Company, 100 Foster City Blvd., Foster City, CA 94404. (415) 573-8041, fax: (415) 574-8226. Operating in California, Arizona, New Mexico, Colorado, and Utah, this fully insured plan includes integrated, holistic health disciplines such as acupuncture, biofeedback, massage, and other therapies. Allopathic medicine is covered as well, but the main focus is on consumer education and prevention. The company hopes to expand into Hawaii, Illinois, Michigan, Oregon, and Washington.

John Alden Life Insurance Company, North Star Marketing, 5500 Glendon Ct., Suite 100, Dublin, OH 43016. (800) 366-6762. This company pays benefits for chiropractic and acupuncture in California and other states that mandate recognition of acupuncturists.

Oxford Health Plans, Inc., Westchester One, 44 South Broadway, White Plains, NY 10601. (203) 852-1442. http:www.oxhp.com/. This Norwalk, Connecticut, health-maintenance organization in October 1996 unveiled the first official alternative provider network to be associated with a large HMO. Oxford, one of the nation's largest and most influential managed-care plans, established a network of 1,000 providers to complement its existing network of 33,000 conventional physicians, to cover acupuncture, massage therapy, Chinese herbology, naturopathy, and more. The alternative services as of this writing are available in New York, New Jersey, and Connecticut.

Mutual of Omaha, Mutual of Omaha Plaza, Omaha, NE 68175. (402) 572-3368. Impressed by the results, this company has approved benefits for an alternative lifestyle-based heart-disease reversal program created by Dean Ornish, M.D.

SPECIFIC SUPPORT GROUPS AND MATERIALS

The **American Menopause Foundation, Inc.,** Empire State Building, 350 Fifth Avenue, Suite 2822, New York, NY 10118. (212) 714-2398. Operates a national network of support groups that deal with alternative treatments, among other issues. They can give you information on a group in your area.

As We Change, A Marketplace for Women, (800) 203-5585. Information, products, and services for menopausal women.

Equinox Press, 144 St. John's Place, Brooklyn, NY 11217. (800) 929-WELL. Publishes *The Cancer Chronicles,* an alternative-treatment newsletter edited by Ralph W. Moss, Ph.D., and resource catalogs of books and tapes about healing and wellness.

The **Foundation for the Advancement in Cancer Therapy,** P. O. Box 1242, Old Chelsea Station, NY, NY 10113. (212) 741-2790.

National Alliance of Breast Cancer Organizations, (212) 889-0606.

Natural Healthcare Hotline, (303) 449-2265.

The **North American Menopause Society,** c/o Department of OB/GYN, University Hospitals of Cleveland, 11100 Euclid Ave., Cleveland, OH 44106. (216) 844-1000. Offers a mainstream perspective on menopause treatment, with lists of suggested readings and physicians in your area specializing in menopause.

People Against Cancer, P. O. Box 10, Otho, IA, 50569. (515) 972-4444.

Physicians Committee for Responsible Medicine, 5100 Wisconsin Avenue, Suite 404, Washington, D.C. 20016; or P. O. Box 6322, Washington, D.C. 20015. (202) 686-2210.

Recommended Reading

ote: Some authors have more books than we had space to list. Also, inclusion on this list does not mean we agree with every single word of a book. Some have idiosyncrasies or small, occasional inaccuracies that fly in the face of what is now common knowledge, or what has been my experience personally or Karta Purkh's clinically. However, all of these books are listed because we believe them to be valuable overall.

Our favorites are in bold type. Three asterisks denotes a "must-read."

Take the rest of your life to become an expert on your body and the medicines of the world, and enjoy!

HERBS

Carroll, David. *Complete Book of Natural Medicines.*
Castleman, Michael. *Nature's Cures.*
Castleman, Michael. *The Healing Herbs.*
Foster, Steven. *Herbal Renaissance.*
Freudberg, David (producer). *The Medicine Garden.*
   (Public radio documentary available on audiocassette)***
Grieve, M. *A Modern Herbal.*
Griggs, Barbara. *Green Pharmacy.*
Hobbs, Christopher. *Echinacea.*
Hobbs, Christopher. *Ginkgo.*
Hobbs, Christopher. *The Ginsengs.*
Hobbs, Christopher. *Handbook for Herbal Healing.*

Hobbs, Christopher. *Milk Thistle*.
Hobbs, Christopher. *Valerian*.
Hoffman, David. *The Elements of Herbalism*.
Hoffman, David. *The New Holistic Herbal*.
Jensen, Bernard. *Nature Has a Remedy*.
Lust, John. *The Herb Book*.
Lust, John, and Michael Tierra, C.A., N.D. *The Natural Remedy Bible*.
Moore, Michael. *Medicinal Plants of the Desert and Canyon West*.
Mowrey, Daniel, Ph.D. *Scientific Validation of Herbal Medicine*.
Mowrey, Daniel, Ph.D. *Herbal Tonic Therapies*.
Null, Gary. *Healing Your Body Naturally*.
Ody, Penelope. *The Complete Medicinal Herbal*.
Rector-Page, Linda, N.D., Ph.D. *Power Plants:*
     Building Immunity with Herbs.
Santillo, Humberto. *Natural Healing with Herbs*.
Tierra, Lesley. *The Herbs of Life*.***
Tierra, Michael, C.A., N.D. *The Way of Herbs*.
Vogel, Virgil J. *American Indian Medicine*.
Willard, Terry. *The Wild Rose Scientific Herbal*.
American Herbalist Guild. *Essays on Herbalism*.

NATURAL MEDICINE AND HEALING

Christopher, John. *School of Natural Healing*.
Gottlieb, Bill, ed. *New Choices in Natural Healing*.
Haas, Elson, M.D. *Staying Healthy with Nutrition*.
Mayell, Mark. *Off the Shelf Natural Health*.
Murray, Michael, N.D., and Pizzorno, Joseph, N.D.
     Encyclopedia of Natural Medicine*.**
Murray, Michael, N.D. *The Healing Power of Herbs*.
Murray, Michael T. *Natural Alternatives to Prescription Drugs*
     and OTC Medications.
Pedersen, Mark. *Nutritional Herbology*.
Weil, Andrew, M.D. *Natural Health, Natural Medicine*.
Weil, Andrew, M.D. *Spontaneous Healing*.***
Wolf, Peggy S., N.D. *Botanical Compendium of Dosages and Products*.

CHINESE MEDICINE

Beinfeld, Harriet, L.Ac. and Efrem Korngold, L.Ac., OMD. *Between Heaven and Earth.*

Foster, Steven. *Herbal Emissaries: Bringing Chinese Herbs to the West.*

Kaptchuk, Ted. *Web That Has No Weaver.*

Lu, Henry. *Legendary Chinese Healing Herbs.*

Pang, T. Y. *Chinese Herbal.*

Reid, Daniel. *Chinese Herbal Medicine.*

Teeguarden, Ron. *Chinese Tonic Herbs.*

AYURVEDA

Bhajan, Yogi. *Foods for Health and Healing.*

Bhajan, Yogi. *The Ancient Science of Self-Healing.*

Chopra, Deepak. *Perfect Health.*

Frawley, David. *Ayurvedic Healing.*

Gerson, Scott. *Ayurveda.*

Lad, Vasant. *Ayurveda.*

Lad, Vasant, and David Frawley. *The Yoga of Herbs.*

Svoboda, Robert. *Prakruti, Your Ayurvedic Constitution.*

Svoboda, Robert. *Ayurveda: Life, Health, and Longevity.*

WOMEN'S HEALTH

Airola, Paavo. *Every Woman's Book.*

Curtis, Susan. *Natural Healing for Women.*

Flaws, Bob. *My Sister, the Moon.*

Gladstar, Rosemary. *Herbal Healing for Women.*

Greenwood, Sadja. *Menopause, Naturally.*

Hudson, Tori, N.D. *Gynecology and Natural Medicine: A Treatment Manual.*

Kamen, Betty. *Hormone Replacement Therapy, Yes or No?*

Ojeda, Linda. *Menopause without Medicine.*

Ryneveld, Edna Copelan. *Secrets of a Natural Menopause: A Positive Drug-Free Approach.*

Sharon, Farida. *Creative Menopause.*

Weed, Susun. *Healing Wise.*

MEN'S HEALTH

Green, James. *Male Herbal: Herbal Health Care for Men and Boys.*
Murray, Michael T. *Male Sexual Vitality.*
Rector-Page, Linda, N.D., Ph.D. *Renewing Male Health and Energy.*

CHILDREN'S HEALTH

Kemper, Kathi J., M.D., Ph.D. *The Holistic Pediatrician.*
Mendelsohn, Robert S., M.D. *How to Raise a Healthy Child—In Spite of Your Doctor.*
Romm, Aviva Jill. *Natural Healing for Babies and Children.*
Schmidt, Michael. *Childhood Ear Infections.*
Smith, Lendon. *Feed Your Kids Right.*
Smith, Lendon. *Hyper Kids.*

IMMUNE-RELATED

Badgley, Laurence. *Healing AIDS Naturally.*
Castleman, Michael. *Cold Cures.*
Fisher, Gregg. *Chronic Fatigue Syndrome.*
Scott, Jimmy. *Cure Your Own Allergies.*
Schulick, Paul. *Ginger, Common Spice and Wonder Drug.*
Sharma, Hari. *Freedom from Disease.*
Swank, Roy Laver, M.D. *The Multiple Sclerosis Diet Book.*

CANCER

Abel, Ulrich, and Der Spiegel. *Chemotherapy of Advanced Epithelial Cancer: A Critical Analysis.*
Austin, Steve, N.D., and Cathy Hitchcock, M.S.W. *Breast Cancer: What You Should Know (But May Not Be Told) About Prevention, Diagnosis, and Treatment.*
Boik, John. *Cancer and Natural Medicine.*
Clark, Hulda Regehr, Ph.D., N.D. *The Cure for All Cancers.*
Fischer, William L. *How to Fight Cancer and Win.*
Kradjian, Robert, M.D. *Save Yourself From Breast Cancer.*

Lynes, Barry. *The Healing of Cancer.*

Moss, Ralph. *The Cancer Industry.*

Moss, Ralph. *Cancer Therapy: The Independent Consumer's Guide to Non-Toxic Treatment and Prevention.*

Quillin, Patrick with Noreen Quillin. *Beating Cancer with Nutrition.*

Rector-Page, Linda, N.D., Ph.D. *Cancer: Can Alternative Therapies Really Help?*

Simone, Charles B. *Cancer and Nutrition.*

MEDICINE AND SCIENCE

Carter, James P. *Racketeering in Medicine: The Suppression of Alternatives.*

Coulter, Harris L. *Divided Legacy—Volume I* (A History of the Schism in Medical Thought).

Coulter, Harris L. *Divided Legacy—Volume II* (The Origins of Western Medicine).

Coulter, Harris L. *Divided Legacy—Volume III* (The Conflict Between Homeopathy and the AMA).

Coulter, Harris L. *Divided Legacy—Volume IV* (Twentieth-Century Medicine: The Bacteriological Era).

Fisher, Jeffrey, M.D. *The Plague Makers.*

Heimlich, Jane. *What Your Doctor Won't Tell You.*

Hovinan, Ralph. *Medical Dark Ages.*

Kuhn, Thomas. *The Structure of Scientific Revolutions.*

Mendelsohn, Robert S., et. al. *Dissent in Medicine: Nine Doctors Speak Out.*

Robin, Eugene D., M.D. *Medical Care Can Be Dangerous to Your Health.*

Silverman, Milton Morris, and Philip R. Lee. *Pills, Profits, and Politics.*

Walker, Martin J. *Dirty Medicine.*

MIND/BODY HEALING

Bhajan, Yogi, *The Teachings of Yogi Bhajan.*

Borysenko, Joan. *Fire in the Soul.*

Borysenko, Joan. *Minding the Body, Mending the Mind.*

Borysenko, Joan, and Miroslav Borysenko. *The Power of the Mind to Heal.*

Dossey, Larry. *Healing Words.****

Dreher, Henry. *The Immune Power Personality.*
Epstein, Gerald N. *Healing Visualizations.*
Justice, Blair, Ph.D. *Who Gets Sick.*
Kabat-Zinn, Jon. *Full Catastrophe Living.*
Kabat-Zinn, Jon. *Wherever You Go, There You Are.*
Moyers, Bill. *Healing and the Mind.*
Siegel, Bernie. *Love, Medicine, and Miracles.*
Siegel, Bernie. *Peace, Love, and Healing.*

FOOD, GENERAL

Barnard, Neal, M.D. *Eat Right, Live Longer.*
Carper, Jean. *Food: Your Miracle Medicine.*
Clark, Nancy, M.S., R.D. *Nancy Clark's Sports Nutrition Guidebook.*
Landis, Robyn. *BodyFueling.*®
Robbins, John. *Diet for a New America.*
Werbach, Melvin, M.D. *Healing with Food.*
Center for Study of Responsive Law. *Eating Clean: Overcoming Food Hazards.*

PERIODICALS

HerbalGram. Published by the American Botanical Council.
Northrup, Dr. Christiane. *Health Wisdom for Women.*
Weil, Dr. Andrew. *Self Healing.*

Bibliography

BOOKS

Beinfeld, Harriet, L.Ac, and Efrem Korngold, L.Ac., OMD. *Between Heaven and Earth*. New York: Ballantine, 1991.

Bensky, Dan, and Andrew Gamble. *Chinese Herbal Medicine Materia Medica*. Seattle: Eastland, 1986.

Brown, J. P. "Role of Gut Bacterial Flora in Nutrition and Health: A Review of Recent Advances in Bacteriological Techniques, Metabolism, and Factors Affecting Flora Composition." *CRC Reviews in Food Science and Nutrition*, 8:229–336, 1977.

Carper, Jean. *Food: Your Miracle Medicine*. New York: HarperCollins, 1993.

Castleman, Michael. *Cold Cures*. New York: Fawcett/Columbine, 1987.

Chakravarti, Sree. *A Healer's Journey*. Cambridge: Rudra, 1991.

Crook, William G., M.D. *The Yeast Connection*. New York: Random House, 1983.

Dharmananda, S., Ph.D. *Your Nature, Your Health*. Portland: Institute for Traditional Medicine and Preventive Health Care, 1986.

Dossey, Larry. *Healing Words: The Power of Prayer and the Practice of Medicine*. San Francisco: HarperSanFrancisco, 1993.

Erasmus, Udo. *Fats That Heal, Fats That Kill*. Burnaby, B.C., Canada: Alive Books, 1993.

Evans, W. C. *Trease and Evans' Pharmacognosy*. London: Balliere Tindall, 1989.

Frawley, David. *Ayurvedic Healing*. Salt Lake City: Passage, 1989.

Golan, Ralph, M.D. *Optimal Wellness*. New York: Ballantine Books, 1995.

Haas, Elson, M.D. *Staying Healthy with Nutrition.* Berkeley, CA: Celestial Arts, 1992.

Heinerman, John. *The Complete Book of Spices.* New Canaan: Keats, 1983.

Heinerman, John. *First Aid with Herbs: Tried and True Health Care in Emergencies and Minor Illnesses.* New Canaan: Keats, 1983.

Heinerman, John. *Heinerman's Encyclopedia of Healing Juices.* West Nyack: Parker Publishing Co., 1994.

Hoffman, David. *The Elements of Herbalism.* Rockport, MA: Element Books, 1991.

Hoffman, David. *The New Holistic Herbal.* Longmead, Shaftesbury, Dorset: Element, 1983.

Kapour, L. D. *CRC Handbook of Ayurvedic Medical Plants.* Boca Raton: CRC Press, 1990.

Khalsa, Karta Purkh Singh, and Bill Camp. *Kinesionics, A Pattern for Life and Health.* Seattle: Sunbeam, 1990.

Lad, Vasant, and David Frawley. *The Yoga of Herbs.* Santa Fe: Lotus, 1986.

Leung, A. Y. *Encyclopedia of Common Natural Ingredients Used in Food, Drugs, and Cosmetics.* New York: J. Wiley and Sons, 1980.

Lust, John. *The Herb Book.* New York: Bantam, 1976.

Mendelsohn, Robert S., M.D. *How to Raise a Healthy Child—In Spite of Your Doctor.* New York: Ballantine, 1984.

Moss, Ralph, *Cancer Therapy: The Independent Consumer's Guide to Non-Toxic Treatment and Prevention.* New York: Equinox Press, 1995.

Moyers, Bill. *Healing and the Mind,* edited by Betty Sue Flowers, exec. producer, David Grubin. New York: Doubleday, 1993.

Murray, Michael T., N.D. *Natural Alternatives to Over-the-Counter and Prescription Drugs.* New York: William Morrow Co., 1994.

Murray, Michael T., N.D., and Joseph E. Pizzorno, N.D. *Encyclopedia of Natural Medicine.* Rocklin, CA: Prima, 1991.

Murray, Michael T., N.D., and Joseph E. Pizzorno, N.D. *Textbook of Natural Medicine.* Seattle, WA: John Bastyr College Publications, 1985.

Nissim, Rina. *Natural Healing in Gynecology: A Manual for Women.* New York: Pandora, 1986. (Translated from the French by Roxanne Claire.)

Ody, Penelope. *The Complete Medicinal Herbal.* London: Dorling Kindersley, 1993.

Rector-Page, Linda, N.D., Ph.D. *Cancer: Can Alternative Therapies Really Help?* Sonora, CA: Health Healing Publications, 1995.

Rector-Page, Linda, N.D., Ph.D. *Power Plants: Building Immunity with Herbs.* Sonora, CA: Health Healing Publications, 1995.

Rector-Page, Linda, N.D., Ph.D. *Renewing Male Health and Energy.* Sonora, CA: Health Healing Publications, 1995.

Schmidt, Michael. *Childhood Ear Infection: What Every Parent and Doctor Should Know About Prevention, Home Cure, and Alternative Treatment.* Berkeley, CA: North Atlantic Books, Homeopathic Educational Services, 1990.

Schulick, Paul. *Ginger, Common Spice and Wonder Drug.* Battleboro: Herbal Free Press, 1994.

Smith, Lendon. *Feed Your Kids Right.* New York: McGraw Hill, 1979.

Smith, Lendon. *Hyper Kids.* Santa Monica: Shaw/Spelling, 1990.

Svoboda, Robert. *Ayurveda—Life, Health, and Longevity.* London: Arkana, 1992.

Svoboda, Robert. *Prakruti, Your Ayurvedic Constitution.* Albuquerque: Geocom, 1988.

Teeguarden, Ron. *Chinese Tonic Herbs.* Tokyo/New York: Japan Publications, 1984.

Tierra, Lesley. *The Herbs of Life.* Freedom: Crossing, 1992.

Tierra, Michael, C.A., N.D. *Planetary Herbology.* Twin Lakes: Lotus, 1992.

Tierra, Michael, C.A., N.D. *The Way of Herbs: Fully Updated—With the Latest Developments.* New York: Simon and Schuster, 1990.

Tyler, Varro E. *Herbs of Choice: Therapeutic Use of Phytomedicinals.* New York: Pharmaceutical Products Press, 1994.

Van Straten, Michael. *Guarana.* Essex: C. W. Daniel, 1994.

Weed, Susun. *Wise Woman Herbal Healing.* Woodstock, NY: Ash Tree Publishing, 1989.

Weil, Andrew, M.D. *Spontaneous Healing: How to Discover and Enhance Your Body's Natural Ability to Maintain and Heal Itself.* New York: Knopf, 1995.

Weiner, Michael. *The Herbal Bible: A Family Guide to Herbal Home Remedies.* San Rafael, CA: Quantum Books, 1992.

Weiner, Michael. *Weiner's Herbal.* New York: Stein and Day, 1980.

Weiss, Rudolf., M.D. *Herbal Medicine.* Beaconsfield: Beaconsfield Publishing, 1988.

Werbach, Dr. Melvin, M.D. *Healing with Food.* New York: HarperCollins, 1994.

PERIODICALS

Abraham, G. E. "The Calcium Controversy." *Journal of Applied Nutrition*, 34:2 69–73, 1982.

Aeosph, Lauri M., N.D., "Cold or Flu: Which Do You Have?" *Delicious!*, December 1995.

Aesoph, Lauri M., N.D. "Plants as Medicines." *Delicious!*, October 1995.

Aesoph, Lauri M., N.D. "The Facts About Brain-Boosting Nutrients." *Delicious!*, May 1995.

Ammon, HRT, Safayhi, H., et al. "Mechanisms of Anti-Inflammatory Actions of Curcumin and Boswellic Acids." *Journal of Ethnopharmacology*, 38:113–19, 1993.

Ammon, HRT, and M. A. Wahl. "Pharmacology of *Curcuma longa*." *Planta Medica*, 57:1–7, 1991.

Arnold, Kathryn. "The Joy of Soy." *Delicious!*, February 1995.

Arora, R., N. Basu, V. Kapour, and A. Jain. "Anti-Inflammatory Studies on *Curcuma longa* (Turmeric)." *Indian Journal of Medical Research*, 59:1,289–95, 1971.

Beil, W., Birkholz, and K. F. Sewing. "Effects of Flavonoids on Parietal Cell Acid Secretion, Gastric Mucosal Prostaglandin Production, and *Helicobacter pylori* Growth." *Arnzeim Forsch*, 45:697–700, 1995.

Bland, Jeffrey S., Ph.D. "Drugs and Liver Overload." *Delicious!*, February 1996.

Bland, Jeffrey S., Ph.D. "Back to Basics." *Let's Live*, October 1995.

Bland, Jeffrey, Ph.D. "Envisioning the Ideal Health Care System." *Delicious!*, March 1995.

Bone, Kerry, Ph.D. "New Research on HIV-1: Implications for Phytotherapy." *Townsend Letters for Doctors*, July 1995.

Bradburn, Elizabeth. "Holistic Health Insurance." *Longevity*, May 1995.

Brevoort, Peggy. "The U.S. Botanical Market—An Overview." *HerbalGram* 36, Spring 1996.

Brody, Jane. "Personal Health: Underactive Thyroids Are Treatable But Often Missed." *New York Times*, 29 March 1995.

Brown, Don. "Research Reviews: Essential Oils for Headache Treatment." *HerbalGram* 38, Fall 1996.

Buttram, Harold, M.D. "Current Childhood Vaccination Programs: Do They Cause More Disease than They Prevent?" *Townsend Letter for Doctors and Patients*, November 1995.

Carrow, Donald J., M.D., and Mitchell Chavez, C.N. "Research Perspectives on Asthma." *Townsend Letter for Doctors and Patients,* August/September 1994.

Castleman, Michael. "Recent Findings in Healing Herbs." *Herb Quarterly,* Fall 1995.

Challem, Jack. "Beta-Carotene Studies Evoke Questions, Criticisms." *Nutrition Science News,* March 1996.

Challem, Jack. "Interpreting Research: What's Good and Bad in Recent Studies." *Nutrition Science News,* April 1996.

Challem, Jack. "Keeping Your Marbles." *Natural Health,* January/February 1995.

Challem, Jack. "Mixed Carotenoids Starting to Overshadow Beta-Carotene." *Nutrition Science News,* June 1995.

Challem, Jack. "Natural Beta-Carotene Looks Good: Could Synthetic Be the Problem?" *The Nutrition Reporter,* vol. 7, no. 9, September 1996.

Challem, Jack. "Studies Explore How Antioxidants Prevent DNA Damage, Breast Cancer Metastasis." *The Nutrition Reporter,* vol. 7, no. 9, September 1996.

Challem, Jack. "Zinc Lozenges Ease Cold Symptoms." *The Nutrition Reporter,* vol. 7, no. 9, September 1996.

Chandra, D., and S. Gupta. "Anti-Inflammatory and Anti-Arthritic Activity of Volatile Oil of *Curcuma longa* (Haldi)." *Indian Journal of Medical Research,* 60:138–42, 1972.

Charles, V., and S. X. Charles. "The Use and Efficacy of *Azadirachta indica* ADR ('Neem') and *Curcuma longa* ('Turmeric') in Scabies: A Pilot Study." *Tropical & Geographical Medicine,* 44 (1–2): 178–81, 1992.

Chowka, Peter Barry. "Prayer Is Good Medicine." *Yoga Journal,* July/August 1996.

Christy, C. J. "Vitamin E in Menopause." *American Journal of Obstetrics and Gynecology,* 50:84–87, 1945. Cited in *American Journal of Natural Medicine,* vol. 2, no. 9, November 1995.

Cohen, Jessica. "The Healing Touch." *Longevity,* July 1994.

Costello, C. H. and E. V. Lynn. "Estrogenic Substances From Plants: I. Glycyrrhiza." *Journal of the American Pharmaceutical Society,* 39:177–180, 1950. Cited in *American Journal of Natural Medicine,* vol. 2, no. 9, November 1995.

Cowley, Geoffrey. "Are Supplements Still Worth Taking?" *Newsweek*, April 25, 1994.

Crutcher, John. "An Interview with Andrew Weil, M.D." *Common Ground of Puget Sound*, June 1995.

Duke, James A., Ph.D. "The Botanical Viewpoint." *HerbalGram* 28, 1993.

Fulder, Stephen, Ph.D., and Meir Tenne, D.Sc. "Ginger as an Anti-Nausea Remedy in Pregnancy: The Issue of Safety." *HerbalGram* 38, Fall 1996.

Gessner, B., A. Voelp, and M. Klasser. "Study of the Long-Term Action of a *Ginkgo Biloba* Extract on Vigilance and Mental Performance as Determined by Means of Quantitative Pharmaco-EEG and Psychometric Measurements." *Arzneim Forsch* 35:1,459–65, 1985.

Glick, L. "Deglycyrrhizinated Liquorice in Peptic Ulcer." *Lancet* ii:817, 1982.

Goodwin, Jan. "Healing Herbs," *New Woman*, May 1995.

Gorman, Christine. "Need a New Drug? You May Get One Now that the FDA Is Primed to Clear More Medicines for Over-the-Counter Sale." *Time*, July 31, 1995.

Gormley, James J. "Ashwagandha: An Anti-Cancer, Anti-Arthritis, Anti-Ulcer 'Adaptogen.'" *Better Nutrition for Today's Living*, February 1996.

Griffin, Katherine. "Alternative Care: Finally Some Coverage." *Health*, October 1995.

Groop, P. H., A. Aro, et. al. "Long-Term Effects of Guar Gum in Subjects with Non-Insulin-Dependent Diabetes Mellitus." *American Journal of Clinical Nutrition* 58:513–18, 1993.

Hamlin, Suzanne. "Take 2 Bowls Zinc-Garlic Pasta, Then Call Me in the Morning." *New York Times*, January, 25, 1995.

Hardy, A. M., and M. G. Fowler. "Child Care Arrangements and Repeated Ear Infections in Young Children." *American Journal of Public Health* 83 (9):1,321–25, September 1993.

Hindmarch, I., and Z. Subhan. "The Psychopharmacological Effects of *Ginkgo biloba* Extract in Normal Healthy Volunteers." *International Journal of Clinical Pharmacology Research* 4:89–93, 1984.

Hochwald, Lambeth. "Reinventing the Vegetable: Scientists Are Shrinking Foods to Create 'Nutraceuticals,' a New Kind of Supplement That Offers the Power of Plants—In a Pill." *Natural Health*, April 1996.

Hofferberth, B. "The Efficacy of Egb761 in Patients with Senile Dementia of the Alzheimer Type: A Double-Blind, Placebo-Controlled Study on

Different Levels of Investigation." *Human Psychopharmacology* 9:215–22, 1994.

Horne, Steven. "Herbal Glycerites for Children." *Proceedings of Fifth Annual Symposium of American Herbalists Guild,* 1994.

Huang, H. C., T. R. Jan, and S. F. Yeh. "Inhibitors Effect of Curcumin, an Anti-Inflammatory Agent, on Vascular Smooth Muscle Cell Proliferation." *European Journal of Pharmacology* 221:381–84, 1992.

Iacono, G., et al, "Chronic Constipation as a Symptom of Cow's Milk Allergy," *Journal of Pediatrics,* 126:34–39, 1995.

Jaret, Peter. "Foods That Fight Cancer." *Health,* March/April 1995.

Keville, Kathi. "Anthocyanidins and Proanthocyanidins." *The Herb Report, The American Herb Association,* vol. 11:3, 1995.

Khalsa, Karta Purkh Singh. "Allergy." *Herb Quarterly,* Fall 1996.

Khalsa, Karta Purkh Singh. "An Herbal Approach to *Candida albicans.*" *Journal of the Northeast Herbal Association,* Winter 1994.

Khalsa, Karta Purkh Singh. "Ayurvedic Herbology in North America." *The Herbalist—Newsletter of the American Herbalists Guild,* Winter/February 1995.

Khalsa, Karta Purkh Singh. "Candida's Curse." *Herb Quarterly,* Summer 1996.

Khalsa, Karta Purkh Singh. "Case Study: Fibromyalgia." *Journal of the American Herb Association,* vol. 10, no. 4:14–15, 1994.

Khalsa, Karta Purkh Singh. "Keeping Children Healthy." *Yoga Journal,* September 1996.

Khalsa, Karta Purkh Singh. "Detoxifying Herbs." *Let's Live,* September 1996.

Khalsa, Karta Purkh Singh. "Diabetes Today." *Herb Quarterly,* Spring 1996.

Khalsa, Karta Purkh Singh. "Natural Remedies for Diabetes." *Yoga Journal,* July 1996.

Khalsa, Karta Purkh Singh. "Enhancing Wellness with Ayurvedic Herbs." *ASK-US Journal,* October 1994.

Khalsa, Karta Purkh Singh. "Herbal Healing: Hyperactivity and Childhood Allergies." *Whole Self Times,* November 1994.

Khalsa, Karta Purkh Singh. "Modern Ayurvedic Herbology." *Ancient Healing Ways,* Winter 1994.

Khalsa, Karta Purkh Singh. "Ms. L.'s Case Study." *Journal of the American Herb Association,* vol. 11, no. 4:19, 1995.

Khalsa, Karta Purkh Singh. "Turmeric—The Medicine Cabinet in a Jar." *Herb Quarterly,* Spring 1996.

Kiso, Y., Y. Suzuki, N. Watanabe, et al: "Antihepatotoxic Principles of *Curcuma longa* Rhizomes." *Planta Medica,* 49: 185–87, 1983.

Kleijnen, J., and P. Knipschild. "*Ginkgo biloba* for Cerebral Insufficiency." *British Journal of Clinical Pharmacology* 34:352–58, 1992.

Kolata, Gina. "Cancer Link Contradicted by New Hormone Study." *New York Times,* July 12, 1995.

Krajick, Kevin. "Will Your Long Life Be a Good Life?" *Longevity,* September 1995.

Kumagai, A., et al. "Effect of Glycyrrhizin on Estrogen Action." *Endocrinologia Japonica* 14:34–38, 1967. Cited in *American Journal of Natural Medicine,* vol. 2, no. 9, November 1995.

Lagnado, Lucette. "Oxford to Create Alternative Medicine Network." *Wall Street Journal,* October 7, 1996.

Leibovitz, Brian. "Polyphenols." *Townsend Letter for Doctors,* May 1994.

LeRoy, Bob. "Milk: What's the Controversy?" *Vegetarian Voice,* vol. 21, no. 2, 1996.

LeRoy, Bob. "So Much Hype, So Little Truth." *Vegetarian Voice,* vol. 21, no. 2, 1996.

LeRoy, Bob. "On the Path to Stronger Bones." *Vegetarian Voice,* vol. 21, no. 3, 1996.

Leviton, Richard. "The Herbalist's Art." *Yoga Journal,* March/April 1993.

Li, C. J., L. J. Zhang, et al: "Three Inhibitors of Type One Human Immunodeficiency Virus Long Terminal Repeat—Directed Gene Expression and Virus Replication." Proceedings of the National Academy of Sciences USA 90:1,839–42, 1993.

Long, Patricia. "The Naturals." *Health,* May/June 1995.

Mayell, M. "Bilberry Update." *East West,* 1990, p. 59.

Mayell, Mark. "Your Nutritional Essentials." *Natural Health,* April 1996.

Mars, Brigitte. "Herbal Kingdom: Calm Down with Chamomile." *Delicious!,* November 1995.

Mars, Brigitte. "From Spice Shelf to Medicine Shelf." *Delicious!,* August 1995.

Mars, Brigitte. "Valerian: A Kinder, Gentler Herb." *Delicious!,* May 1995.

Marshall, Melinda. "Warning: Antibiotics Could Endanger Your Child." *Reader's Digest,* December 1996.

McCaleb, Rob. "Chasteberry: A Tonic for Menstrual Problems." *Delicious!*, September 1995.

McCaleb, Rob. "Garlic: The World's Tastiest Medicine." *Delicious!*, February 1995.

McCaleb, Rob. "Ginkgo: Nature's Circulation Booster." *Delicious!*, May 1995.

McCaleb, Rob. "Herbal Kingdom: Feeling Anxious? Take Valerian." *Delicious!*, December 1995.

McCaleb, Rob. "Increase Your Endurance with High-Performance Herbs." *Delicious!*, July 1995.

McCaleb, Rob. "The Fruits of Healing." *Delicious!*, February 1996.

McCaleb, Rob. "Ten Best Herbs to Keep You Healthy." *Delicious!*, August 1995.

McCaleb, Rob. "Upset Stomach? Try Ginger." *Delicious!*, June 1995.

McCaleb, Rob. "Two Immune-Enhancing Herbs." *Delicious!*, December 1995.

Mead, Nathaniel. "Boost Melatonin Naturally." *Natural Health*, March/April 1996.

Morris, Kathryn, M.D., and Sue Ungar, M.S., N.P. "Natural Progesterone Surpasses Provera." *Women's Health Forum*, vol. 4, no. 3, May 1995.

Mowrey, Daniel B., Ph.D. "Tonic Herbs." *Let's Live*, December 1995.

Mukundan, M.A., M. C. Chacko, et al. "Effect of Turmeric and Curcumin on BP-DNA Adducts." *Carcinogenesis*, 14:493–96, 1993.

Murray, Frank. "Editor's Note." *Better Nutrition for Today's Living*, November 1995.

Murray, Michael T., N.D. "Allergies: Natural Relief for Asthma and Hay Fever." *Health Counselor*, vol. 4, no. 3.

Murray, Michael T., N.D. "Chronic Fatigue Syndrome." *American Journal of Natural Medicine*, vol. 2, no. 6, July/August 1995.

Murray, Michael T., N.D. "Cimicifuga Extract (Black Cohosh): A Natural Alternative to Estrogen for Menopause." *Health Counselor*, vol. 8, no. 2.

Murray, Michael T., N.D. "Curcumin: A Potent Anti-Inflammatory Agent." *American Journal of Natural Medicine*, vol. 1, no. 4, December, 1994.

Murray, Michael T., N.D. "Hawthorn: Nature's Cardiotonic." *American Journal of Natural Medicine*, vol. 2, no. 7, September 1995.

Murray, Michael T., N.D. "Lifestyle and Dietary Factors in Depression." *American Journal of Natural Medicine,* vol. 2, no. 10, December 1995.

Murray, Michael T., N.D. "Menopause: Is Estrogen Necessary?" *American Journal of Natural Medicine,* November 1995.

Murray, Michael T., N.D. "New Uses for Ginger: Botanical Report." *Health Counselor,* vol 4. no. 4.

Murray, Michael T., N.D. "Saw Palmetto: Nature's Answer to an Enlarged Prostate." *Health Counselor,* vol. 6, no. 4.

Murray, Michael T. "The Clinical Use of *Hypericum perforatum.*" *American Journal of Natural Medicine,* vol. 2, issue 3, 1995.

Murray, Michael T., N.D. "The Importance of Dietary Fiber." *Phyto-Pharmica Review,* vol. 4, no. 1, 1990.

Murray, Michael T., N.D. "The Natural Approach to Ulcers." *Health Counselor,* vol. 7, no. 6.

Nagabhushan, M., and S. V. Bhide. "Curcumin as an Inhibitor of Cancer." *Journal of the American College of Nutrition,* 11:192–198, 1992.

Northrup, Christiane, M.D. "Achieving a Healthy Balance." *Delicious!,* March 1995.

Northrup, Christiane, M.D. *Women's Health.* A special supplement to Dr. Christiane Northrup's *Health Wisdom for Women* newsletter. n.d.

Pati, Dr. K. "Gymnema sylvestre," *New Editions Health World,* June 1996.

Patterson, Eric. "Standardized Extracts: Herbal Medicine of the Future?" *Herb Market Review,* 1996.

Pizzorno, Lara, M.A., L.M.P. "Fifty Ways to Take Charge of Your Health." *Delicious!,* February, 1996.

Pizzorno, Lara, M.A., L.M.P. "Power Up Your Immune System." *Delicious!,* October 1995.

Pizzorno, Lara, M.A., L.M.P. "Your Thoughts Can Heal." *Delicious!,* May 1995.

Quillin, Patrick M., "Re-Engineering the War on Cancer," *Alternative and Complimentary Therapies,* September/October 1995.

Qureshi, S., et al. "Toxicity Studies on *Alpinia galanga* and *Curcuma longa.*" *Planta Medica* 58:124, 1992.

Radetsky, Peter. "Killing Cancer Naturally." *Longevity,* March 1995.

Rogers, Sherry A., M.D. "Doctor's Dialogue: One of the Best-Kept Secrets in Medicine: Osteoarthritis Is Reparable." *Let's Live,* October 1995.

Rogers, Sherry A. "How the Sick Get Sicker, Quicker, By Following Current Medical Protocol." *Townsend Letter for Doctors,* October 1993.

Rogers, Sherry A. "Macrobiotic Diet Proven to Improve Cancer Survival." *Townsend Letter for Doctors,* February/March 1994.

Rogers, Sherry A., M.D. "Penny-Wise and Pound Foolish—How Cost Effective Is Environmental Medicine?" *Townsend Letter for Doctors,* April 1995.

Sahey, Billie Jay, Ph.D. "Of GABA, Tranquilizers, and Anxiety." *Townsend Letter for Doctors and Patients,* no. 149:86.

Sardi, Bill. "Eradicating Cataracts." *Townsend Letter for Doctors,* June 1995.

Seddon, Johanna M., M.D., et al. "Dietary Carotenoids, Vitamins A, C, and E and Advanced Age-Related Macular Degeneration." *Journal of the American Medical Association* 272 (18): 1,413–20, November 9, 1994. Cited in *Better Nutrition for Today's Living,* February 1996.

Sharma, O. P. "Antioxidant Properties of Curcumin and Related Compounds." *Biochemistry and Pharmacology* 25:1,811–25, 1976.

Skobeloff, E. M., W. H. Spivey, R. M. McNamara, and L. Greenspon. "Intravenous Magnesium Sulfate for the Treatment of Acute Asthma in the Emergency Department." *Journal of the American Medical Association* 262 (9):1,210–13, 1989.

Smith, Ed. "A Case for Full Herbal Extracts." *Natural Foods Merchandiser,* February 1996.

Smith, Linda Wasmer. "Forever Young." *Veggie Life,* May 1995.

Sodhi, Virender, M.D. (Ayurved), N.D. "Ashwaghanda for Rejuvenation." *New Editions Health World,* n.d.

Stock, Melissa T., and Kellye Hunter. "The Healing Power of Peppers." *The Natural Way,* March/April 1996.

Tewari, S. N., and A. K. Wilson. "Deglycyrrhizinated Liquorice in Duodenal Ulcer." *Practitioner* 210:820–25, 1972.

Thomson, Bill. "The Medical Revolution." *Natural Health,* April 1996.

Trenkle, Peeka. "Vaccinations, An Alternative Perspective." *Journal of the Northeast Herb Association,* Winter 1995.

Turpie, A. G., J. Runcie, and T. J. Thomson. "Clinical Trial of Deglycyrrhizinate Liquorice in Gastric Ulcer." *Gut* 10:299–303, 1969.

Ubbink, Johan, et. al. "Vitamin Requirements for the Treatment of Hyperhomocysteinemia in Humans." *Journal of Nutrition* 124:1,927–33, 1994.

Wachter, Sarah. "All-Natural Stress Soothers." *Longevity*, January 1995.

Wallace, Edward, N.D., D.C. "Homeopathy." *Delicious!*, February 1996.

Wallace, Edward, N.D., D.C., "What to Do When Your Head Aches," *Delicious!*, March 1996.

Webb, Ginger, and Mark Blumenthal. "Milk Thistle Fruits for Treatment of Death Cap Mushroom Poisoning." *HerbalGram* 37.

Webb, Ginger. "Valerian Safety Confirmed in Overdose Research Reviews." *HerbalGram* 36.

Weil, Andrew, M.D. "Ask Dr. Weil." *Natural Health*, March/April 1996.

Weil, Andrew, M.D. "Estrogen Therapy: Balancing the Cancer Risks and Heart Benefits." *Self Healing*, vol. 1, issue 1.

Weil, Andrew, M.D. "Five Steps to Migraine Relief." *Self Healing*, vol. 1, issue 6, May 1996.

Weil, Andrew, M.D. "Is It Necessary to Take Supplements if You Eat a Healthy Diet?" *Self Healing*, vol. 1, issue 1.

Weil, Andrew, M.D. "Living with Arthritis." *Self Healing*, vol. 1, issue 4.

Weil, Andrew, M.D. "Relieving Hay Fever." *Self Healing*, vol. 1, issue 1.

Weil, Andrew, M.D. "The Body's Healing Systems: The Future of Medical Education." *Alternative & Complementary Therapies*, September/October 1995.

Werbach, Dr. Melvin, M.D. "Bronchial Asthma and Magnesium." *Townsend Letter for Doctors and Patients*, November 1993.

Whitcomb, D. C., and G. D. Block. "Association of Acetaminophen Hepatotoxicity with Fasting and Ethanol Use." *JAMA* 272 (23): 1,845–50, December 21, 1994.

Whitelegg, Margaret, B.A. "In Defense of Comfrey." National Institute of Medical Herbalists' *The Herbalist*, August 1994.

Wolfe, Tom. "Three Commonly Asked Questions about Herbs." *Herb Market Review*, February 1995.

Wright, Karen. "Menopause, Naturally," *Health*, January 1996.

Zimmerman, Marcia, M.Ed., C.N. "Immune Building Wonder Herbs." *Delicious!*, October 1995.

Zimmerman, Marcia, M.Ed., C.N. "Phytochemicals and Disease Prevention." *Alternative & Complementary Therapies*, April/May 1995.

Zucker, Martin. "Diet and Breast Cancer: What's the Connection?" *Let's Live*, May 1996.

No Authors

"AHPA Rescinds Chaparral Ban: Creates Hotline for Adverse Effects." *HerbalGram* 35.

"Are 'Safe' Drugs Really Safe?" *Longevity*, September 1994.

"Benefits of Standardized Herbal Extracts." *The Energy Times*, May/June 1995.

"Berberine-Containing Plants in Psoriasis." *American Journal of Natural Medicine*, vol. 3, no. 1, January/February 1996.

"Can Aspirin Protect You from Cancer?" *Berkeley Wellness Letter*, vol. 12, issue 3, December 1995.

"Capsules: Newsbreaks in Herb Research." *Herbs for Health*, March 1996.

"'Complementary' Medicine: Is It Good for What Ails You?" *Business Week*, November 27, 1995.

"Curcumin: A Potent Anti-Inflammatory Agent." *The American Journal of Natural Medicine*, vol. 1, no. 4, December 1994.

"Devil's Claw Proven Useful in Easing Some Patients' Arthritis Pain." *Better Nutrition for Today's Living*, February 1996.

"DGL May Inhibit *Helicobacter pylori*." *American Journal of Natural Medicine*, vol. 2, no. 10, December 1995.

"Faster, Cheaper Treatment of UTIs." *Elle*, May 1995.

"Fibromyalgia." *Nutritional Pearls*, vol. 17, August/September 1993.

"Healthscene." *Health Counselor*, vol. 7, no. 6.

"Kava Makes You Calm," *Health Counselor*, vol. 7, no. 6, citing *The British Journal of Phytotherapy*, vol. 3, no. 4, 1993/94.

"Lutein and Other Antioxidants Aid in Protecting Your Eyes." *Better Nutrition for Today's Living*, February 1996.

"Nebraska Law Criminalizes Ma Huang." *HerbalGram* 38, Fall 1996.

"Nutritional Research Bulletin." *American Journal of Natural Medicine*, vol. 2, no. 10, December 1995.

"Questions and Answers: Ask the Editors." *Herbs for Health*, March 1996.

"St. John's Wort: Effective Medicine for Depression, Infection, and More." *Better Nutrition for Today's Living*, February 1996.

"The Unique Pharmacology of *Coleus forskohlii*." *The American Journal of Natural Medicine*, vol. 1, no. 3, November 1994.

"Vitamin C and Magnesium in Diabetes." *American Journal of Natural Medicine*, vol. 3, no. 1, January/February 1996.

"Zantac and Tagamet vs. DGL." *American Journal of Natural Medicine*, October 1994, vol. 1, no. 2.

MULTIMEDIA

Freudberg, David. *The Medicine Garden*. Written and produced for public radio by David Freudberg. Cambridge, MA: Far Reaching Communications, 1996.

Hoffman, David. *Therapeutic Herbalism*. A correspondence course in phytotherapy. Santa Rosa: David Hoffman, n.d.

McCaleb, Rob. "Boosting Immunity with Herbs." At Herb Research Foundation's Internet World Wide Web site (http://sunsite.unc.edu/hrf/).

McCaleb, Rob. "The Herbally Aware Traveler." At Herb Research Foundation's Internet World Wide Web site (http://sunsite.unc.edu/hrf/).

Moore, Michael, *The Herbalist*, May 1995, posted at
gopher://president.oit.unc.edu:70/11/../.pub/academic/medicine/
alternative-healthcare/Southwest-School-of-Botanical-Medicine OR
sunsite.unc.edu/pub/academic/medicine/alternative-healthcare/
Southwest-School-of-Botanical-Medicine

"Always Natural, Always Healthy?" Town Meeting, KOMO-TV 4 (ABC) Seattle, May 19, 1995.

"Herbal Teas and Toxicity," Copyright 1995 Health ResponseAbility Systems, Inc., posted on America Online, Better Health and Medical Network (keyword: Better Health or HRS)>Alternative and Complementary Medicine>Alternative Health Articles.

Notes

CHAPTER 1: HERBS: THE ORIGINAL MEDICINE

[1]Goodwin, Jan, "Healing Herbs," *New Woman*, May 1995.

[2]Quillin, Patrick M., "Re-Engineering the War on Cancer," *Alternative and Complimentary Therapies*, September/October 1995, pages 279–280.

[3]Beinfeld, Harriet, L.Ac., and Efrem Korngold, L.Ac., OMD. *Between Heaven and Earth* (New York: Ballantine, 1991), p. 23.

[4]Crutcher, John, "An Interview with Andrew Weil, M.D.," *Common Ground of Puget Sound*, June 1995.

[5]Webb, Ginger, "Valerian Safety Confirmed in Overdose Research Reviews," *HerbalGram* 36, citing Willey, Leanna B., "Valerian Overdose: A Case Report," *Veterinary and Human Toxicology*, vol. 37, no. 4, August 1995, pages 364–365.

[6]*The Medicine Garden*, written and produced for public radio by David Freudberg, 1996.

[7]Ibid.

[8]Ibid.

[9]Weil, Andrew, M.D., "Is It Necessary to Take Supplements if You Eat a Healthy Diet?" *Self Healing*, vol. 1, issue 1, p. 3.

[10]Weiner, Michael, *Weiner's Herbal* (Mill Valley, CA: Quantum Books, 1990).

CHAPTER 3: PERSPECTIVES ON RESEARCH

[1]Wolfe, Tom, "Three Commonly Asked Questions about Herbs," *Herb Market Review,* February 1995.

[2]Dossey, Dr. Larry, *Healing Words: The Power of Prayer and the Practice of Medicine* (San Francisco: HarperSanFrancisco, 1993), p. xv (preface).

[3]"Can Aspirin Protect You from Cancer?" *Berkeley Wellness Letter,* vol. 12, issue 3, December 1995, p.1.

[4]Moyers, Bill, *Healing and the Mind* (New York: Doubleday, 1993), pp. 98–99.

[5]Northrup, Christiane, M.D., *Women's Health,* a special supplement to Dr. Christiane Northrup's *Health Wisdom for Women* newsletter. N.d.

[6]Chowka, Peter Barry, "Prayer Is Good Medicine," *Yoga Journal,* July/August 1996, p. 157.

[7]Duke, James A., "The Botanical Alternative," *HerbalGram* 28, 1993, p. 48.

[8]Long, Patricia, "The Naturals," *Health,* May/June 1995.

[9]Duke, James A., "The Botanical Alternative," *HerbalGram* 28, 1993, p. 48.

[10]Ibid.

[11]Dossey, Dr. Larry, *Healing Words: The Power of Prayer and the Practice of Medicine* (San Francisco: HarperSanFrancisco, 1993), p. 203.

[12]Quillin, Patrick M., "Re-Engineering the War on Cancer," *Alternative and Complimentary Therapies,* September/October 1995.

[13]Bradburn, Elizabeth. "Holistic Health Insurance," *Longevity,* May 1994.

[14]Kolata, Gina, "Cancer Link Contradicted by New Hormone Study," *New York Times,* July 12, 1995.

[15]Krajick, Kevin, "Will Your Long Life Be a Good Life?" *Longevity,* September 1995.

[16]Crutcher, John, "An Interview with Andrew Weil, M.D.," *Common Ground of Puget Sound,* June 1995.

[17]Bland, Jeffrey, Ph.D., "Envisioning the Ideal Health Care System," *Delicious!,* March 1995, p. 60.

CHAPTER 4: IMMUNE SYSTEM 101

[1]*Let's Live,* December 1995, quoting Andrew Gaeddert, *Chinese Herbs in the Western Clinic* (Dublin, CA: Get Well Foundation, 1994).

[2]Pizzorno, Lara, "Power Up Your Immune System," *Delicious!,* October 1995.

CHAPTER 5: PREVENTION 101:
IMMUNE-BOOSTING BASICS

[1]Murray, Michael T., N.D., "The Importance of Dietary Fiber," *Phyto-Pharmica Review*, vol. 4, no. 1, 1990.

[2]*American Journal of Clinical Nutrition*, vol. 26, 1973.

[3]Pizzorno, Lara, "Power Up Your Immune System," *Delicious!*, October 1995.

[4]Jaret, Peter, "Foods That Fight Cancer," *Health*, March/April 1995.

[5]Ibid.

[6]Ibid.

[7]Challem, Jack, "Studies Explore How Antioxidants Prevent DNA Damage, Breast Cancer Metastasis," *The Nutrition Reporter*, vol. 7, no. 9, September 1996.

[8]Challem, Jack, "Natural Beta-Carotene Looks Good. Could Synthetic Be the Problem?" *The Nutrition Reporter*, vol. 7, no. 9, September 1996.

[9]Pizzorno, Lara, "Power Up Your Immune System," *Delicious!*, October 1995.

[10]Pizzorno, Lara, "Power Up Your Immune System," *Delicious!*, October 1995, citing Hardy, A. M., and M. G. Fowler, "Child Care Arrangements and Repeated Ear Infections in Young Children," *American Journal of Public Health* 83 (9):1,321–25, September 1993.

CHAPTER 6:
HEALTH-BUILDING HERBS, FOODS, AND NUTRIENTS

[1]Mowrey, Daniel B., Ph. D., "Tonic Herbs," *Let's Live*, December 1995, p. 39.

[2]McCaleb, Rob, "Boosting Immunity with Herbs," at Herb Research Foundation's Internet World Wide Web site (http://sunsite.unc.edu/hrf/).

[3]McCaleb, Rob, "Two Immune-Enhancing Herbs," *Delicious!*, December 1995.

[4]Sharma, O. P., "Antioxidant Properties of Curcumin and Related Compounds," *Biochemistry and Pharmacology*, 25:1,811–25, 1976.

[5]Li, C. J., L. J. Zhang, et al., "Three Inhibitors of Type One Human Immunodeficiency Virus Long Terminal Repeat—Directed Gene Expression and Virus Replication," *Proceedings of the National Academy of Sciences USA*, 90:1,839–42, 1993.

[6]Huang, H. C., T. R. Jan, and S. F. Yeh, "Inhibitors Effect of Curcumin, An Anti-Inflammatory Agent, on Vascular Smooth Muscle Cell Proliferation," *European Journal of Pharmacology*, 221:381–84, 1992.

[7]Mukundan, M.A., M. C. Chacko, et al., "Effect of Turmeric and Curcumin on BP-DNA Adducts," *Carcinogenesis*, 14:493–96, 1993.

[8]Nagabhushan, M., and S. V. Bhide, "Curcumin as an Inhibitor of Cancer," *Journal of the American College of Nutrition* 11:192–198, 1992.

[9]"Capsules: Newsbreaks in Herb Research," *Herbs for Health*, March 1996.

[10]Rogers, Sherry A., "How the Sick Get Sicker, Quicker, by Following Current Medical Protocol," *Townsend Letter for Doctors*, October 1993.

[11]Golan, Ralph, M.D., *Optimal Wellness* (New York: Ballantine Books, 1995), p. 166.

CHAPTER 7:
COLDS AND FLU:
DODGING THE IMMUNE BREAKDOWN EPIDEMIC

[1]Hamlin, Suzanne, "Take 2 Bowls Zinc-Garlic Pasta, Then Call Me in the Morning," *New York Times*, January 25, 1995.

[2]Weil, Andrew, M.D., "Ask Dr. Weil," *Natural Health*, March/April 1996.

[3]Castleman, Michael, "Recent Findings in Healing Herbs," *Herb Quarterly*, Fall 1995.

[4]McCaleb, Rob, "Two Immune-Enhancing Herbs," *Delicious!*, December 1995.

[5]Ibid.

[6]Tyler, Varro E., *Herbs of Choice: Therapeutic Use of Phytomedicinals* (New York: Pharmaceutical Products Press, 1994).

[7]McCaleb, Rob, "Upset Stomach? Try Ginger," *Delicious!*, June 1995.

CHAPTER 8:
ESPECIALLY FOR WOMEN:
NATURAL HEALING FOR A WOMAN'S LIFETIME

[1]Tyler, Varro E., *Herbs of Choice: Therapeutic Use of Phytomedicinals* (New York: Pharmaceutical Products Press, 1994).

[2]McCaleb, Rob, "Chasteberry: A Tonic for Menstrual Problems," *Delicious!*, September 1995.

[3]Fulder, Stephen, Ph.D., and Meir Tenne, D.Sc., "Ginger as an Anti-Nausea Remedy in Pregnancy: The Issue of Safety," *HerbalGram* 38, Fall 1996.

[4]Ibid.

[5]Ibid.

[6]Northrup, Christiane, M.D., *Women's Health,* a special supplement to Dr. Christiane Northrup's *Health Wisdom for Women* newsletter. n.d.

[7]Weil, Andrew, M.D., "Estrogen Therapy: Balancing the Cancer Risks and Heart Benefits," *Self Healing,* vol. 1, issue 1, p. 4.

[8]Wright, Karen, "Menopause, Naturally," *Health,* January 1996.

[9]Kolata, Gina, "Cancer Link Contradicted by New Hormone Study," *New York Times,* July 12, 1995.

[10]Murray, Michael T., N.D., "Menopause: Is Estrogen Necessary?" *American Journal of Natural Medicine,* November 1995.

[11]Murray, Michael T., N.D., "Cimicifuga Extract (Black Cohosh): A Natural Alternative to Estrogen for Menopause," *Health Counselor,* vol. 8, no. 2.

[12]Ibid.

[13]Ibid.

[14]Ibid.

[15]Wright, Karen, "Menopause, Naturally," *Health,* January 1996.

[16]Murray, Michael T., N.D. "Menopause: Is Estrogen Necessary?" *American Journal of Natural Medicine,* November 1995.

[17]Wright, Karen, "Menopause, Naturally," *Health,* January 1996.

[18]"Faster, Cheaper Treatment of UTIs," *Elle,* May 1995.

CHAPTER 9:
ESPECIALLY FOR MEN:
NATURAL HEALING FOR A MAN'S LIFETIME

[1]Murray, Michael T., N.D., "Saw Palmetto: Nature's Answer to an Enlarged Prostate," *Health Counselor,* vol. 6, no. 4.

[2]*American Journal of Natural Medicine,* vol. 1, September 1994.

[3]Murray, Michael T., N.D., "Saw Palmetto: Nature's Answer to an Enlarged Prostate," *Health Counselor,* vol. 6, no. 4.

[4]Ibid.

[5]Jaret, Peter, "Foods That Fight Cancer," *Health,* March/April 1995.

[6]Moss, Ralph W., Ph.D., *Cancer Therapy: The Independent Consumer's Guide to Non-Toxic Treatment and Prevention* (New York: Equinox Press, 1995).

[7]*American Journal of Natural Medicine,* vol. 2, no. 10, December 1995.

[8]"Healthscene," *Health Counselor,* vol. 7, no. 6., quoting Michael T. Murray, N.D., *Male Sexual Vitality.*

CHAPTER 10:
HERBS FOR BABIES AND CHILDREN

[1]Aesoph, Lauri, N.D., "Cold or Flu: Which Do You Have?" *Delicious!,* December 1995.

[2]LeRoy, Bob, "Milk: What's the Controversy?" *Vegetarian Voice,* vol. 21, no. 2, 1996.

[3]Ibid.

[4]Murray, Frank, "Editor's Note," *Better Nutrition for Today's Living,* November 1995.

[5]Ibid.

[6]*New England Journal of Medicine,* 327:302, 1992, as cited in LeRoy, Bob, "Milk: What's the Controversy?" *Vegetarian Voice,* vol. 21, no. 2, 1996.

[7]*Diabetes,* 42:228, 1993, as cited in LeRoy, Bob, "Milk: What's the Controversy?" *Vegetarian Voice,* vol. 21, no. 2, 1996.

[8]Journal of the American Dietetic Association, 94:3:314, 1994, as cited in LeRoy, Bob, "Milk: What's the Controversy?" *Vegetarian Voice,* vol. 21, no. 2, 1996.

[9]American Journal of Clinical Nutrition, 51:489, 1990, as cited in LeRoy, Bob, "Milk: What's the Controversy?" *Vegetarian Voice,* vol. 21, no. 2, 1996.

[10]Mendelsohn, Robert S., M.D., *How to Raise a Healthy Child—In Spite of Your Doctor* (New York: Ballantine, 1984).

[11]Schmidt, Michael, *Childhood Ear Infection: What Every Parent and Doctor Should Know About Prevention, Home Cure, and Alternative Treatment* (Berkeley: North Atlantic Books, 1993).

[12]Marshall, Melinda, "Warning: Antibiotics Could Endanger Your Child," *Reader's Digest,* December 1996.

[13]Ibid.

[14]*Nutrition Science News,* January 1996.

[15]Mendelsohn, Robert S., M.D., *How to Raise a Healthy Child—In Spite of Your Doctor* (New York: Ballantine, 1984).

[16]Iacono, G., et al, "Chronic Constipation as a Symptom of Cow's Milk Allergy," *Journal of Pediatrics*, 126:34–39, 1995.

CHAPTER 11: ENERGIZING HERBS

[1]McCaleb, Rob, "Increase Your Endurance with High-Performance Herbs," *Delicious!*, July 1995.
[2]Van Straten, Michael, *Guarana* (Essex: C. W. Daniel, 1994), p. 101.

CHAPTER 12:
HERBS FOR DEPRESSION, ADDICTIONS, ANXIETY, AND INSOMNIA

[1]Murray, Michael T., "The Clinical Use of *Hypericum perforatum*," *American Journal of Natural Medicine*, vol. 2, issue 3, 1995.
[2]"The Unique Pharmacology of Coleus forskohlii," *The American Journal of Natural Medicine*, vol. 1, no. 3, November 1994, citing Wachtel, H. and Loschmann, P. A., "Effects of Forskolin and Cyclic Nucleotides in Animal Models Predictive of Antidepressant Activity: Interactions with Rolipram," *Psychopharmacology*, 90:430–35, 1986.
[3]Murray, Michael T., N.D., "Lifestyle and Dietary Factors in Depression," *American Journal of Natural Medicine*, vol. 2, no. 10, December 1995.
[4]Ibid.
[5]"Nutritional Research Bulletin," *American Journal of Natural Medicine*, vol. 2, no. 10, December 1995, citing Benjamin J., et al: "Inositol Treatment in Psychiatry," *Psychopharmacology Bulletin*, 31:167–75, 1995.
[6]John Heinerman, *Heinerman's Encyclopedia of Healing Juices* (West Nyack: Parker Publishing Co., 1994).
[7]Webb, Ginger, "Valerian Safety Confirmed in Overdose Research Reviews," *HerbalGram* 36, citing Willey, Leanna B., "Valerian Overdose: A Case Report," *Veterinary and Human Toxicology*, vol. 37, no. 4, August 1995, pages 364–365.
[8]"Kava Makes You Calm," *Health Counselor*, vol. 7, no. 6, citing *The British Journal of Phytotherapy*, vol. 3, no. 4, 1993/94.
[9]Mead, Nathaniel, "Boost Melatonin Naturally," *Natural Health*, March/April 1996, p. 54, quoting Reiter, Russel J., Ph.D., and Jo

Robinson, *Melatonin: Your Body's Natural Wonder Drug* (New York: Bantam Doubleday Dell, 1995).

[10]Mead, Nathaniel, "Boost Melatonin Naturally," *Natural Health*, March/April 1996.

[11]Dr. Billie Jay Sahley, Ph.D., *Townsend Letter for Doctors and Patients*, December 1995.

CHAPTER 13:
KEEPING YOUR HEAD (AND YOUR BODY): HERBS FOR LONGEVITY

[1]Challem, Jack, "Keeping Your Marbles," *Natural Health*, January/February 1995.

[2]Ibid.

[3]"Forever Young," Linda Wasmer Smith, *Veggie Life*, May 1995.

[4]McCaleb, Rob, "Ginkgo: Nature's Circulation Booster," *Delicious!*, May 1995.

[5]Aesoph, Lauri, M., N.D., "The Facts about Brain-Boosting Nutrients," *Delicious!*, May 1995.

[6]Challem, Jack, "Keeping Your Marbles," *Natural Health*, January/February 1995.

CHAPTER 14:
HERBAL RENEWAL: CLEANSE, DETOX, REBUILD

[1]Sherry A. Rogers, M.D., "Macrobiotic Diet Proven to Improve Cancer Survival," *Townsend Letter for Doctors*, February/March 1994, p. 147.

[2]Webb, Ginger, and Mark Blumenthal, "Milk Thistle Fruits for Treatment of Death Cap Mushroom Poisoning," *HerbalGram* 37. McCaleb, Rob, "Ten Best Herbs to Keep You Healthy," *Delicious!*, August 1995.

[3]Webb, Ginger, and Mark Blumenthal, "Milk Thistle Fruits for Treatment of Death Cap Mushroom Poisoning," *HerbalGram* 37.

[4]Ibid.

[5]Kiso, Y., Y. Suzuki, N. Watanabe, et al, "Antihepatotoxic Principles of *Curcuma longa* Rhizomes," *Planta Medica* 49: 185–87, 1983.

[6]Golan, Ralph, M.D., *Optimal Wellness* (New York: Ballantine Books, 1995), p. 166.

CHAPTER 15: HERBS FOR SKIN

[1]Leibovitz, Brian, "Polyphenols and Bioflavonoids: The Medicines of Tomorrow," *Townsend Letter for Doctors*, May 1994.
[2]Charles, V., and S. X. Charles. "The Use and Efficacy of *Azadirachta indica* ADR ("Neem") and *Curcuma longa* ("Turmeric") in Scabies: A Pilot Study," *Tropical & Geographical Medicine*, 44(1–2):178–81, 1992.
[3]"Berberine-Containing Plants in Psoriasis," *American Journal of Natural Medicine*, vol. 3, no. 1, January/February 1996, citing Muller, K., Ziereis, K., and Gawklik, I., "The Antipsoriatic Mahonia aquifolium and Its Active Constituents: II. Antiproliferative Activity against Cell Growth of Human Keratinocytes," *Planta Medica*, 61(1):74–75, 1995.
[4]Mars, Brigitte, "Herbal Kingdom: Calm Down with Chamomile," *Delicious!*, November 1995, quoting *Hautker*, vol. 62, 1987.

CHAPTER 16: HERBS FOR ALLERGIES

[1]Weil, Andrew, M.D., "Relieving Hay Fever," *Self Healing*, vol. 1, issue 1, p. 6.
[2]Golan, Ralph, M.D., *Optimal Wellness* (New York: Ballantine Books, 1995), p. 260.
[3]*The Medicine Garden*, written and produced for public radio by David Freudberg, 1996.
[4]"The Unique Pharmacology of *Coleus forskohlii*," *The American Journal of Natural Medicine*, vol. 1, no. 3, November 1994.
[5]Werbach, Melvin, M.D., "Bronchial Asthma and Magnesium," *Townsend Letter for Doctors and Patients*, November 1993.
[6]Skobeloff, E. M., W. H. Spivey, R. M. McNamara, and L. Greenspon, "Intravenous Magnesium Sulfate for the Treatment of Acute Asthma in the Emergency Department," *Journal of the American Medical Association* 262(9):1,210–13, 1989.
[7]Donald J. Carrow, M.D., and Mitchell Chavez, C.N., "Research Perspectives on Asthma," *Townsend Letter for Doctors and Patients*, August/September 1994.

CHAPTER 17: HERBS FOR ARTHRITIS

[1]Weil, Andrew, M.D., "Living with Arthritis," *Self Healing,* vol. 1, issue 4, p. 6.

[2]Ibid.

[3]Ammon, H.R.T., H. Safayhi, et al., "Mechanisms of Anti-Inflammatory Actions of Curcumin and Boswellic Acids," *Journal of Ethnopharmacology,* 38:113–19, 1993.

Arora, R., N. Basu, V. Kapour, and A. Jain, "Anti-Inflammatory Studies on *Curcuma longa* (Turmeric)," *Indian Journal of Medical Research,* 59:1,289–95, 1971.

Chandra, D., and S. Gupta, "Anti-Inflammatory and Anti-Arthritic Activity of Volatile Oil of *Curcuma longa* (Haldi)," *Indian Journal of Medical Research,* 60:138–42, 1972.

Murray, Michael T., N.D., "Curcumin: A Potent Anti-Inflammatory Agent," *The American Journal of Natural Medicine,* vol. 1, no. 4, December 1994.

[4]Qureshi, S., et al., "Toxicity Studies on *Alpinia galanga* and *Curcuma longa,*" *Planta Medica,* 58:124, 1992.

[5]"Curcumin, A Potent Anti-inflammatory Agent," *The American Journal of Natural Medicine,* vol. 1, no. 4, December 1994.

[6]Murray, Michael T., N.D., "New Uses for Ginger: Botanical Report," *Health Counselor,* vol. 4, no. 4., p. 18.

[7]Sodhi, Virender, M.D., "Ashwaganda for Rejuvenation," *New Editions Health World,* n.d.

[8]Smith, Linda Wasmer, "Forever Young," *Veggie Life,* May 1995.

[9]Ibid.

[10]Pizzorno, Lara, "50 Ways to Take Charge of Your Health," *Delicious!,* February 1996.

[11]*Annals of Internal Medicine* 1993, vol. 119, no. 9, cited by Pizzorno, Lara, "50 Ways to Take Charge of Your Health," *Delicious!,* February 1996.

[12]Weil, Andrew, M.D., "Living with Arthritis," *Self Healing,* vol. 1, issue 4, p. 1.

[13]"Acetabular Bone Destruction Related to Non-Steroidal Anti-Inflammatory Drugs," *The Lancet* ii:11–13, 1985. Brandt, K. D., "Effects of Non-Steroidal Anti-Inflammatory Drugs on Chrondroctye Metabolism in Vitro and In Vivo," *American Journal of Medicine,* 5A:29–34, 1987, cited in Rogers, Sherry A., M.D., "Doctor's Dialogue: One of

the Best-Kept Secrets in Medicine: Osteoarthritis Is Reparable," *Let's Live*, October 1995.

[14]Smith, Linda Wasmer, "Forever Young," *Veggie Life*, May 1995.

CHAPTER 19: HERBS FOR DIABETES

[1]Murray, Michael T., N.D., and Joseph E. Pizzorno, N.D., *Encyclopedia of Natural Medicine* (Rocklin, CA: Prima, 1991), citing Jenkins, D.J.A., Wolever, T.M.S., Bacon, S., et al., "Diabetic Diets: High Carbohydrate Combined with High Fiber," *American Journal of Clinical Nutrition*, 33:1,729–33, 1980.

[2]Groop, P. H., A. Aro, et al., "Long-term Effects of Guar Gum in Subjects with Non-Insulin-Dependent Diabetes Mellitus," *American Journal of Clinical Nutrition*, 58:513–18, 1993, cited in *Townsend Letter for Doctors and Patients*, April 1994.

[3]Pati, Dr. K., "Gymnema sylvestre," *New Editions Health World*, May 1995, June 1996.

[4]Ibid.

[5]Raghuram, T. C., R. D. Sharma, et. al. "Effect of fenugreek seeds on intravenous glucose disposition in non-insulin dependent diabetic patients," *Phytotherapy Research*, 8:83–6, 1994.

[6]"Vitamin C and Magnesium in Diabetes," *American Journal of Natural Medicine*, vol. 3, no. 1, January/February 1996.

CHAPTER 20: HERBS FOR THE HEART

[1]McCaleb, Rob, "The Fruits of Healing," *Delicious!*, 1996.

[2]Ibid.

[3]Ubbink, Johan, et. al, "Vitamin Requirements for the Treatment of Hyperhomocysteinemia in Humans," *Journal of Nutrition*, 124:1,927–33, 1994, cited in *Better Nutrition for Today's Living*, November 1995.

CHAPTER 21:
HERBS FOR HEADACHES AND OTHER ACHES

[1]Wachter, Sarah, "All-Natural Stress Soothers," *Longevity*, January 1995.

[2]Brown, Don, "Research Reviews: Essential Oils for Headache Treatment," *HerbalGram* 38, Fall 1996, quoting Gobel, H., G. Schmidt, M. Dworshak, et. al. "Essential plant oils and headache mechanisms," *Phytomedicine* 2(2):93–102, 1995.

[3]Pizzorno, Lara, "50 Ways to Take Charge of Your Health," *Delicious!*, February 1996.

[4]Weil, Andrew, M.D., "Five Steps to Migraine Relief," *Self Healing*, vol. 1, issue 6, May 1996, p. 4.

[5]Wachter, Sarah, "All-Natural Stress Soothers," *Longevity*, January 1995.

[6]Pizzorno, Lara, "50 Ways to Take Charge of Your Health," *Delicious!*, February 1996.

CHAPTER 22: HERBS FOR DIGESTION

[1]Gorman, Christine, "Need a New Drug? You May Get One Now that the FDA Is Primed to Clear More Medicines for Over-the-Counter Sale," *Time*, July 31, 1995.

[2]"Zantac and Tagamet vs. DGL," *American Journal of Natural Medicine*, vol. 1, no. 2., October 1994, pages 8–9.

[3]"Questions and Answers: Ask the Editors," *Herbs for Health*, March 1996.

[4]Murray, Michael T., N.D., "The Natural Approach to Ulcers," *Health Counselor*, vol. 7, no. 6., p. 14.

[5]Weil, Andrew, "Living with Arthritis," *Self Healing*, vol. 1, issue 4, p. 6.

[6]Reuters, San Francisco, September 29, as posted on America Online.

[7]Murray, Michael T., N.D., "The Natural Approach to Ulcers," *Health Counselor*, vol. 7, no. 6, p. 15.

[8]Ibid.

[9]"Zantac and Tagamet vs. DGL," *American Journal of Natural Medicine*, vol. 1, no. 2, October 1994, pages 8–9.

[10]Golan, Dr. Ralph, M.D., *Optimal Wellness* (New York: Ballantine Books, 1995), p. 420. "DGL May Inhibit *Helicobacter pylori*," *American Journal of Natural Medicine*, vol. 2, no. 10, December 1995, p. 16. "Zantac and Tagamet vs. DGL," *American Journal of Natural Medicine*, vol. 1, no. 2, October 1994, pages 8–9.

[11]"DGL May Inhibit *Helicobacter pylori*," *American Journal of Natural Medicine*

vol. 2, no. 10, December 1995, p. 16. "Zantac and Tagamet vs. DGL," *American Journal of Natural Medicine,* vol. 1, no. 2, October 1994, pages 8–9. Beil, W., Birkholz, and K. F. Sewing, "Effects of Flavonoids on Parietal Cell Acid Secretion, Gastric Mucosal Prostaglandin Production and *Helicobacter pylori* Growth," *Arnzeim Forsch Drug Research,* 45:697–700, 1995, cited in "DGL May Inhibit *Helicobacter pylori,*" *American Journal of Natural Medicine,* vol. 2, no. 10, December 1995, p. 16.

[12]"Zantac and Tagamet vs. DGL," *American Journal of Natural Medicine,* vol. 1, no. 2, October 1994, pages 8–9.

[13]Stock, Melissa T,. and Kellye Hunter, "The Healing Power of Peppers," *The Natural Way,* March/April 1996.

CHAPTER 23: LIVING IT: HERBS IN PRACTICE

[1]Horne, Steven, "Herbal Glycerites for Children," *Proceedings of Fifth Annual Symposium of American Herbalists Guild,* 1994.

[2]Ibid.

[3]Ibid.

[4]Rector-Page, Linda, N.D., Ph.D., *Power Plants: Building Immunity with Herbs* (Sonora, CA: Health Healing Publications, 1995).

[5]Smith, Ed, "A Case for Full Herbal Extracts," *Natural Foods Merchandiser,* February 1996.

[6]Moore, Michael, *The Herbalist,* May 1995, posted at gopher://president.oit.unc.edu:70/11/../.pub/academic/medicine/ alternative-healthcare/Southwest-School-of-Botanical-Medicine OR sunsite.unc.edu/pub/academic/medicine/alternative-healthcare/ Southwest-School-of-Botanical-Medicine

[7]Ibid.

[8]Ibid.

CHAPTER 24: URBAN MYTHS AND SIDEWALK TALK

[1]Moore, Michael, *The Herbalist,* May 1995, posted at gopher://president.oit.unc.edu:70/11/../.pub/academic/medicine/ alternative-healthcare/Southwest-School-of-Botanical-Medicine OR

sunsite.unc.edu/pub/academic/medicine/alternative-healthcare/ Southwest-School-of-Botanical-Medicine

[2]Ibid.

[3]Long, Patricia, "The Naturals," *Health,* May/June 1995, p. 90.

[4]Ibid., p. 89.

[5]Bergner, Paul, "Echinacea Myth: Phagocytosis not Diminished after Ten Days," *Medical Herbalism,* 1994, no. 6(1):1.

[6]Mowrey, Daniel, Ph.D., "Tonic Herbs," *Let's Live,* December 1995.

[7]Bone, Kerry, Ph.D., "New Research on HIV-1: Implications for Phytotherapy," *Townsend Letter for Doctors,* July 1995, citing Coeugniet, E. G. and R. Kühnast, *Therapiewoche* 36:3,352, 1986.

[8]Herb Research Foundation's Internet World Wide Web site (http://sunsite,unc.edu/hrf/).

[9]Ibid.

[10]Bergner, P., "Hepatotoxicity of Pyrrolizidine Alkaloids," *Medical Herbalism,* no. 6 (1):10, 1994.

[11]"Herbal Teas and Toxicity," Copyright 1995 Health ResponseAbility Systems, Inc., posted on America Online, Better Health and Medical Network (keywords: Better Health or HRS)>Alternative and Complementary Medicine>Alternative Health Articles.

[12]Whitelegg, Margaret, "In Defense of Comfrey," National Institute of Medical Herbalists' *The Herbalist,* August 1994.

[13]Ibid.

[14]"Always Natural, Always Healthy?" Town Meeting, May 1995.

[15]Ibid.

[16]Blumenthal, Mark, and Penny King, "The Agony of the Ecstacy: Herbal High Products Get Media Attention," *HerbalGram* 37, p. 23.

[17]Ibid.

[18]Duke, James A., Ph.D., "Viewpoint," *HerbalGram* 28, 1993, citing *Chemical Marketing Reporter,* June 4, 1990.

[19]Duke, James A., Ph.D., "Viewpoint," *HerbalGram* 28, 1993.

[20]Ibid., citing *Journal of the American Medical Association,* Nov. 27, 1987, p. 2, 891.

[21]Kolata, Gina, "Cancer Link Contradicted by New Hormone Study," *New York Times,* July 12, 1995.

[22]"Are 'Safe' Drugs Really Safe?" *Longevity,* September 1994.

[23]Whitcomb, D.C., and G. D. Block, "Association of Acetaminophen

Hepatotoxicity with Fasting and Ethanol Use," *Journal of the American Medical Association* 272 (23):1,845–50, December 21, 1994.

[24]Wallace, Edward, N.D., D.C., "What to Do When Your Head Aches," *Delicious!*, March 1996.

Index